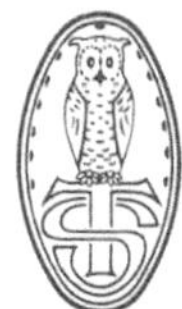 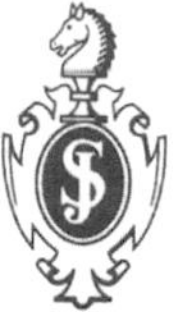

Proceedings of the Symposium on Current Concepts on the
Use of Aortic and Pulmonary Allografts for Heart Valve
Substitutes

Berlin (West), September 7—9, 1987

A. C. Yankah, R. Hetzer, D. C. Miller,
D. N. Ross, J. Somerville,
M. H. Yacoub (Eds.)

Cardiac Valve Allografts 1962–1987

Current Concepts on the Use of Aortic and Pulmonary Allografts for Heart Valve Substitutes

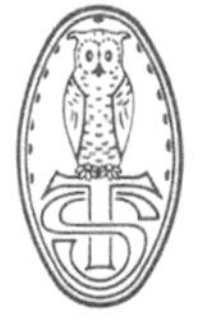

Steinkopff Verlag Darmstadt
Springer-Verlag New York

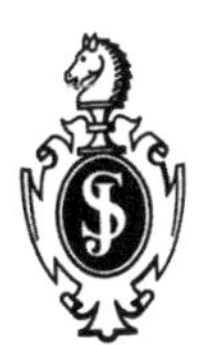

A. Charles Yankah, M.D.
Consultant
German Heart Center Berlin
Clinic for Cardiothoracic
and Vascular Surgery
D-1000 Berlin (West) 65
Germany

Roland Hetzer, M.D.
Professor, Chairman and
Director
Clinic for Cardiothoracic
and Vascular Surgery
German Heart Center Berlin
D-1000 Berlin (West) 65
Germany

D. Craig Miller, M.D.
Ass. Professor of Cardiac
Surgery
Stanford University
Dept. of Cardiovascular Surgery
Stanford
California 94305,
USA

Donald Ross, M.D.
Consultant Cardiac Surgeon
Director or Surgery
National Heart Hospital
Westmoreland Street
London WIM 8BA
UK.

Jane Somerville, M.D.
Consultant Cardiologist
National Heart Hospital
Westmoreland Street
London WIM 8BA
UK.

Magdi H. Yacoub, M.D.
Professor & Consultant Cardiac
Surgeon
Harefield Hospital,
National Heart and Brompton
Hospital, London
UK.

CIP-Titelaufnahme der Deutschen Bibliothek

Cardiac valve allografts: 1962–1987; current concepts on the use of aort. and pulmonary allografts
for heart valve substitutes; [proceedings of the Symposium on Current Concepts on the Use of Aort.
and Pulmonary Allografts for Heart Valve Substitutes, Berlin (West), September 7–9, 1987] / A. C.
Yankah . . . (eds.). — Darmstadt: Steinkopff; New York: Springer, 1988.
ISBN-13: 978-3-642-72422-0   e-ISBN-13: 978-3-642-72420-6
DOI: 10.1007/978-3-642-72420-6
NE: Yankah, A. C. [Hrsg.]; Symposium on Current Concepts on the Use of Aortic and Pulmonary
Allografts for Heart Valve Substitutes < 1987, Berlin, West >

Foreword

It was the genius of Gordon Murray in Toronto that introduced the use of allografts into cardiac surgery in the 1950s. Soon after this on opposite sides of the world, Sir Brian Barratt-Boyes in Auckland, New Zealand, and Mr. Donald Ross in London, undertook to use allografts for the replacement of diseased aortic valves. Since that time the global interest in allografts has been patchy, episodic, and without a consensus. Nonetheless, for the last 20 years at least three groups in the world have steadfastly pursued the development of new and relevant information concerning the use of allograft valves in humans. These are the centres of Sir Brian Barratt-Boyes, Mr. Donald Ross, and Mark O'Brien in Brisbane. More recently, talented investigators, including Drs. Yankah, Yacoub, and others, have been developing information concerning the immunological aspects of the use of allografts, as well as their clinical use. No doubt, at present, cardiac valve allografts of one sort or another are the devices of choice for conduits and have an important place in the surgery of aortic valve replacement. Even so, in the mind of this writer at least, the future usefulness of allografts for the replacement of diseased cardiac valves and conduits between a ventricle and the pulmonary artery, remains problematic, and depends upon improvements in other devices for this purpose and upon improvements that may be made in preparing and using allografts.

The question for the future, then, is whether developments in bioprostheses and mechanical valves will eventuate in devices so superior to those currently available that there will be little or no place for the logistically and technically more difficult task of using allograft valves. Improvements may be made in the performance and behavior of allograft valves as well, of course, but it seems less likely that these will result in dramatic improvements.

This book brings together the most important current work in this interesting and always changing field. Dr. Yankah and his colleagues are to be congratulated for conceiving the idea of this project and providing such an important scientific stimulus to it. Careful study of this book will provide timely and important information for the reader.

John W. Kirklin

Preface

In the face of the very limited experience we had, as compared to the other centers, the German Heart Center organized this Symposium on the current concepts on the use of aortic and pulmonary allografts for heart valve substitutes in Berlin from Sept. 7–9, 1987 most egoistically, with the primary aim of learning as much as possible from the great number of experts with much larger experience and knowledge in this field. The Symposium also marked the 25th anniversary of the first clinical use of aortic valve allograft in the subcoronary position, a pioneer work which was achieved by two prominent surgeons, Mr. Donald N. Ross, Senior Surgeon, National Heart Hospital, London, UK and Sir Brian Barratt-Boyes, Surgeon-in-Chief, Green Lane Hospital, Auckland, New Zealand, who were the honorary guests at the meeting. We congratulate Dr. Gordon Murray who paved the way, experimentally and clinically in the 1950s to this success. We consider the development of this particular field as exemplary for cardiac surgery on the whole, where after various technical developments and changing opinions in preservation techniques and immunological aspects, the original method has survived with greater and better understanding, with more precise indications and the possibility of reliable comparison.

The symposium as its theme suggests, was exclusively devoted to the use of cardiac valve allografts in the subcoronary and pulmonary positions. The use of allografts in the mitral and tricuspid positions was cautiously discussed but not in detail.

The Berlin symposium which took place during the 750th anniversary of the city of Berlin, brought together cardiologists, cryobiologists, engineers, pathologists, practitioners and surgeons from Austria, Australia, Belgium, People's Republic of China, France, the Federal Republic of Germany, German Democratic Republic, Hungary, Italy, Netherlands, Portugal, Poland, Spain, Taiwan, R.O.C., United Kingdom, USA who listened to the 41 presentations and a panel discussion over 2 days and participated actively in the lively discussions.

The live video transmission of subcoronary transplantation of aortic allograft from the operating room of the German Heart Center to the International Congress Center Berlin where the faculty of experts answered questions from the audience and elaborated on the surgical techniques, was accepted as an interesting new way of scientific communication.

Opportunity was given to surgeons who were interested in using allograft valves for valve replacement, on their return home, to practice the transplantation techniques under the supervision of allograft experts, during the special laboratory session provided by the organizers.

Now that the interest in allograft surgery is growing, the problems of procuring adequate donor allografts of different sizes arise.

Currently, our major source of allograft valve harvesting is from the recipients' hearts at the time of cardiac transplantation. We have now performed 93 heart transplantations since April 1986 here in Berlin. This shows the number of valves we could have at our disposal. Organized regional procurement centers in collaboration with organ transplant centers, intensive ease and trauma units might help in developing regional or hospital-based allograft valve banks.

It was most appropriate to start the Symposium with Mr. Donald N. Ross, London and let it end with Sir Brian Barratt-Boyes who have contributed continuously and scientifically to the "state of the art". The faculty members were very cooperative with the collection of the manuscripts. The editing of this book has been a challenging and memorable experience without constraints and we are very happy being able to present the proceedings within such a short time after the symposium.

We would also like to thank the members of the editorial board for their cooperation. Finally, but not least, we are greatly indebted to the City of Berlin, Mrs. Roder and her hard-working team and all the sponsors who provided the funds to make this symposium possible.

This book entails the work of cryobiologists, immunologists, pathologists, cardiologists and surgeons who are experts on cardiac valve allografts and it was a great pleasure to host the Berlin Symposium, and we hope that the reader will get more valuable information out of the proceedings for the benefit of his patients.

Berlin, December 1987

Roland Hetzer
A. Charles Yankah

To our families and loved ones,
whose religious understanding of the demands
of our surgical and scientific lives
made this book possible.

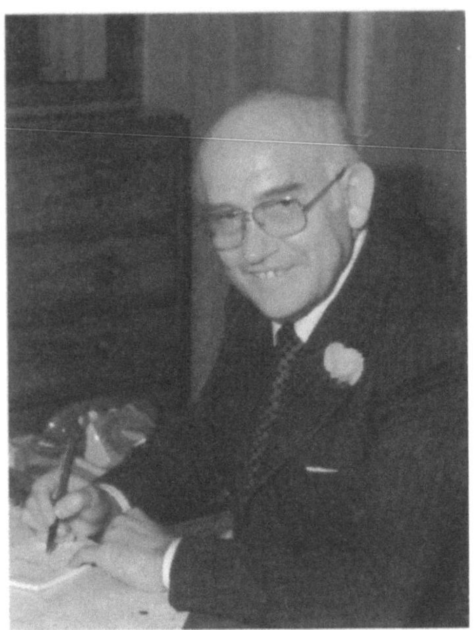

Mr. Donald N. Ross
Senior Surgeon
National Heart Hospital
London, U.K.

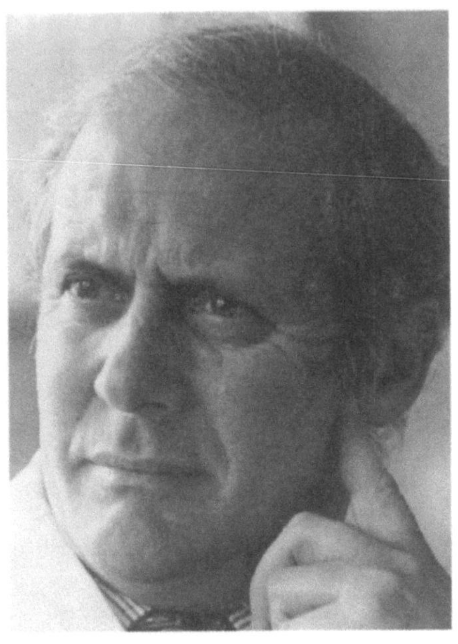

Sir Brian G. Barratt-Boyes
Surgeon-in-chief
Green Lane Hospital
Auckland, New Zealand

The two pioneer surgeons who independently and successfully inserted the first aortic allografts in the subcoronary position in June and August 1962.

Contents

XII

Long-term results of antibiotic-treated (4 °C) allograft valves and valved conduits

Intermediate and long-term results of cryopreserved allografts

Faculty, contributors and invited discussants

Sally P. Allwork
London, UK

William W. Angell
La Jolla, California, USA

Harvey L. Bank
Charleston, South Carolina, USA

Sir Brian Barratt-Boyes
Auckland, New Zealand

John G. Baust
Binghamton, New York, USA

Douglas Behrendt
Iowa City, Iowa, USA

E. Berreklouw
Eindhoven, Netherlands

Endre Bodnar
London, UK

Aldo R. Castaneda
Boston, Massachusetts, USA

Ing-Sh Chiu
Taipei, Taiwan

David R. Clarke
Denver, Colorado, USA

J. Terrance Davis
Toledo, Ohio, USA

Antoni Dziatkowiak
Crakow, Poland

Martin Elliott
London, UK

Eckhart Fleck
Berlin (West), Germany

Francis Fontan
Bordeaux, France

Y. A. Goffin
Leeds, UK

Lorenzo Gonzalez-Lavin
New Brunswick, New Jersey, USA

A. J. Gunning
Oxford, UK

Roland Hetzer
Berlin (West), Germany

Richard A. Jonas
Boston, Massachusetts, USA

Phillip H. Kay
London, UK

F. Keller
Berlin (West), Germany

James K. Kirklin
Birmingham, Alabama, USA

P. Lange
Kiel, FRG

S. Randolph May
Houston, Texas, USA

Hans Meisner
München, FRG

D. Craig Miller
Stanford, California, USA

J. E. Molina
Minnesota, USA

A. E. Moulton
Omaha, USA

Hans-Konrad Müller-Hermelink
Würzburg, FRG

W. Müller-Ruchholtz
Kiel, FRG

Mark F. O'Brien
Brisbane, Australia

Donald N. Ross
London, UK

Jane Somerville
London, UK

Rosemary Radley-Smith
Harefield, UK

Stephan Schüler
Berlin (West), Germany

David Sikarskie
Hougthon, Michigan, USA

Jaroslav Stark
London, UK

M. Trenkner
Gdansk, Poland

Kevin Turley
San Francisco, USA

Arnim Wessel
Kiel, FRG

Magdi H. Yacoub
Harefield and London, UK

A. Charles Yankah
Berlin (West), Germany

G. Ziemer
Hannover, FRG

Evolution of the biological concept in cardiac surgery: A Pilgrim's Progress

D. N. Ross

The National Heart Hospital, Westmoreland Street, London, U.K.

It is an honour and a great pleasure to contribute to the celebration of 25 years of adherence to the biological valve principle.

In addressing the readers of this book dedicated to biological and more particularly human or allograft tissue, I must assume that I am preaching to the converted. As such I also expect you all to know the story of the Pilgrim's Progress and Christian the hero's exposure to the temptations of life on his journey to perfection.

However, it would be too simple to assume that the Pilgrim's Progress which we travel as surgeons throughout our careers arrives at a clear-cut division in our path leading either to righteousness, on the one hand, or to damnation on the other; in other words setting us firmly on the biological or the mechanical pathway depending on our inherent convictions.

Like Christian (no relation to Barnard) the hero in the classical Pilgrim's Progress, there are many temptations and byways straddling our way making compromise easy or often leading us up a blind alley.

Speculating idly about myself and Albert Starr as two pilgrims starting on that valve pilgrimage in 1962, I would like to believe that our deeply rooted conviction and steadfast persistence has had its rewards and that 25 years later I and my biological cohorts, and he and his mechanical divisions, were both about to enter the Kingdom of Heaven, pure and unsullied and with the biological waverers and bioprosthetic compromisers regaled to the flames of external damnation.

Alas, as in the classical story, it is only a dream and to quote Shakespeare to bring us back to reality:

"We are such stuff as dreams are made on and our little life is rounded with a sleep".

After that diversion into the world of fantasy, back to the harsh world of decisions in which we must decide what the biological concept means to us.

First, let me make the point that the use of biological tissue in surgery in no way represents a re-invention of the wheel. This attitude of re-inventing the wheel is a common failing among cardiac surgeons who quite recently have felt they had done this in returning to the long-established concept of conservative mitral valve surgery which, in fact, has been regularly practised since the start of cardiac surgery.

My own surgical heritage has been deeply influenced by the biological as opposed to the mechanical, plastic or petro-chemical approach, largely as a result of my early training with Lord Brock. He epitomised the biological concept both from a deep-seated conviction and partly from a lack of the plastic and mechanical alternatives freely available to us today. Consequently, we espoused the use of biological tissue, both from conviction and necessity. Initially this involved mainly the use of autologous pericardium, then homograft blood vessel segments, and finally valves.

However, before stepping into the cosy bioprosthetic world of beautifully boxed, glutaraldehyde-preserved complex amalgams of denatured tissue, plastic and steel, it is timely to review the biological scene as we know it and in its historical perspective.

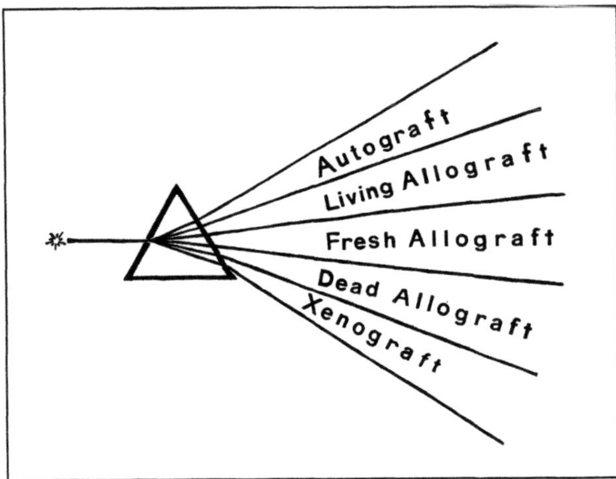

Fig. 1. The available biological valves cover a wide spectrum.

Included in our loose concept of biological tissue is a wide spectrum ranging from fully viable, freshly removed autogenous tissue, to dead inert and denatured animal tissue converted into flexible tanned leather by means of the ubiquitous glutaraldehyde solution (Fig. 1). In between lies a whole range of biological alternatives.

In descending order of acceptability from the recipient's point of view, we must put the fresh living autograft at the top of the tree and it must surely rank as our "biological gold standard", having a full complement of histo-compatible living cells unmodified by any sterilisation or storage process which could denature the collagen matrix and damage the cells.

Ranking next in importance must be allografts or homografts with the entirely fresh untreated homograft removed from a donor and immediately placed in recipient position at the top of this section. This is analogous to fresh organ transplantation and merits the title of a homovital graft (cornea is a good example but the description applies equally to the freshly removed aortic valve homograft — perhaps removed from a transplant recipient).

These truly living allografts enjoy the advantages and incur the constraints inherent in all living organ transplants and, in order to retain those properties which almost elevate them to the status of the fresh autografts, they may or may not require immunosuppressive depending on the degree of antigenicity of the tissue.

Next, in order of preference, are the conventional stored homografts which have been used throughout the years with varying degrees of viability of the different cellular components. These valves rate in order to acceptability depending on the time delay from death to processing and their subsequent storage-time before use.

2

Also the type of processing and consequent denaturing of the protein is a very relevant consideration.

Stored allograft tissues include not only valves but homologous skin, dura mater and pericardium, and viability is no longer a primary consideration but an index of structural integrity which is now becoming increasingly important. In fact, it is very unlikely that any allograft valves remain viable, since all living cells must be antigenic and evoke a rejection process.

Finally, and not strictly part of this book, we have the commercially produced group of xenografts rendered to a large extent immunologically inert by conversion into flexible leather, but often retaining the ability to stimulate a vigorous tissue reaction or rejection process. This applies to glutaraldehyde preserved pericardium, calf pericardial valves and porcine xenografts.

Table 1. Range of biological tissues used in valve replacement.

Fresh living autograft	—	Biological gold standard
Fresh living allografts	—	Homovital
Stored allografts	—	Variable viability Structurally "intact"
Commercial xenografts	—	Flexible "leather" denatured protein

In this discussion we must confine our remarks to valves and particularly to the first two categories, namely autografts and homografts (or allografts). This gives us the opportunity to look backwards to their past history and forward to what we anticipate to be a bright future.

To quote the poet John Keats:

"Then felt I like some watcher of the skies when a new planet swims into his ken".

To us, the use of an aortic valve homograft was indeed like a new star in our surgical firmament and entirely in accord with our biological principles.

To set the record straight, the use of a homograft valve was first tried in the descending aorta of dogs in 1952 by Lam (1) of Detroit. He was pessimistic since the nonfunctional aortic leaflets became shrunken and fibrosed (Fig. 2).

However, while I was a surgical research fellow in 1953 at Guy's Hospital, Brock put us to work to repeat Lam's studies and we demonstrated that the homograft cusps would persist, but only if they were subjected to a fully pulsatile functional workload.

Gordon Murray (2) of Toronto proved this clinically in 1956 by inserting fresh and fully living homografts into the descending thoracic aorta of patients with aortic regurgitation and the valves were reported by Heimbecker to be functional 20 years later — clearly a strong argument in favour of fully viable untreated valves (Fig. 3). From our dog homograft valve experience, we then took a wrong turning in our pilgrim's progress into chemical and destructive methods of sterilizing and preserving aortic segments and valves, and we favoured ethylene oxide sterilisation followed by freeze-drying. These valves were tested for durability in a crude pulse duplicator but the emphasis was on sterilisation and preservation methods.

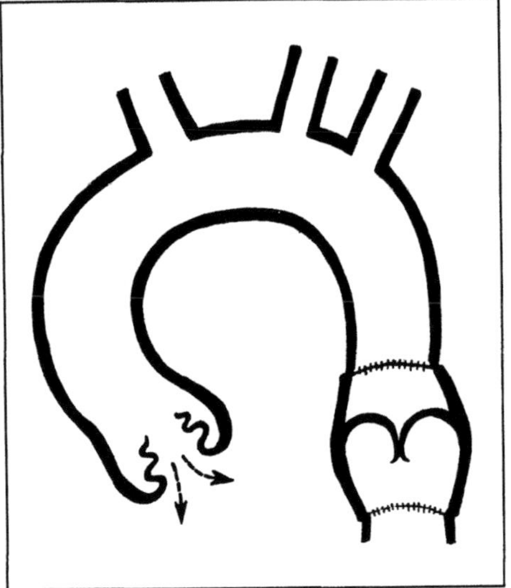

Fig. 2. Homograft valve cusps will only persist if they have a pulsatile workload.

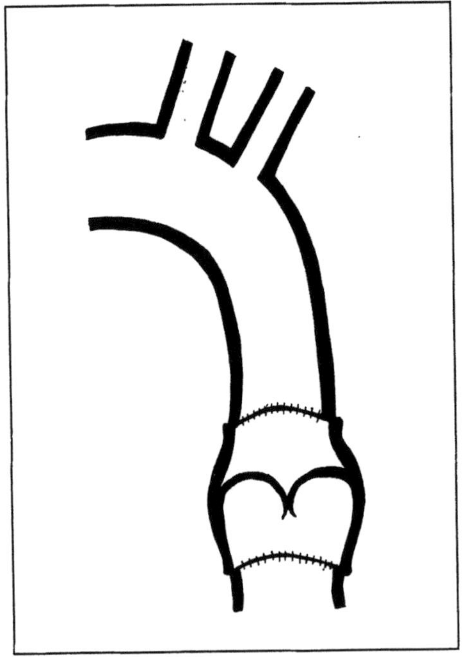

Fig. 3. Site of insertion of the homograft valve in Murray's clinical cases.

Such was our state of unpreparedness that in June 1962 (2), an aortic valve that I was decalcifying disappeared down the sucker tubing at a time when Starr valves were only a distant rumour. We had no alternative but to reconstitute one of our freeze-dried aortic homograft valves and sew it in with a single suture layer — a technique which fortunately had already been suggested to us by our colleagues Gunning and Duran (4) of Oxford.

4

The rest is history. You can imagine our delight when the first valve was not rejected and continued to function in that patient for 4 1/2 years. We forgot about the newly available mechanical valves — a state of amnesia which I must confess persists to this day. The homograft valve became an established surgical technique although eventually with only a few persistent and courageous exponents of the method, largely in the Antipodes.

Now when we review the outcome of those early ventures, I believe we can fairly claim that the aortic homograft represents the best available aortic valve replacement, irrespective of age, sex, and degree of disability. Their utilisation is increasing rapidly and we have supplied them to surgeons all over the world (Table 2).

Unlike the mechanical valve and the bioprosthetic valve which are subject to various so-called failure modes, its only real problem relates to degeneration, probably starting around 7 years (7 year itch!) and resulting from simple wear and tear and, to a lesser extent, calcification. Other features like embolism, thrombosis, haemolysis, perivalvular leak and sudden death do not apply and the incidence of infection is certainly no greater and possibly less than for a prosthetic valve replacement (Table 3).

In other words we are simply faced with a durability problem — questions of design are not relevant and cannot be faulted.

There is little time to dilate on our homograft experience which will be analysed in greater detail by others in this book. In summary, our homograft department has processed nearly 5000 valves, of which approximately 3000 have been inserted. I have used 1270 of these, distributed through all four valve areas, but mainly the aortic.

Table 2. Summary of advantages of the homograft valve.

1.	Best available aortic valve replacement
2.	Ideal for pulmonary valve replacement and right ventricular outflow reconstruction
3.	Suitable for children
4.	Applications to all four valve sites
5.	Can be used for any age
6.	Clear advantages in infective endocarditis

Table 3. Comparison of failure modes for homografts and other valves.

Other valves	Homografts
Embolism	(Infection)
Thrombosis	Degeneration
Haemorrhage	
Perivalve leak	
Sudden death	
Infection	
Degeneration	

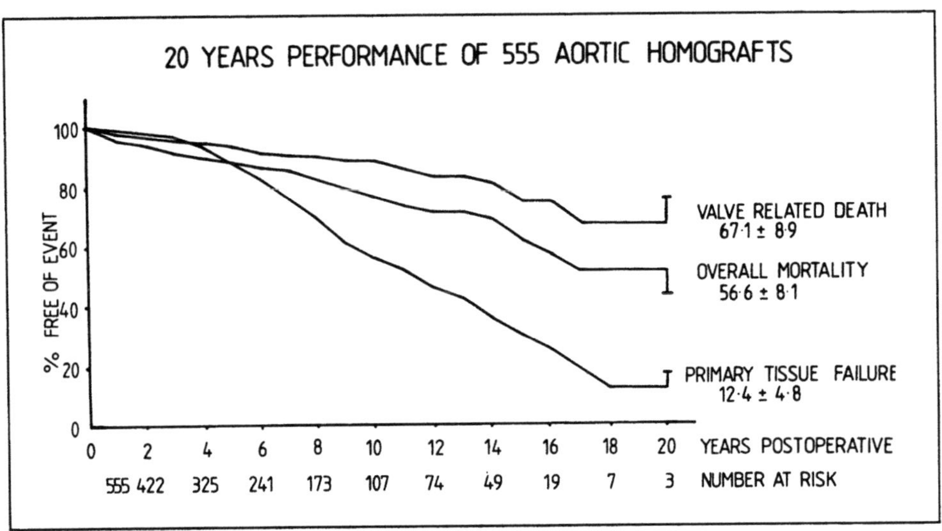

Fig. 4. Actuarial survival for 555 isolated aortic homografts over 20 years. Primary tissue failure is the outstanding problem.

In order to draw some valid conclusions we have selected a fairly homogenous group of 555 surviving isolated aortic valve replacements carried out in one hospital and all by the same surgeon over a 20-year period.

At 10 years, 89% of patients are free of valve-related deaths and over 80% are surviving. By 20 years, the figures are 67% and 56% respectively, figures which bear comparison with any other reported valve series stretching over 20 years (Fig. 4).

The message that is clear from the third actuarial curve is that primary tissue failure is the outstanding residual problem that we face.

In confirmation of this statement is the fact that over the past 5 years, that is before tissue failure emerges as a problem, 120 aortic homografts have been inserted with no deaths and no complications. In other words, if results are reported before the end of 5 years, all types of biological valves will have excellent results.

We have not been able to establish that one form of valve preservation is better than another, although our early freeze-dried series certainly showed more intrinsic calcification of the cusps than subsequent frozen and fresh valves. Also, our frozen series is relatively small.

What can we do to make our flexible freehand-inserted homografts still more effective or long lasting? Following general principles, they should ideally be fresh, with little or no delay from the time of harvesting to clinic use, fully viable (endothelium, fibroblasts and collagen) and with the protein not denatured by storage and preservatives. In hard, practical, real-life terms, these criteria are difficult if not impossible to achieve on a regular basis.

Some form of antibiotic or chemical sterilisation must clearly be used if we are to have a readily available cadaver supply. To minimise degenerative autolysis they should be available I believe within 7—10 days of harvesting and used within 21 days. Alternatively they should be frozen immediately after sterilisation to arrest autolysis (Table 4).

6

Table 4. Minimal requirements for preservation of cusp structure and integrity (homograft aortic valves).

1.	Some method of sterilisation
2.	Release as sterile within 7—10 days of harvesting or Freeze immediately after sterilising
3.	Use fresh valves within 3 weeks of storage

There are certainly valid arguments in favour of immediate freezing but equally persuasive arguments for having a selection of so-called fresh valves. I and many of my colleagues still prefer to have a selection of fresh antibiotic-preserved valves at operation rather than one frozen valve and with no alternative choice, but a certain degree of wastage is inevitable.

From aortic valve homografts we progressed in 1966 (5) to their use in right ventricular outflow reconstruction and I still believe this was one of the most important and wide-ranging developments in complex congenital heart disease. The striking feature of this type of reconstruction is that although the homograft aortic wall calcifies early, especially in children, the conduit does not stenose and the cusps remain functional for many years.

I believe our introduction of pulmonary rather than aortic homografts in 1983 (6) for the right ventricular outflow tract was long overdue. It is a logical development and with good scientific backup, particularly in regard to calcification, as presented by my Italian associate Dr. Ugo Livi (7).

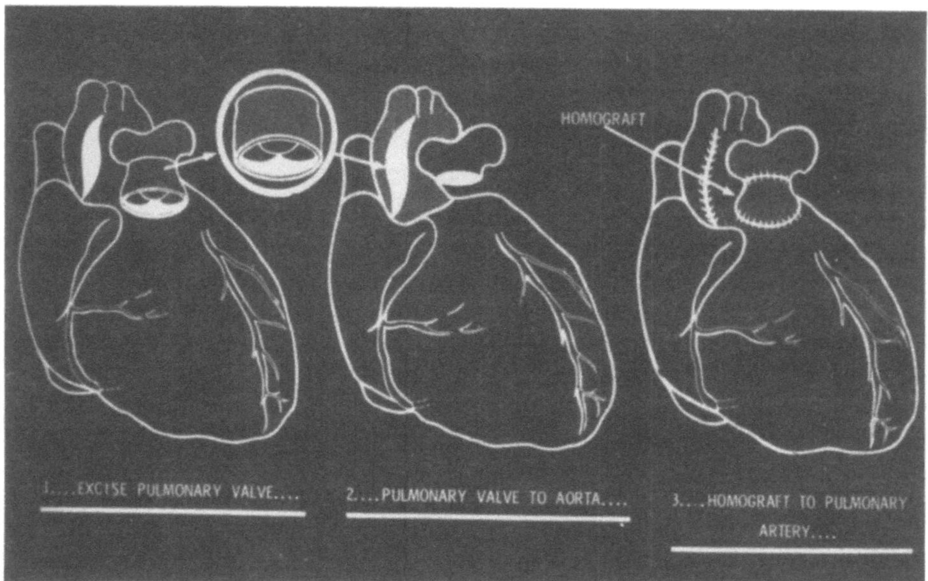

Fig. 5. Steps in the operation to transplant the pulmonary valve to the aortic site.

Encouraged by this work, I have recently even used pulmonary homografts for aortic valve replacement.

The acme of our biosurgical achievement came, I believe, in 1967 (8) when we auto-transplanted the patient's own pulmonary valve to the aortic position and, less well-known but equally important, to the mitral position also. Shumway's team had reported some experimental moves in this direction (9) but this was the first clinical experience offering the prospect of a truly permanent living valve replacement (Fig. 5).

When you consider that the autogenous living pulmonary valve is immediately transferred to the aortic area, inserted freehand without delay or any form of chemical treatment, that is, conforming to our ideal criteria, you will not be surprised that these autografts function as you might expect when living cells are placed in their natural environment and with perfect design characteristics. In other words, they persist and function perfectly and do not show signs of degeneration.

Our only initial anxiety was that the cusps would not support aortic pressure — let me reassure you; there has never been an acute valve failure in over 250 cases. Furthermore, late degenerative failure such as other biological valves experience is again virtually unknown in the autograft and many are now coming up to 20 years' follow-up.

Considering briefly my National Heart Hospital results, 241 patients had an autograft in the 20-year period between 1967 and 1987. There is an overall mortality of 6.6% (16 patients) but no deaths over the last 10 years. The deaths were during the early learning period, usually from damage to the first septal coronary artery (10).

Table 5. Early and late results after pulmonary autografts (20 years' experience).

241 Patients	—	N.N.H. London	
16 Deaths (6.6%)			
No deaths in last 11 years			
225 Survivors			
First 10 years			Second 10 years
Technical failures	13		4
Tissue failure	7		0
Valve related deaths	7		0
All deaths	15		0

I.E. no operative deaths, late deaths and no tissue failure over past 10 years

The 225 hospital survivors have been followed for 20 years. In the first 10 years there were 13 technical or tissue failures but only four in the last 10 years (Table 5). Early "tissue failures" were probably the result of malinsertion, trauma or in some cases clinical or subclinical endocarditis. However, there have been no operative deaths, no late deaths and no documented valve failures over the past 10 years.

At first we recognised a number of self-imposed restrictions limiting their application to single valve disease and initially at least to young people. We now cover most age groups and have an increasing interest in the valve's growth potential for very young patients.

8

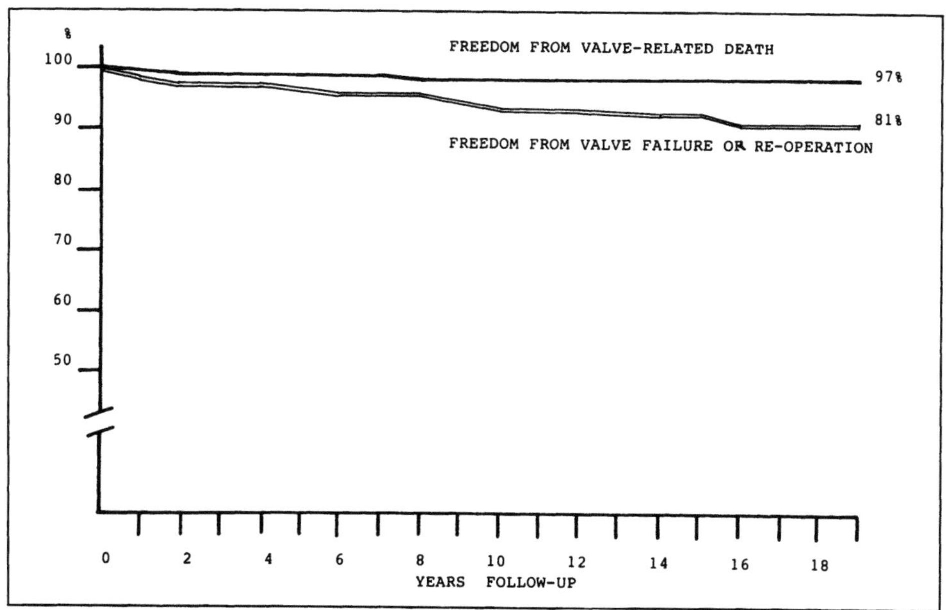

Fig. 6. The reconstruction of the right ventricle presents little risk to the patient.

The only criticism that can be levelled at this procedure relates to right ventricular reconstruction with a homograft or more recently a pulmonary homograft. As with cyanotic congenital cases, the function of the homograft valve in this low pressure area is excellent and valve dysfunction, if it occurs, presents virtually no threat to life (Fig. 6).

If I have digressed slightly from the theme of the book by enthusing about autografts, it is because I believe they represent our gold standard and there are many fascinating attributes in living tissue which we cannot ignore. For example, we cannot with impunity expect living reactive tissue to adapt to an alien environment, but the potential is there if we can exploit it successfully. Hence, we saw living autogenous fascia lata removed from the leg subjected to the stresses of the mitral area, and trying to adapt a tricuspid to a bicuspid configuration before becoming haemodyamically incompetent.

The abundantly available autogenous pericardium freely available at our operations undoubtedly has great strength and potential adaptability, if we can exploit it successfully, and I am surprised that it has not been used more often rather than the expensive commercially prepared glutaraldehyde variety commonly used.

As I see it, if we accept, as I believe we do, that three-cusp freehand inserted aortic and pulmonary valves are ideal for aortic and pulmonary valve replacement, we are left with the challenge of the mitral and tricuspid area as sites for homograft and autograft replacement.

As I have mentioned, we have already used pulmonary autografts as mitral valve replacements with encouraging results. One such valve survived for 14 years in spite of an episode of endocarditis which was successfully treated medically. Another, used as a mitral replacement in a young girl, has seen her through a successful pregnancy and has been inplace for 18 years.

The non-viable aortic homograft and pulmonary homograft fixed on frames have been less successful in the mitral area. However, this is not necessarily a valid criticism of the valve but rather of our use of a three-cusp configuration, together with a rigid or semi-rigid prosthesis, in an area with very different pressure loads and flow characteristics. Also, if the homograft valves had been professionally mounted they would, I am sure, have given better service.

I would like to see the re-introduction of homografts and autografts mounted on fully flexible supports as mitral replacements, especially for children, and the somewhat larger pulmonary homograft should function admirably for the low pressure tricuspid area.

On first principles, the ideal mitral valve replacement has to be another mitral valve, complete with chordae and papillary muscles. Such a concept is not new (12). We and several other surgeons, including Professor Bernhard of Kiel, have some experience of the technique. It seems that the time is ripe for like-minded biologically oriented surgeons to review this possibility rather than go on unthinkingly putting in inverted aortic valves in the mitral position and simply changing the name on the box. By doing so we flout every physical, anatomical and physiological concept of the normal mitral valve. We may be deceiving ourselves but I do not think we are deceiving the heart.

Only fools speculate about the future and I am no exception in that I have been trying to see the way ahead in valve surgery for a long time, but with only limited success. If I have to speculate, I believe that replacement of the whole aortic root with a competent adult-sized valve structure offers an important step forward for the relief of left ventricular outflow obstruction (13) and for the infected aortic root (14), particularly after prosthetic endocarditis with abscess formation. As an autograft root, it may ultimately be the best method of aortic valve replacement, certainly in growing children, becaue of its growth potential.

We reaffirm our faith in the biological tissue principle which we espoused over 25 years ago. I believe we have remained faithful to this concept throughout all the vagaries of fashion and the all-pervading subtle commercial pressures. During this period, certain principles have been observed, others have emerged and at times it has been difficult to recognise when we are ignoring or even inadvertantly transgressing them.

Undoubtedly there are new fields to be explored and new paths for us to tread in our Pilgrim's Progress. So I take up my journey again with my friend Christian on his Pilgrim's Progress and take comfort from Ulysses complaint (which Tennyson puts into mouth):

"Yet all experience is an arch wherethrough gleams that untravelled world whose margin fades forever and forever when I move"

References

1. Lam CR, Aram HH, Munnell ER (1952) An experimental study of aortic valve homografts. Surg Gynaecol Obstets 94: 129

2. Murray G (1956) Homologous aortic valve segment transplants as surgical treatment of aortic and mitral insufficiency. Angiology 7: 446
3. Ross DN (1962) Homograft replacement of aortic valve. Lancet 2: 487
4. Gunning A, Duran CG (1962) A method of placing a total aortic valve in the subcoronary position. Lancet 2: 488
5. Ross DN, Somerville J (1966) Correction of pulmonary atresia with a homograft aortic valve. Lancet 2: 1446
6. Kay PH, Livi U, Robles A, Ross DN (1986) In: Bodnar E, Yacoub M (eds) Pulmonary homograft biologic bioprosthetic valves. Yorke Medical Books, p 58
7. Livi U, Abdulla AK, Parker R, Olsen E, Ross DN (1987) Viability and morphology of aortic and pulmonary homografts. J Thorac Cardiovasc Surg 93: 755
8. Ross DN (1969) Replacement of aortic and mitral valves with a pulmonary autograft. Lancet 2: 956
9. Pillsbury RC, Shumway NE (1966) Replacement of the aortic valve with the autogenous pulmonary valve. Surg Forum 17: 176
10. Geens M, Gonzalez-Lavin L, Dawbarn C, Ross DN (1971) Surgical anatomy of the pulmonary artery root in relation to pulmonary valve autograft and surgery of the RV outflow tract. J Thorac Cardiovasc Surg 262
11. Oh N, Somerville J, Ross DN, Ross JK, Emanuel R (1973) Mitral valve replacement with preserved cadaveric aortic homografts. J Thorac Cardiovasc Surg 65: 712
12. Berghuis J, Rastelli GC, Van Riet PD, Titus JL, Swan HJC, Ellis FH (1964) Homotransplantation of the mitral valve. Circulation 29: 1—47
13. Somerville J, Ross DN (1982) Homograft replacement of aortic root with re-implantation of the coronary arteries. Brit J 47: 473
14. Donaldson RM, Ross DN (1982) Homograft aortic root replacement for complicated prosthetic valve endocarditis. Circulation 70 (Suppl 1) 178—182
15. Oh W, Somerville J, Ross DN, Ross JK, Emanuel R (1973) Mitral valve replacement with preserved cadaveric aortic homografts. J Thorac Cardiovasc Surg 65: 712

Author's address:
D. N. Ross, M.D.
The National Heart Hospital
Westmoreland Street
London, W.1., U.K.

Allogeneic valve procurement in cardiac transplantation

S. Schüler, A. C. Yankah, R. Hetzer

German Heart Center Berlin (West), Germany

Introduction

Although clinical experience in the transplantation of heart valve allografts is rapidly increasing, the shortage of vital valves is still a key-point in the extension of allogeneic valve surgery. In the past, organ donors who were not suitable for cardiac transplantation provided a significant source for allogeneic valve procurement; however, with the increasing number of cardiac transplant procedures and the extension of the classical criteria for the selection of cardiac donors (1) this number is further decreasing.

In order to increase this small number of valve donors, we have started to use explanted hearts from heart transplant recipients, harvested during the operation for immediate preservation. A similar procedure has also been reported by others (2).

Patients and Methods

Between April 1986 and September 1987, 98 patients underwent orthotopic heart transplantation. Their ages ranged between 4 and 62 years with a mean of 40 years. The main preoperative diagnosis was congestive cardiomyopathy and end-stage coronary artery disease. The mean operative frequency was 5.8 operations per month (Fig. 1). In October 1986, an allogeneic valve surgery program was initiated. Due to the very small number of potential valve donors, explanted heart valves from transplant recipients were used.

The allograft preparation technique in transplant recipient's hearts had to be slightly modified. In contrast to normal valve donors, in transplant recipient's hearts, only a short vascular segment of the aorta and the pulmonary artery can be resected (Fig. 2) because the distal ending of the recipient's aorta and pulmonary artery have to be long enough for the classical transplantation procedure, as employed by Lower and Shumway (2) (Fig. 3).

Results

During an 11-month period, a total number of 75 hearts have been procured for allogeneic valves. 67 of those were harvested during transplantation procedures. Only eight donor hearts not suitable for cardiac transplantation were obtained. Out of the 134 allogeneic valves, 109 could be preserved for implantation; however, 25

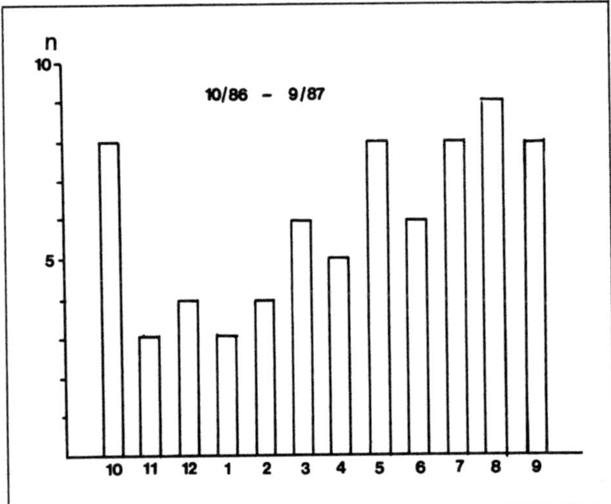

Fig. 1. Number of heart transplantation procedures per month between October 1986 and September 1987.

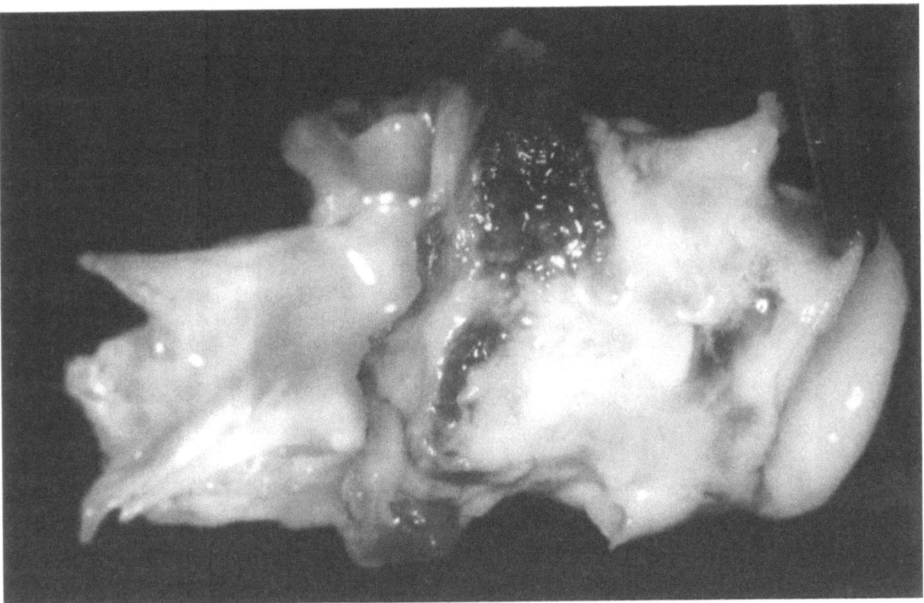

Fig. 2. Aortic conduit obtained from a transplant recipient's heart.

valves had to be excluded for various reasons; in nine hearts from recipients with end-stage coronary artery disease the aortic valve had to be rejected because of gross calcification. Five aortic valves from patients with congestive cardiomyopathy had to be discarded because of significant valve insufficiency. In seven aortic valves, gross calcifications could be found. In addition, four valves had to be excluded due to technical problems (Table 1). The interval between the explantation of the heart

14

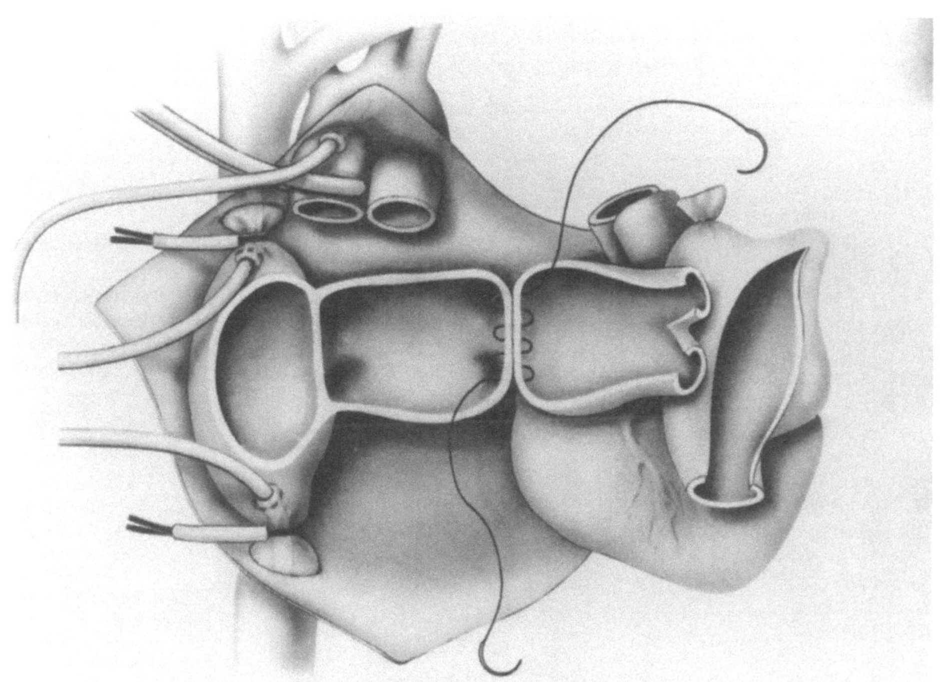

Fig. 3. Operative technique of orthotopic heart transplantation. Following resection of the recipient's heart, the remnants of the atria and ascending parts of the great vessels are anastomosed to the corresponding structures of the donor heart. Therefore, the allograft segment is significantly shorter compared to the classical technique in normal valve donors.

Table 1. Reasons for the unsuitability of 25 allogeneic valves.

Gross calcifications	9 aortic valves
Valve insufficiency	5 aortic valves
Atherosclerotic lesions	7 aortic valves
Technical problems	1 aortic valve
	3 pulmonary valves

and the beginning of the preservation procedure was 1 h in the majority of allografts. In seven hearts this period had to be extended up to 30 h for logistic reasons.

Conclusion

Explanted hearts of transplant recipients present a major source of allogeneic valve procurement. Therefore, an active transplantation program offers an ideal condition for allogeneic valve surgery. In the majority of explanted hearts, the valves were found to be normal. Less than 10% of all explanted valves had to be discarded, mainly due to gross calcifications or incompetence in hearts from patients with end-stage coronary artery disease or with congestive cardiomyopathy.

The major advantage of using hearts of transplant recipients is the immediate preservation of vital valves which might reduce tissue damage due to prolonged warm ischaemia.

References

1. Schüler S, Warnecke H, Matheis G, Hetzer R (1988) Extended donor criteria for cardiac transplantation. J Heart Transpl, in press
2. Dhalla N, Khaghani A, Radley-Smith R, Yacoub M (1986) Early and long-term performance of aortic homograft root replacement in biologic bioprosthetic valves. In: Bodnar E, Yacoub M (eds) Biologic Bioprosthetic Valves. Yorke Medical Books, p 7
3. Lower RR, Shumway NE (1960) Studies on orthotopic transplantation of the canine heart. Surg Forum 11: 11

Authors' address:
Stephan Schüler, M.D.
German Heart Center
Augustenburger Platz 1
1000 Berlin (West) 65
Germany

Antibiotic sterilisation in the preparation of homovital homograft valves: Is it necessary?

L. Gonzalez-Lavin, L. McGrath, M. Alvarez, D. Graf

Deborah Research Institute, Deborah Heart and Lung Center, Brown Mills, New Jersey, and Robert Wood Johnson Medical School — UMDNJ, New Brunswick, New Jersey, U.S.A.

Introduction

Homograft aortic heart valves collected at autopsy and treated with antibiotic solution before implantation have been found to be clinically superior to those sterilised by other methods (7, 9, 12, 20). Antibiotic sterilised aortic valves were first used clinically in 1968 at Green Lane Hospital. Since then, many antibiotic formulae have been devised.

Although valve preparation with this method has resulted in clinically superior results, antibiotic immersion has been shown to affect negatively the two factors thought to influence long-term valve survival: fibroblast viability, and host ingrowth into and onto the implanted leaflets (14—16, 18—19, 25). The source of homograft valves has expanded to include hearts obtained under sterile conditions from brain-dead, multi-organ donors, hence the term "homovital". It has been postulated that homovital valves are sterile and may be immediately implanted, cryopreserved, or stored in nutrient media alone. The present investigation was undertaken in order to examine this possibility.

Materials and methods

17 homovital aortic and pulmonary valved conduits were procured from hearts retrieved during sterile, multiorgan harvests from brain-dead, heart beating cadavers. In all cases, the cause of brain death was head trauma, ruptured cerebral aneurysm, or asphyxia. Donors were maintained on life support systems for 1—10 days (mean 3.4 $\pm$ 1). All blood cultures had been negative within 48 h prior to harvest. 62.5 % of donors received broad spectrum of intravenous antibiotics at some time during hospitalisation. The hearts were not acceptable for transplantation due to either a prolonged period of hypotension, a significant amount of inotropic support, or lack of a suitable recipient.

Upon removal from the donor mediastinum, each heart was rinsed in cold heparinised lactated Ringer's solution and double bagged in sterile plastic bags containing 200 ml of the same solution. The bags were sealed in a sterile nalgene jar and transported on ice to the homograft laboratory. Time between donor harvest and valve dissection ranged from 9—17 h (mean 12.4 $\pm$ 1).

Valve dissection was aseptically performed under a laminar flow hood. Several small pieces of distal pulmonary artery or aorta approximately 2×2 mm were taken for

culture following removal of excess adventitia and pericardium. Dissected valves were then placed in sealed sterile jars of antibiotic nutrient medium at 4 °C for 48 h (Table 1). Following this sterilisation period, the homografts were aseptically rinsed of antibiotic solution and again cultured prior to being prepared for cryopreservation.

Cultures for aerobic and anaerobic organisms were performed in liquid thioglycolate, and subcultured every third day. They were observed for a period of 10 days. Fungal cultures were performed in liquid Saboraud and Saboraud slant, and observed for a period of 1 month.

Table 1. Antibiotic nutrient medium.

250 ml RPMI # 1640, 10% fetal calf serum	
Cefoxilin	240 mcg/ml
Ticarcillin	2.5 mg/ml
Polymixin	100 mcg/ml
Neomycin	250 mcg/ml
Nystatin	500 U/ml

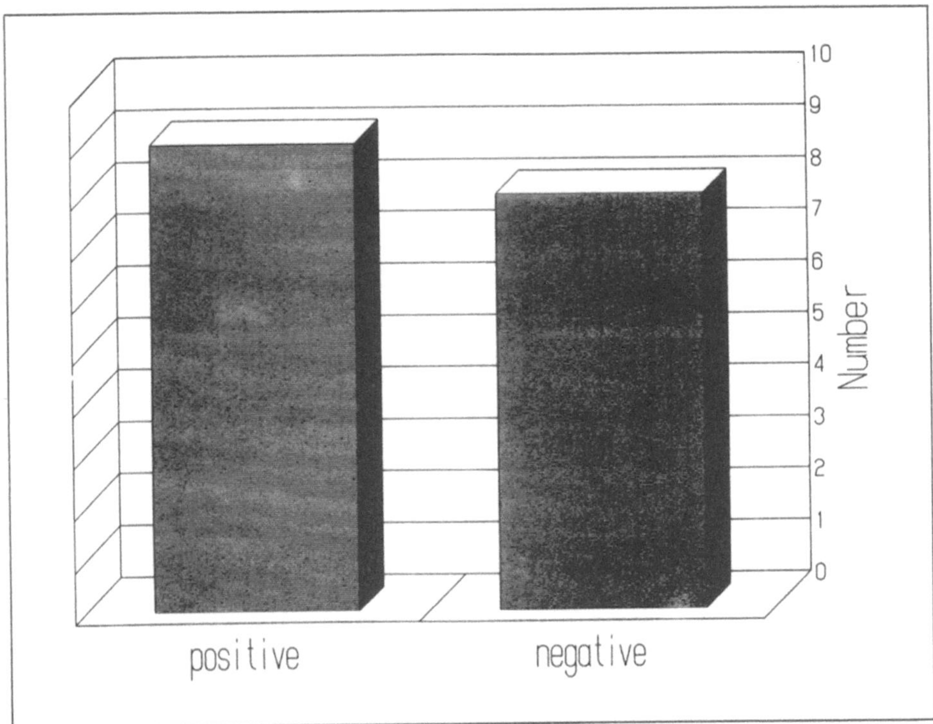

Fig. 1. Culture results, which were positive in 53 % of valves.

18

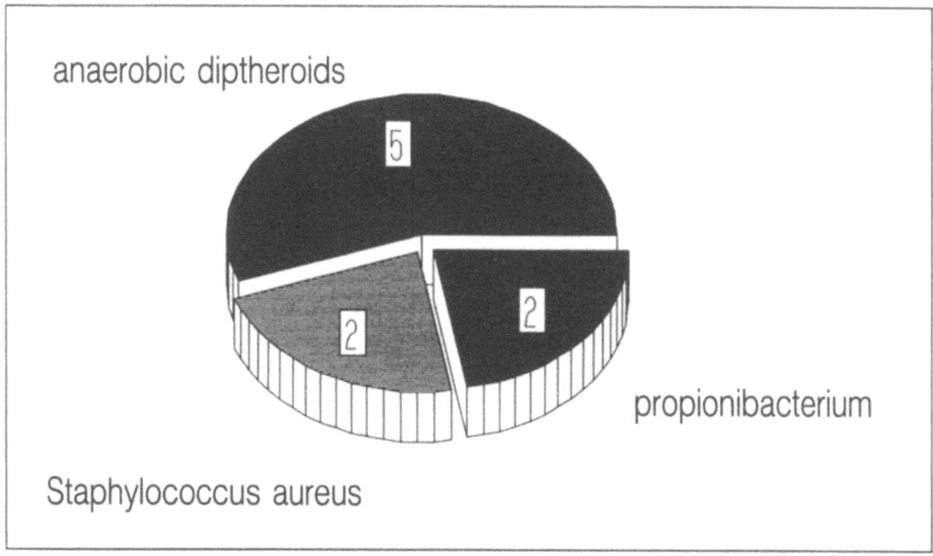

Fig. 2. Organisms isolated from positive cultures.

Results

Nine homografts has positive cultures at dissection from the donor heart (53 %) (Fig. 1). All positive cultures were evident during the first 48-h observation period. Contaminating organisms included anaerobic diphtheroids, Staphylococcus aureus, and propionibacterium (Fig. 2). All fungal cultures were negative.

Following 48-h antibiotic immersion, seven of the previously contaminated homografts had negative cultures, while two valves continued to grow anaerobic diptheroids.

We have implanted 13 homovital homograft valves. All cultures taken at the time of implantation were negative. One patient developed a mediastinal abscess which required resternotomy and drainage; he subsequently recovered and was discharged. There have been no instances of late infection.

Discussion

Homograft aortic valves were first used for clinical aortic valve replacement in 1962 (24). The need for sterilisation during the preparation and storage of homografts was immediately recognized, as it was not logistically possible to collect valves at autopsy under sterile conditions. In addition, it was shown that post mortem blood cultures were positive in 95 % of cadavers (29).

Initial methods of sterilisation included ethylene oxide, beta propriolactone, formalin, gamma irradiation, and freeze drying. However, the incidence of valve failure secondary to cusp rupture or calcification detracted from otherwise good clinical results (11, 21, 23, 26). It was felt that structural changes occurred in denatured valves and perhaps viable donor fibroblasts were an important factor which would contribute to long-term function (4, 10, 20).

Antibiotic immersion was introduced in 1969 by Barratt-Boyes (8), followed by numerous methods to assess fibroblast viability of the treated valves (1, 2, 5, 13, 15, 17, 19, 28). Initial clinical results with antibiotic-treated valves showed a very low incidence of valve failure (7, 9, 12, 20). Barratt-Boyes suggested that long-term valve survival was related to growth of host tissue into and onto the implanted leaflets, with more extensive ingrowth resulting in longer valve function (14—16). Both of those factors, fibroblast viability and host ingrowth have been shown to be adversely affected by antibiotic immersion (14—16, 18, 19, 25). Many different formulae have been advocated since 1968 to overcome these problems (3, 6, 22, 25).

The technique of antibiotic immersion has been cited as unreliable, and the belief that it is less damaging to valve structural integrity has been questioned (16, 27).

Antibiotic immersion has been shown to decrease the Class I antigens in endothelial and interstitial and Class II antigens in interstitial cells which may be associated with accelerated homograft degeneration in some patients (30).

During the last decade, more aggressive medical treatment and advances in the field of organ transplantation have resulted in an increase in the number of multiorgan donors, and therefore homovital homograft valves. Some homograft banks depend entirely on homovital, while for others, homovital tissue constitutes a very small percentage of their inventory. The possibility exists that valves could be stored untreated until culture results are known, after which contaminated valves could be discarded. This practice, however, would result in a considerable waste of homografts, as is demonstrated here.

The source of homovital homograft contamination is not readily apparent; however, time spent by the donor on life support systems, and the sequence of organ removal at the time of harvest may be considered. It is of interest to note that homograft valves removed from recipient hearts during heart transplantation are always sterile, and may be implanted untreated without consequence.

In conclusion, homograft valves procured from brain dead multiorgan donors should be considered contaminated. Even if the source of contamination is identified, it is not likely that donor management or procurement procedures would be changed, so antibiotic sterilisation is essential and should not be disregarded.

References

1. Al-Janabi N, Gibson K, Rose J, Ross D (1973) Protein synthesis in fresh aortic and pulmonary allografts as an additional test for viability. Cardiovasc Res 7: 247
2. Al-Janabi N, Gonzalez-Lavin L, Neirotti R, Ross D (1972) Viability of fresh aortic valve homografts: A quantitative assessment. Thorax 27: 83
3. Al-Janabi N, Ross D (1973) Enhanced viability of fresh aortic homografts stored in nutrient medium. Cardiovasc Res 7: 817
4. Angell W, Shumway N, Kosek J (1972) A five year study of viable aortic valve homografts. Thorac Cardiovasc Surg 64: 329
5. Angell W, Wuerflein R, Chun C, Shumway N (1973) Antibiotic sterilization of aortic homografts. N Z Med J 77: 31
6. Armiger L, Gavin J, Barratt-Boyes B (1983) Histological assessment of orthotopic aortic valve leaflet allografts: Its role in selecting graft pretreatment. Pathology 15: 67
7. Barratt-Boyes B (1971) Long-term followup of aortic valvular grafts. Br Heart J, Suppl I, 33: 60

8. Barratt-Boyes B, Roche A (1969) A review of aortic valve homografts over a six and one half year period. Annal Surg 170: 483
9. Barratt-Boyes B, Roche A, Brandt P, Smith J, Lowe J (1969) Aortic Homograft Valve Replacement. A long-term followup of an initial series of 101 patients. Circulation XL: 763
10. Barratt-Boyes B, Roche A, Whitlock R (1977) Six year review of the results of freehand aortic valve replacement using an antibiotic sterilized homograft valve. Circulation 55: 353
11. Beach M, Bowman F, Kaiser G et al (1972) Aortic valve replacement with frozen irradiated homografts. A long-term evaluation. Circulation Suppl I, XLV, XLVI: I-29
12. Bodnar E, Wain W, Martelli V, et al (1979) Long-term performance of 580 homografts and autograft valves used for aortic valve replacement. Thorac Cardiovasc Surg 27: 31
13. Chalcroft S, Gavin J, Seelye R (1974) A method for evaluating the effects of allograft sterilization procedures on the viability of human fibroblasts. Thorax 29: 539
14. Gavin J, Barratt-Boyes B, Hitchcock G, Herson P (1973) Histopathology of "fresh" human aortic valve allografts. Thorax 28: 482
15. Gavin J, Herson P, Barratt-Boyes B (1972) The pathology of chemically sterilized heart valve allografts. Pathology 4: 175
16. Gavin J, Herdson P, Monro J, Barratt-Boyes B (1973) Pathology of antibiotic treated human heart valve allografts. Thorax 28: 473
17. Gavin J, Monro J, Wall F, Chalcroft S (1973) Fine structural changes in the fibroblasts of canine homograft valves prepared for grafting. Thorax 28: 748
18. Girinath M, Gavin J, Strickett M, Barratt-Boyes B (1974) The effets of antibiotics and storage on the viability and ultrastructure of fibroblasts in canine heart valves prepared for grafting. Aust N Z J Surg 44: 170
19. Gonzalez-Lavin L, Al-Janabi N, Lockey E, Ross D (1973) Fibroblast viability in antibiotic treated valves. N Z Med J 77: 36
20. Gonzalez-Lavin L, Al-Janabi N, Ross D (1972) Long-term results after aortic valve replacement with preserved aortic homografts. Ann Thorac Surg 13: 594
21. Gonzalez-Lavin L, Ross D (1971) Late results after aortic valve replacement with homologous valves. Thorac Cardiovasc Surg 19: 308
22. Lockey E, Al-Janabi N, Gonzalez-Lavin L, Ross D (1972) A method of sterilizing and preserving fresh allograft heart valves. Thorax 27: 398
23. Missen G, Roberts C (1970) Calcification and cusp rupture in human aortic valve homografts sterilized by ethylene oxide and freeze dried. Lancet 2: 962
24. Ross D (1962) Homograft Replacement of the aortic valve. Lancet 2: 487
25. Strickett M, Barratt-Boyes B, MacCulloch D (1983) Disinfection of human heart valve allografts with antibiotics in low concentration. Pathology 15: 457
26. Wallace R, Londe S, Titus J (1974) Aortic valve replacement with preserved aortic valve homografts. Thorac Cardiovasc Surg 67: 44, 1974
27. Waterworth P, Lockey E, Berry E, Pearce H (1974) A critical investigation into the antibiotic sterilization of heart valve homografts. Thorax 29: 432
28. Watts L, Duffy P, Field R, Stafford E, O'Brien M (1976) Establishment of a viable homograft cardiac valve bank: A rapid method of determining homograft viability. Ann Thorac Surg 21: 230
29. Yacoub M, Kittle C (1970) Sterilization of valve homografts by antibiotic solutions. Circulation Suppl II, 41, 42: 29
30. Yacoub M, Suitters A, Khaghani A, Rose M (1986) Localization of major histocompatibility complex (HLA, ABC, and DR) antigens in aortic homografts. in: Bodnar and Yacoub (eds) Biologic bioprosthetic valves, proceedings of the III International Symposium. Yorke Medical Books, p 65

Authors' address:
Lorenzo Gonzalez-Lavin, M.D.
Chairman, Department of Surgery
Deborah Heart and Lung Center
Browns Mills, New Jersey 08015
U.S.A.

Procurement and viability of cardiac valve allografts

A. C. Yankah*, R. Hetzer

German Heart Center Berlin, Berlin (West), Germany

Introduction

The intermediate and long-term advantages of allografts in subcoronary and right ventricular outflow tracts outlined by the contributors of this book, and in previous reports (1, 3—9) suggest their superiority over other implantable prosthetic valves. Unfortunately the use of allograft is restricted, owing to procurement problems; therefore, allografts can be used as alternative valve substitutes for defined indications. In a state of perfection, one should aim at improving the longevity and durability of allograft valves by identifying the factors which influence them in vitro and in vivo (2, 10). The purpose of this communication, therefore, is to define viable and nonviable allografts (cellular components) which are generally in use in clinical practice and to establish some guidelines for future assessment.

Material and Methods

Seven fresh aortic valves (7 × 3 cusps) and ten pulmonary valves (10 × 3 cusps) were used for the study. Alcian blue dye exclusion test was used to test for viability of monolayer endothelial cells and fibroblasts of the allografts after 2 h at room temperature and 1, 2, 10, 20 and 30 h at 4 °C storage temperature, before treating them with antibiotics for final storage at 4 °C and − 80 °C for 7—14 days and 3—9 months, respectively (Table 1). The valves were stored in nutrient medium RPMI 1640 and human serum albumin. The technique for obtaining monolayer cells and dye exclusion test are described elsewhere (3, 6). The viable cells are unstained or slightly

Table 1. Antibiotic solutions used for treating contaminated cardiac valve allografts.

	I	II	III
Antibiotic solutions	1982—1984 RPMI 1640 + FCS	1985—1986 RPMI 1640 + FCS	Since Oct. 1986 RPMI 1640 + Human serum
Gentamycin	160 MG/L	40 MG/L	40 MG/L
Azlocillin	4000 MG/L	1000 MG/L	1000 MG/L
Flucloxacillin	2000 MG/L	1000 MG/L	1000 MG/L
Metronidazol	200 MG/L	200 MG/L	200 MG/L
Amphotericin B	100 MG/L	100 MG/L	100 MG/L

FCS = Fetal calf serum; I + II: University of Kiel*.

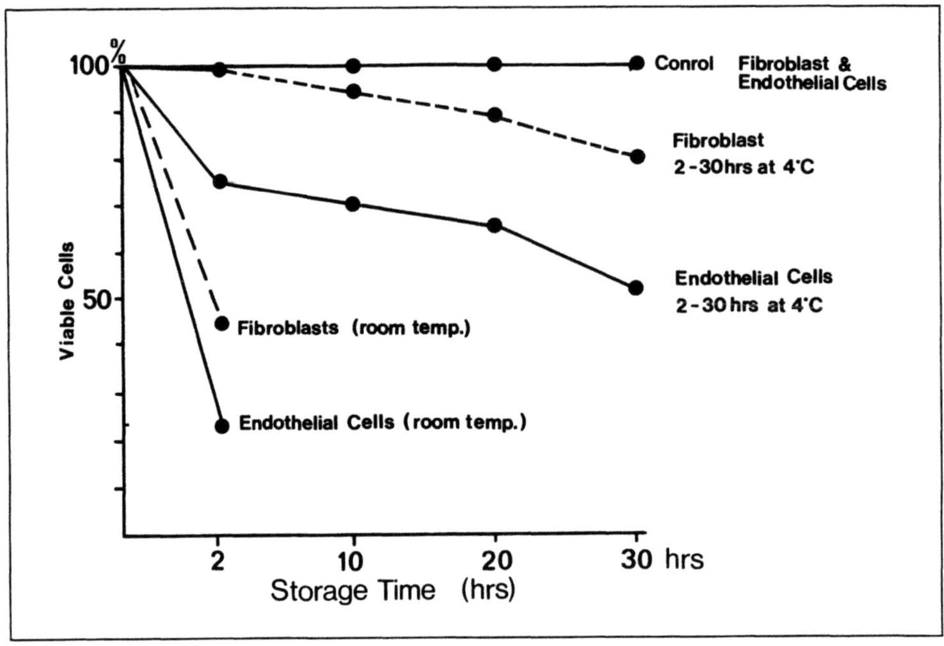

Fig. 1. Procurement of cardiac valve allografts: relationship between viability and temperature.

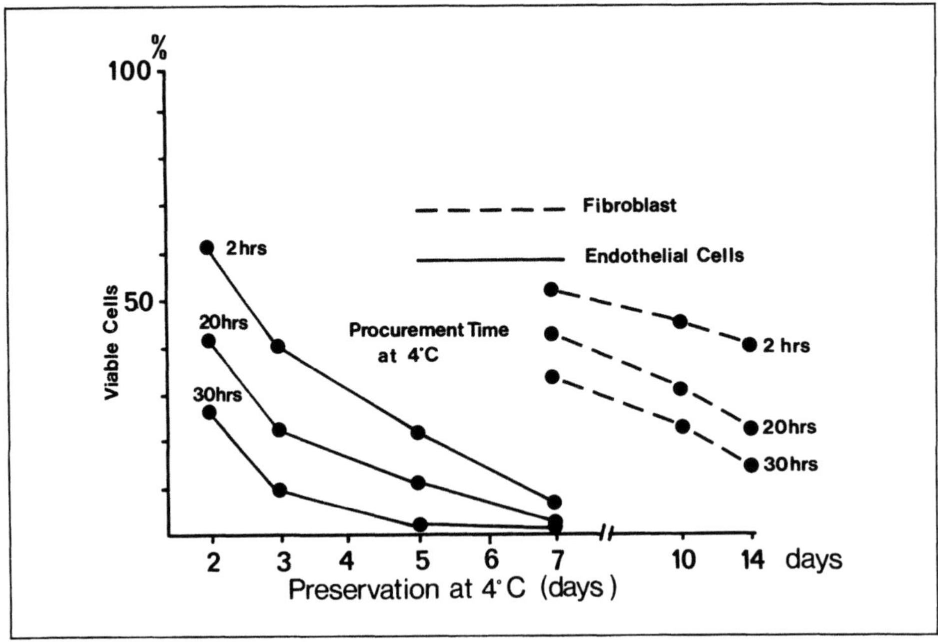

Fig. 2. Viability of cellular components after procurement and preservation.

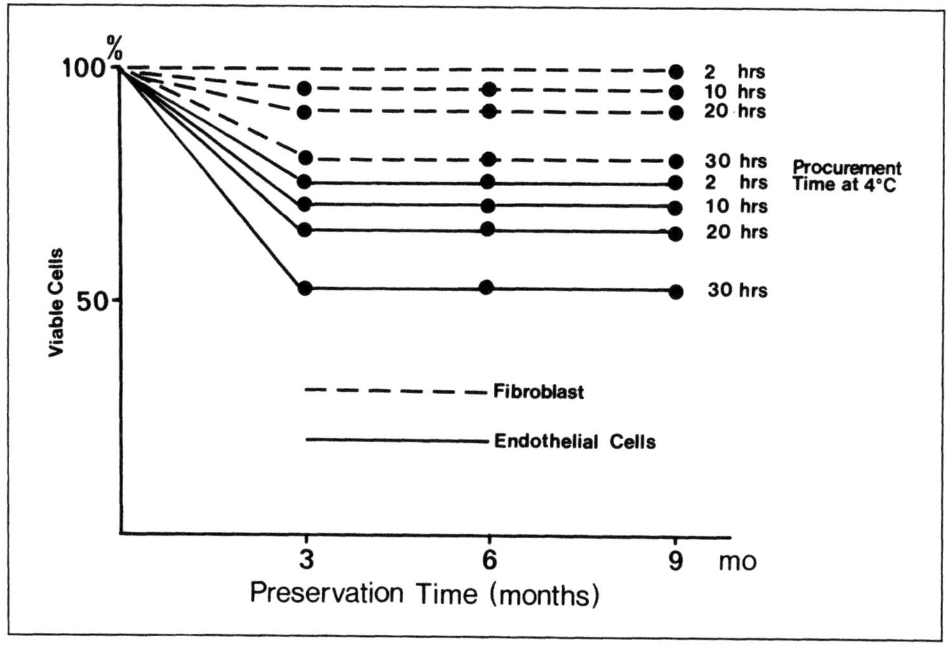

Fig. 3. Viability of cryopreserved allografts under defined procurement conditions (time and temperature).

stained, while the dead cells are recognized by deep blue staining. The percentage viability is the ratio of the number of unstained cells to the total number of cells identified microscopically ($\times$ 100).

Results

The control valve specimens obtained within 5 min post-cardiac explant showed 100% viable endothelial cells and fibroblasts. 24% of the endothelial cells and 45% of the fibroblasts were alive after 2 h exposure at room temperature as compared to 76% and 100% viability after 2 h storage at 4 °C, respectively. After 20 h storage at 4 °C, 65% and 90% viable endothelial cells and fibroblasts were identified, respectively. The viable cells decreased to 53% and 80% after 30 h in favour of endothelial cells and fibroblasts, respectively (Fig. 1).

Having now defined the time- and temperature-related viability status of the procured allografts, they were subjected to routine preservation in antibiotic solution and nutrient medium for 12 h, after which final storage at 4 °C for 7—14 days and — 80 °C for 3—9 months was made.

The viability of cellular components reduced insignificantly after 12 h antibiotic treatment; however, there was a significant viability loss after further storage at 4 °C thereafter until 14 days (Fig. 2). Unlike the cryopreserved allografts, the viability loss of cellular components was non-significant (Fig. 3).

Conclusions

Heart explants obtained within 30 h after circulatory arrest, and maintained at 4 °C are acceptable, although they might have different survival and longevity rates. Obligatory antibiotic treatment at 12 h showed a minimum effect on viability. Warm ischaemia was the major cause of ongoing viability loss during preservation at 4 °C. Cryopreservation is therefore preferable for long-term storage. Maintenance of viable endothelial cells in vitro raises the question of histocompatibility in allograft surgery in order to protect further viability loss of cellular components in vivo.

Acknowledgement

We are grateful to Mrs. Lee for her technical assistance in the preparation of the manuscript.

References

1. Angell WW, Angell JD, Oury JH, et al (1987) Long-term follow-up of viable frozen aortic homografts. A viable homograft bank. J Thorac Cardiovasc Surg 93: 815—822
2. Bank HL, Brockbank KGM (1987) Basic principles of cyrobiology. J Cardiac Surg I No. 3 Suppl: 137—143
3. Barratt-Boyes BG (1979) Cardiothoracic surgery in the antipodes. J Thorac Cardiovasc Surg 78: 804—822
4. Kirklin JK, Kirklin JW, Pacifico AD (1985) Homograft replacement of the aortic valve. Cardiol Clin 3: 329—341
5. Miller C, Shumway E (1987) Fresh aortic allografts: Long-term results with free-hand aortic valve replacement. J Cardiac Surg I, No. 3 Suppl: 185—191
6. O'Brien MF, Stafford G, Gardner M, et al (1987) The viable cryopreserved allograft aortic valve. J Cardiac Surg I, No 3 Suppl: 153—167
7. Penta A, Qureshi S, Radley-Smith R, Yacoub MH (1984) Patient status 10 years or more after fresh homograft replacement of aortic valve. Circulation 70, Suppl I: I-182
8. Ross D (1987) Application of homografts in clinical surgery. J Cardiac Surg I, No 3, Suppl: 175—183
9. Somerville J, Ross D (1985) (May) Fate of the aortic homograft used for reconstruction of the right ventricular outflow tract (Abstract). Proceedings of the Third International Symposium on Biologic and Bioprosthetic valves. London
10. Yankah AC, Wottge HU, Müller-Hermelink HK, et al (1987) Transplantation of aortic and pulmonary allografts, enhanced viability of endothelial cells by cryopreservation, importance of histocompatibility. J Cardiac Surg I, No 3 Suppl: 209—220

Authors' address:
A. C. Yankah, M.D.
German Heart Center
Augustenburger Platz 1
1000 Berlin (West) 65
Germany

Cryobiology of tissues

S. R. May[1], J. G. Baust[2]

[1]LifeCell Corporation, Texas, U.S.A.,
[2]Center for Cryobiological Research, State University of New York at Binghamton, U.S.A.

Introduction

There is considerable interest in the transplantation of mammalian tissues for the treatment of disease states and trauma and the correction of tissue malfunction. The logistics of tissue procurement for transplantation are such that some method of tissue preservation is highly desirable. To date, the most common method of preservation has been hypothermic storage, either cold storage above freezing (usually 4 °C) or else cryopreservation and storage in the frozen state (usually − 70 °C to − 196 °C). The advantage of hypothermic storage in the unfrozen state is that ice damage is avoided, but the disadvantage is that there is a limited storage duration of about 1 week or less (11, 19). The advantage of cryopreservation is that truly long-term preservation ranging from months to years can be obtained, while the disadvantage is in the lack of a complete understanding of the mechanism of cryoinjury, so that cryopreservation produces significant damage as a result of ice formation during the freezing process. Nevertheless, cryopreservation has decided advantages over refrigerated storage provided that effective methodologies can be developed for the specific tissue under consideration.

Difficulties in tissue cryopreservation

Certain difficulties are inherent in attempts to cryopreserve tissue, and Table 1 lists some of them. The most important of these are tissue mass and geometry, since these dictate the degree of control which can be maintained over the cooling and warming processes. Excessive supercooling and extended exothermic and endothermic temperature plateaus during cooling and warming, respectively, can occur if the tissue is so thick or of such mass that it prevents rapid equilibration of the surface temperature to yield virtual homogeneity of temperature throughout. Thin tissue cross-sections prevent the establishment of significant temperature gradients between the surface and the interior. It is for this reason that thin tissues such as skin and heart valves have been able to be cryopreserved by technologies which apply cooling or warming to the outside of the tissues (9).
Another difficulty in tissue cryopreservation is the fact that most tissues have a mixture of cell types. Since different cell types demonstrate different sensitivity to cryoinjury, the choice of a particular cryopreservation regimen could result in the preservation of some cell types at the expense of others, which would suffer signif-

Table 1. Variables affecting tissue cryopreservation.

Tissue mass	Cellular density
Tissue geometry	General tissue architecture
Mixed cell types	Vascular components

icant cryoinjury. Such a differential susceptibility to cryoinjury has been shown, for example, in the epithelial and fibroblastic cells of skin (2).

The cellular density of the tissue is also a difficulty. If cells are packed at a density similar to that of organs, for example 80%, then cryosurvival is reduced. The mechanism of this effect is not known, but the degree of packing affects the access of cryoprotectant to the cells, the exchange of water across the membrane, and the formation of ice (14).

Another difficulty, general tissue architecture, refers to the specific structure of the tissue, including layers of different cell types such as occurs in skin, or areas of different cells such as occurs in the Islets of Langerhans in pancreatic tissue. Architectural inhomogeneities may lead to natural fracture planes when the tissue is frozen. Thus, freezing of skin may promote a separation between the dermal and epidermal layer postthaw or posttransplantation (5).

Finally, there is the difficulty of the vascular components in tissue. The vascular system in a tissue has endothelial cells which are exquisitely sensitive to injury, and this includes cryoinjury (3). Thus, if the in situ posttransplantation viability of the cryopreserved tissue depends upon the functioning of its vascular system, rather than simple diffusion to supply nutrients, then sufficient damage might be incurred by the tissue's vascular system during the cryopreservation process to cause subsequent graft failure. A typical example involves the lack of viability of grafted kidneys due to failure of circulation posttransplantation (13).

Cryopreservation variables

The ten primary variables which impinge on the effectiveness of cryopreservation are enumerated in Table 2 in the order of their occurrence during the cryopreservation process. The table also matches each variable with a list of specific concerns or potential negative outcomes associated with the specific choice of procedural variable.

We have already mentioned that the size and geometry of tissue creates problems of thermal inhomogeneity, so that proper control of the cooling and warming rate might be precluded. A relatively large amount of this inhomogeneity due to large tissue mass or thickness will impede the proper control of temperature throughout the tissue, allowing the possibility of potentially damaging exothermic temperature plateaus such as those found in blood cells (17). Anoxia or hypoxia is an important concern from the time the tissue is removed from the donor; a suitable isolation medium must be chosen to balance the nutritional and osmotic needs of the cell, the former to provide adequate energy for the cells' ion pumps and the latter to prevent dialysis of required intracellular solutes. Similar caveats hold for the cryoprotectant medium, which is often delivered to the tissue in a base medium iden-

28

Table 2. Cryopreservation variables and their related problems.

Variable	Concern
Tissue size and geometry	Thermal inhomogeneity
Isolation medium	Anoxia/hypoxia dialysis
Cryoprotectant	Toxicity Osmolarity Dialysis
Prefreeze cooling	Thermal shock Membrane adjustment Changed reaction rates
Cooling	Ice damage Exothermic temperature plateau Solute concentration Membrane effects
Water state	Temperature Time Chemical reactions
Warming	Same as cooling, except the temperature plateau is endothermic.
Restoration medium	Toxicity Osmolarity Dialysis
Removal of cryoprotectant	Osmolarity
Viability	Adequate structure Adequate function

tical to the isolation medium. The cryoprotective agent must be chosen for low toxicity to the particular tissue being cryopreserved, and the exposure of the tissue to the cryoprotectant must be adjusted so as to allow sufficient time for adequate uptake of the agent, while minimizing the length of exposure to the agent's toxic properties. For most tissues, like skin (Ralph Guttman, unpublished data) and embryos (Kenneth Bondioli, unpublished data), a 15-min exposure at 4 °C is sufficient. Osmotic stress on the membranes might be decreased by using a two-step addition of the cryoprotectant, e.g., first 7% glycerol, then 15-min equilibration time, then 15% glycerol, followed by more equilibration time.

The next series of cryopreservation variables to be considered relate to the cooling of the tissue. Prefreeze cooling refers to the change in tissue temperature from 37 °C (donor body temperature) to 4 °C (refrigerator temperature). This is usually accomplished as a single-step transfer, or at most a two-step transfer: from 37 °C to 22 °C (room temperature) and from 22 °C to 4 °C. During this period, there are gross changes in the cell membrane and in the rates of biochemical reactions in the cell; the cell may not be able to produce sufficient energy levels to maintain isotonicity, so this should be compensated for by the use of an isolation and/or storage medium which is isotonic for as many cellular constituents as possible. Sufficient time for membranes shrinkage should be allowed during this temperature transition. This also applies during cooling. Generally, a slow cooling rate of between $-1\,^{\circ}C$ per mintue and $-5\,^{\circ}C$ per minute is employed with tissue (1).

The water state is related to the final storage temperature and the duration of storage. At storage temperatures below the glass transition temperature (at least $-139\,^{\circ}C$ and probably lower, for water) no water movement and recrystallization of ice will occur to yield mechanical damage, and rates of chemical reactions and biophysical processes will be too slow to affect cell survival in a negative way (4). Warming of frozen tissue again presents the opportunity for the formation of a potentially harmful temperature plateau unless adequate control of warming rate is achieved throughout the tissue. That rate must exceed $+100\,^{\circ}C$ per minute (1, 10, 15).

Finally, the choice of restoration or revitalization medium should be made on the basis of the tissue's nutritional and osmotic needs. The cryoprotectant-containing medium must be dialyzed out of the tissue at such a rate so as to preclude osmotic damage, and perhaps a two-step procedure of first transferring a tissue in 15% (v/v) glycerol to a 7% solution and, after equilibration, to a 0% solution should be employed. The definition and assessment of viability should be based upon the preservation of adequate structure and function.

Successfully preserved mammalian tissues

In spite of the myriad complications associated with cryopreservation, nearly a dozen tissues have been reported to be effectively cryopreserved (1). These are listed in Table 3. I have chosen to place these tissues into two categories: those whose posttransplantation role is primarily structural in its functioning and those whose role is mainly biosynthetic in its functioning.

The cryopreservable tissues which are structural in their function appear to have certain similarities, namely, they are characterized by relatively high collagen content, relatively light cell densities or even nearly acellularity, few cell layers with concomitant ease of permeability, relatively few cell types, relatively simple architecture, flat geometry, and they possess relatively active pentose phosphate pathways. It is easy to see why these types of tissues are among the most readily cryopreservable, since many of their specific attributes overcome many of the innate difficulties inherent in the cryopreservation process. It is problematical whether the cells of these tissues are adequately cryopreserved to retain their viability, since their viability may not be required for their structural role, and they might subsequently be colonized by the graft recipient's own cells. Certainly, techniques which could destroy the cellular viability of these tissues, such as excessive heat or chemical toxicity, appear to decrease their longevity and effectiveness posttransplantation. However, no definitive study has shown precisely what level of cellular viability is required for adequate posttransplantation performance. Hopefully, future work will

30

Table 3. Successfully preserved mammalian tissues.

Structural functionality	Biosynthetic functionality
Dura mater	Embryos and fetal tissues
Corneas	Pancreatic tissue
Fascia lata	Parathyroid tissue
Heart valves	Thyroid tissue
Immature teeth	
Skin	
Veins and arteries	

further define the role of cellular viability in these cryopreserved, transplantable tissues with a structural functionality.

The second group of cryopreservable tissues, those with biosynthetic functionality, are a little more difficult to preserve than the first group, and rightly so, for they do not possess many of the above-mentioned attributes. Instead, they rely primarily on small size and concomitantly easy permeability and homogeneity of temperature throughout to promote cryopreservability. Most of these tissues are glandular in function, and only small portions of the entire gland are cryopreserved as individual units. An example of this is the cryopreservation of individual isolated Islets of Langerhans for the pancreas (6). Unlike the structural type of cryopreservable tissue, the biosynthetic tissues appear to require cellular viability and function in order to maintain their biosynthetic capacity.

General cryopreservation scheme

In general terms, tissues are currently cryopreserved by the application of slow cooling rates to material which has equilibrated with relatively high molar concentration (> 0.5 M) of the permeating cryoprotectants glycerol or dimethyl sulphoxide, followed by storage in liquid nitrogen and very rapid warming directly prior to use (Table 4). Cryoprotectants such as glycerol and dimethyl sulphoxide protect slowly frozen cells by one of the following mechanisms: (i) reduction in the increase of salt concentration with the dehydration associated with cooling, (ii) reduction of the temperature-dependent cell shrinkage at a given temperature, and (iii) reduction in the proportion of the solution frozen at a given temperature (12). The technique enumerated is Table 4 is quite suitable for the structural tissues listed in Table 3. Of the items presented in Table 4, the rapidity of the warming rate, the osmolarity of the isolation medium or cryoprotectant base, and the presence and concentration of a cryoprotectant seem to be the most critical components.

The very nature of the scheme presented in Table 4 is such that it is a general method which is partially effective in cryopreserving many tissues; however, it does not appear to be optimized for any given tissue, since some cell death appears to always be detectable post-thaw, due to the fact that all cryoprotectants are cytotoxic to some degree (18). Certain points should be made with regard to the general cryopreser-

Table 4. General cryopreservation scheme for mammalian tissues.

Parameter	Usual choice
Tissue size	Flat tissues, small cell aggregates or individual cells
Isolation medium or cryoprotectant base	Phosphate buffered saline or standard tissue culture medium (e.g. Eagle's Minimal Essential Medium with fetal calf serum)
Cryoprotectant	5—15% v/v glycerol or dimethyl sulfoxide; instilled in 1—2 step dilution
Prefreeze cooling	Single step to 4 °C
Cooling	− 1 °C per minute to − 5 °C per minute
Storage	− 196 °C (liquid nitrogen)
Warming	> 100 °—200 °C per minute
Restorative medium	Phosphate buffered saline or standard tissue culture medium
Removal of cryoprotectant	1—2 Step Dilution
Viability	Tested by graft "take" and sometimes by biochemical markers

vation scheme in Table 4. Firstly, there is a requirement for a flat tissue for the sake of rapid uptake of the cryoprotectant and rapid warming after storage. Secondly, the use of tissue culture medium is good for the maintenance of the cells when the tissue is being stored prior to cryopreservation; however, at 4 °C these media generally change their pH. The rapid (> 100 °C per minute) warming is needed for many cell types, but may be inappropriate for some, such as mammalian embryos, which are optimally rewarmed at rates of 4 °—25 ° per minute (7). The specific cooling and warming rates used must be optimized for the tissue being preserved. Storage is usually in liquid nitrogen to minimize the chance for ice crystal formation and subsequent tissue damage due to temperature rises above − 139 °C during storage (4). The warming rate is quite rapid, and could be even faster, e.g. + 1,000 °C per minute as reported for skin (10). It might be helpful to remove the cryoprotectant in a one- or two-step dilution to minimize osmotic stress to the cells.

Finally, the choice of cryopreservation technique is usually based on subsequent graft "takes", where no statistical comparison between different cryopreservation schemes has been vigorously undertaken. In spite of these many caveats, the scheme presented in Table 4 has been found to work with many tissues.

The future

Several promising new methods of tissue cryopreservation have recently become available. One of these is a technique based on the ultrarapid cooling of the tissue on a metal mirror cooled with liquid nitrogen or liquid helium. This technique precludes the use of cryoprotectants and thus obviates their cytotoxicity and osmotic stresses associated with their use. The rapidity of the ultrarapid cooling produced by this method is sufficient to convert the water in tissue into a glass state, so no damaging ice crystals are formed; this process is called vitrification. After vitrification, the tissue can be slowly dried while the temperature is raised to ultimately allow room-temperature storage of the preserved tissue (8). The technique has been found to be effective in the case of mammalian corneas, and work is in progress on other tissues.

Finally, some experiments have been undertaken with high potassium cryoprotectants (19) or with the use of multiple low-dose cryoprotectants in order to achieve vitrification at a higher temperature and with a reduction in the total amount of cytotoxicity because each cryoprotectant is present in a lower dose than usually required (6, 16).

The surgical need for effective tissue transplants acts as a strong impetus for the improvement of tissue preservation technologies. These improvements are most likely to come in the areas of preservation media and cooling techniques. There is no doubt that the future of tissue cryopreservation holds great promise for the effective preservation of an increased number of clinically useful tissues.

References

1. Ashwood-Smith MJ (1980) Low temperature preservation of cells, tissues and organs. In: Ashwood-Smith MJ, Farrant J (eds) Low temperature preservation in medicine and biology. University Park Press, Baltimore, p 19—44
2. Athreya BH, Grimes EL, Lehr HB, Green AE, Coriell LL (1969) Differential susceptibility of epithelial cells and fibroblasts of human skin to freeze injury. Cryobiology 5: 262—269
3. Belzer FO, Hoffman R, Huang J, Downes G (1972) Endothelial damage in perfused dog kidney and cold sensitivity of vascular Na-K-ATPase. Cryobiology 9: 457—465
4. Grout BWW, Morris GJ (1987) Freezing and cellular organization. In: Grout BWW, Morris GJ (eds) The effects of low temperatures on biological systems. Edward Arnold, London, pp 147—173
5. Heck EL, Bergstresser PR, Baxter CR (1985) Composite skin graft: Frozen dermal allografts support the engraftment and expansion of autologous epidermis. J Trauma 25: 106—112
6. Jutte NHPM, Heyse P, Jansen HG, Bruining GJ, Zeilmaker GH (1987) Vitrification of human islets of Langerhans. Cryobiology 24: 403—411
7. Leibo SP, Mazur P, Jackowski SC (1974) Factors affecting survival of mouse embryos during freezing and thawing. Exp Cell Res 89: 79—88
8. Linner JG, Livesey SA, Harrison DS, Steiner AL (1986) A new technique for removal of amorphous phase tissue water without ice crystal damage: A preparative method for ultrastructural analysis and immunoelectron microscopy. J Histochem Cytochem 34: 1123—1135
9. May SR, DeClement FA (1980) Skin banking methodology: An evaluation of package format, cooling and warming rates, and storage efficiency. Cryobiology 17: 33—45
10. May SR, Wainwright JF (1985) Optimum warming rates to maintain glucose metabolism in porcine skin cryopreserved by slow cooling. Cryobiology 22: 196—202
11. May SR, Wainwright JF (1985) Integrated study of the structural and metabolic degeneration of skin during 4 °C storage in nutrient medium. Cryobiology 22: 18—34
12. Mazur P (1974) Fundamental cryobiology and the preservation of organs by freezing. In: Karow AM Jr, Pegg DE (eds) Organ Preservation for Transplantation. Marcel Dekker, New York, Basel, pp 143—175
13. Pegg DR, Green CJ (1973) The functional state of kidneys perfused at 37 °C with a bloodless fluid. J Surg Res 15: 218
14. Pegg DE, Jacobsen IA, Armitage WJ, Taylor MJ (1979) Mechanisms of cryoinjury in organs. In: Pegg DE, Jacobsen IA (eds) Organ Preservation II. Churchill Livingstone, Edinburgh, p 132

15. Rajotte RV, Stewart HL, Voss WAG, Shnika TK, Dosstor JB (1977) Viability studies on frozen-thawed rat islets of Langerhans. Cryobiology 14: 116—120
16. Rall WF, Fahy GM (1985) Ice-free cryopreservation of mouse embryos at — 196 ˚C by vitrification. Nature 313: 573—575
17. Rowe AW, Rinfret AP (1962) Controlled rate freezing of bone marrow. Blood 20: 636
18. Shlafer M (1974) Pharmacological considerations in cryopreservation. In: Karow AM Jr, Pegg DE (eds) Organ Preservation for Transplantation. Marcel Dekker, New York, Basel, pp 177—212
19. Taylor MJ (1986) Clinical cryobiology of tissues: Preservation of corneas. Cryobiology 23: 323—353

Authors' address:
S. R. May, Ph.D.
LifeCell Corporation
3606-A Research Forest Drive
The Woodlands
Texas 77381
U.S.A.

Cryopreservation of aortic valve homografts

J. K. Kirklin, J. W. Kirklin, A. D. Pacifico, S. J. Phillips

University of Alabama Medical Center, Department of Surgery,
University Station, Birmingham, U.S.A.

The technique of cryopreservation of aortic valve homografts was developed by Dr. Mark O'Brien at Prince Charles Hospital in Brisbane, Australia. This technique has been duplicated with minor modifications at the University of Alabama at Birmingham (UAB). Since 1981, the technique of cryopreservation for storage of aortic valve homografts has been employed at UAB.

At the time of procurement, the heart, ascending aorta, and aortic arch are harvested. The heart and ascending aorta is then placed in a basin containing Ringer's Lactate or normal saline solution at 4 °C. At this time, all blood is rinsed from the heart and ascending aorta. The heart is prepared for transport by placing it in a sterile bowel bag with several hundred cubic centimeters of saline or Ringer's solution. This is placed within a second bowel bag, which is then placed in a cooler packed with ice for transport to the tissue bank.

The *dissection* of the homograft aortic valve and ascending aorta is carried out with sterile technique under a laminar flow hood. The epicardium is dissected from the aorta down to the base of the aortic root. The right and left coronary arteries are transected approximately 33 cm from the ostia, and the aorta is further dissected free from the pulmonary artery. The homograft is dissected free from the underlying cardiac muscle by incising the adjacent portions of the right ventricle, right atrium, and left atrium.

The valve is now moistened and carefully sized and its length measured. The posterior mitral leaflet is removed and sectioned into two pieces which will be used for culture.

The *sterilisation* process is completed by placing the homograft valve and one of the mitral leaflet sections into a special container with antibiotic solution (Table 1). A sample of the shipping solution and the remaining leaflet section are sent for microbiological culture. The specimen container is now placed in a wide-mouthed jar fitted with an air-tight lid and incubated for 24 h at 37 °C.

After this period, the allograft is ready for *packaging*. At this time, the second mitral leaflet section and a sample of the antibiotic solution are sent for fungal and bacterial

Table 1. Antibiotic solution for aortic valve homografts.

Amphotericin B	10 µg/ml RPMI
Streptomycin	50 µg/ml RPMI
Penicillin	50 units/ml RPMI

The above are added to 250 ml of RPMI 1640 (a balanced, buffered salt solution with supplementary amino acids, vitamins, and glucose). The solution is prepared prior to valve dissection and is stored at 4 °C for no longer than 24 h, after which it is discarded.

cultures. The freezing solution contains RPMI 1640 (180 ml) with 10 % fetal calf serum. Dimethylsulphoxide (DMSO) (20 ml) is added to obtain a 10 % DMSO solution. The homograft is placed in 100 ml of the freezing solution and transferred to a sterile polyester pouch which is heat sealed. This pouch is then placed in a larger sterile nylon suran-coated pouch which is also heat sealed. Five to 10 ml of the freezing solution are poured into a sterile container and sent for culture.

The *cryopreservation* process is initiated by placing the homograft in a controlled rate liquid nitrogen freezing chamber (Cryomed*). The homograft is frozen at a rate of 1 °C/min to — 40 °C and then removed from the freezing chamber and placed in a storage box which is then stored in a liquid nitrogen refrigerator at — 192 °C.

The homograft is later discarded if any of the leaflet sections or solutions prove to be contaminated by bacteria or fungi after the antibiotic treatment.

When the surgeon selects the appropriate size of homograft valve in the operating room, the homografts in its sealed pouch is transported from the liquid nitrogen refrigerator to the operating room for the *thawing* and *diluting* process. The outer pouch is cut with sterile scissors and the inner pouch, containing the frozen homograft, is placed in warm saline (42 ° to 50 °C) for 2—3 min. The inner pouch with the homograft is then placed in a second basin with warm saline, to complete the thawing procedure, which is generally accomplished within 4 min. Dilution of the DMSO solution is accomplished by gently rinsing and warming the homograft in four successive solutions containing RPMI plus 10 % fetal calf serum and decreasing concentrations of DSMO. The homograft is rinsed in each of the four solutions for 1 min. After completing the rinsing and diluting process, a small piece of the homograft plus several millimeters of RPMI solution are sent for culture. The homograft is now ready for trimming and implantation.

Authors' address:
James K. Kirklin, M.D.
UAB, Department of Surgery
University Station
739 Zeigler Bldg.,
Birmingham, AL 35294
U.S.A.

---

* Mt. Clemens, MI 48045

Factors affecting the viability of cryopreserved allograft heart valves

A. E. Heacox, R. T. McNally, K. G. M. Brockbank

CryoLife, Inc., Marietta, U.S.A.

Introduction

Allograft heart valves have been used for more than 25 years as replacements for diseased aortic valves and repair of congenital abnormalities. In many instances, particularly paediatric surgery, it is the valve of choice due to its non-obstructive flow, relative freedom from calcification and thromboembolism without anticoagulation therapy. In order to permit valve size matching for recipients, it is necessary to find methods of storage which will maintain cellular viability. The best method which allows infinite, convenient storage is cryopreservation.

The longevity and durability of allograft heart valves is dependent upon cellular viability because living fibroblasts are necessary for the maintenance of the valve matrix (10, 18). This is emphasized by the fact that human aortic valves stored at 4 °C for more than 4 days have low initial viability and are non-viable at explant. These "fresh" valves show a significant increase in incidence of rupture and leaflet perforation as well as a 20% to 30% increase in valve-related death, reoperation and embolism when compared to viable cryopreserved tissue (17).

There are three major reasons why the so-called "fresh" antibiotic 4 °C stored valves will be reduced in quality. Firstly, prolonged exposure to antibiotics will eventually be toxic to the valve cellular elements. Secondly, tissues stored at temperatures above their freezing point but below their physiological temperature requirement become oedematous due to water influx into the extracellular matrix compartment. Finally, there are the effects of ischaemia upon the valve cells. With the onset of ischaemia, cells enter a potentially reversible phase of general metabolic depression. For operational purposes, we consider 24 h of cold ischaemia prior to receipt at our laboratories to be the maximum acceptable interval. Eventually, this period may be extended by incorporation of some of the many modifications attempted in the literature for organ perfusion and transport solutions, such as adenosine and high phosphate, to retard the loss of high energy phosphate bonds, glycolytic inhibitors (citrate and 2-dioxy-glucose-6 phosphate), calcium channel blockers and agents which quench oxygen free radicals.

The highest viability standards must be maintained throughout the entire processing procedure. This includes, in addition to procurement and transportation, sterilisation, freezing, storage, thawing, and eventual transplantation of the allograft valve. In the following paper, we will review some of the current techniques utilised in the cryopreservation of human allograft valves which will affect their viability.

37

Sterilisation

Various methods have been used to sterilise allograft heart valves. In the past, ethylene oxide (22), beta-propiolactone (11), and gamma irradiation (15), were used. However, all of the above render a non-viable and possibly structurally damaged valve; therefore, these methods are no longer used.

Today, the most commonly used and widely accepted method of sterilisation for allograft tissue is broad spectrum antibiotics in a nutrient medium (Table I). Antibiotic treatments should provide sterile tissue in a reproducible manner and simultaneously maintain viability. Generally, all the methods reported in the literature seem to provide adequate sterility; however, the level of cellular viability has, in many cases, never been ascertained.

It is also possible that antibiotic resistant organisms will be encountered. Thus, it is important that post-treatment microbial screening be performed in order to eliminate the possibility of transplanting contaminated tissue. The cell culture media used in these treatments serve as a buffered balanced salt solution, providing energy and essential nutrients in the pre-freeze and post-thaw intervals. These media should extend cellular viability, but they are not adequate for long-term preservation.

The vast majority of antibiotics function by disrupting bacterial cell division or metabolism and therefore require the presence of proliferating organisms in order to be effective. Most antibiotics will be more effective over a shorter time period if the incubation occurs at 37 °C as opposed to 4 °C. The other side of the problem is, of course, toxicity to the cells which are to be preserved. This antibiotic cytotoxicity will depend upon the specific antibiotics used and is a function of both exposure time and temperature. As a rule of thumb, it is safe to say that cell mortality will increase as the temperature and exposure time to any antibiotic mixture increases. Thus, the very time and temperature changes which will best assure sterility (37 °C

Table 1. Antibiotic treatments for allograft heart valves.

Antibiotics	Medium	Incubation time (h)	Temp (°C)	Reference
Gentamycin, Methicillin Erythromycin-Lactobionate, Nystatin	Hanks sol, TC 199 w/ 10% FBS*, Hams F-10	24	4	10, 16
Penicillin, Streptomycin, Kanamycin, Amphotericin B	Hanks sol.	24—72	4	4, 10
Gentamycin, Azlocillin, Flucloxacillin, Metronidazol, Amphotericin B	RPMI-1640 w 20% FBS	Storage Time Indef.	4	23
Cefoxitin, Lincomycin, Polymyxin B, Vancomycin, Amphotericin B	TC 199	48	4	4, 2
Penicillin, Streptomycin, Amphotericin B	Eagles MEM**	24	37	21

FBS*   + fetal bovine serum
MEM** = minimum essential medium

and a long exposure time) may be detrimental to fibroblast viability. If low temperature incubation is chosen, it may be possible to enhance antibiotic effectiveness. It should be pointed out that polymyxin B and amphotericin B have a detergent-like quality and will act on the cell membrane of a resting organism. Although the spectrum of organism they affect is rather narrow, they will likely enhance the effectiveness of antibiotic treatments which are administered at 4 °C providing they do not have a membrane destabilizing effect upon the valve fibroblast.

When designing an effective tissue sterilisation protocol, it is necessary to assay viability as well as sterility. It is difficult to compare the antibiotic treatments mentioned in this paper, with respect to viability, because the authors either chose not to discuss viability or used differing assay techniques. In fact, some of the techniques used appear inappropriate for valve fibroblasts (5). We will avoid discussing various assays and their suitability because they appear elsewhere in this volume (3). However, it should be pointed out that the best assay is the determination of protein synthesis following incubation in radio-labelled amino acids, using scintillation counting (1, 14, 18) coupled with autoradiographic analysis of tissue sections (7, 18, 19). As a final note, we would like to point out that Watts et al. have described a fast qualitative method for determining allograft valve viability by following glucose utilisation and pH change. Because of its non destructive nature, this method might be used, if properly quantified, as a spot-check during processing.

Cryopreservation

Mammalian cells have been successfully frozen in the presence of cryoprotectants at rates between 0.3 and 10 °C/min. In most cases, freezing is done kinetically in the presence of a cryoprotectant such as glycerol or dimethylsulphoxide (DMSO). In these cases, freezing occurs at an optimum rate for the particular cell type or tissue in question. The optimum rates observed are ultimately determined by cell size and permeability, and can be explained by the two factor hypothesis of freezing injury (12). This hypothesis infers that cells frozen at a rate below optimum suffer damage due to solution effects (i.e., dehydration, increased solute concentration, changes in pH, etc.) that occur as water is being removed from the cell. The loss of water is an osmotic response to solutes concentrated in the external medium as water is incorporated into growing ice crystals. When the cooling rate is above optimum, the cells do not have sufficient time to respond to the hyperosmotic external medium and intracellular ice is formed, resulting in cell damage or death. It should be pointed out that the optimum cooling rate is determined by the interaction of many variables, but factors such as type and concentration of cryoprotectant, as well as warming rate, need special consideration.

While it is possible to make mathematical estimates of optimum freezing rates, most researchers choose to take an empirical approach. Such is the case with allograft heart valves. Allograft valves have been successfully cryopreserved using glycerol or DMSO in nutrient media and cooled at rates ranging from 1.0 °C to 1.5 °C/min. The most extensive study in this area is that of van der Kamp et al. (19), who tested various concentrations of glycerol, ethylene glycol, and DMSO, and analysed the results quantitatively by the incorporation of [H^3]-proline into collagen by canine and human valve fibroblasts. This work showed that valves frozen in Ham's F-10 medium supplemented with 15% fetal calf serum showed superior viability (81% of controls) when frozen at 1 °C/min. The valves in this study were thawed "rapidly" but there is no indication of the actual rate. The rate would be largely dependent on the total volume of the sample and the temperature of the water bath used for thawing. Dilution of the cryoprotective agent was done stepwise over a 15-min period. This study only investigated the effects of changes in cryoprotectant and cryoprotectant concentration on fibroblast survival. The effects of changes in the cooling rate and warming rate, which are often more critical, have not been investigated. Because the interactions of cooling rate, warming rate and cryoprotectant influence optimum survival (6, 8), a study investigating the role of these factors in promoting fibroblast or endothelial survival may prove worthwhile.

Storage

Storage of cryopreserved tissue should be at a sufficiently low temperature so that gradual growth of ice crystals over time is prevented. This temperature should be below the glass transition point of the medium in which it is frozen in order to prevent chemical reaction. The glass transition temperature of pure water is − 139 °C and freezing media are commonly in the range of − 120 °C. A convenient storage system is liquid nitrogen at − 196 °C or the vapor phase of a liquid nitrogen freezer (− 170° to − 180 °C). In addition, there are an increasing number of mechanical refrigerators which can safely maintain temperatures below − 135 °C. Most reports on cryopreserved allograft valves indicate that storage was done at − 196 °C. However, Wallace (20) has stored chemically treated valves at − 70 °C without long-term success of implants, and Watts (21) indicated that preserved leaflets stored at − 75° for up to 7 months produced viable cell cultures. In the latter case, however, no quantitative information is available, so deleterious effects of storage at this temperature may have not been properly assessed.

In general, temperatures in the − 70° to − 115 °C range are not suitable for the long-term storage of viable tissues because of damaging ice crystal growth, as well as physical and chemical reactions which can take place slowly with time (24). To minimize such damage, samples should be stored in liquid nitrogen so that temperature fluctuations do not occur during storage. It should be noted that even short exposures to ambient temperatures may cause the sample to warm, permitting ice crystal growth.

Thawing and dilution

As was stated earlier in this paper, cellular viability in cryopreserved tissues is dependent on a number of interactions, warming rate being one of them (6, 8, 9, 13). Changes in warming rate will not only affect the survival of frozen cells, but may shift or broaden the rates at which optimum cooling can take place (8). Fast warming is usually desirable and has been recommended with heart valves. The actual achievable warming rate is dependent upon the total volume of the homograft and solution,

40

the insulating qualities of the packaging, and temperature of the thawing medium. In the allograft literature, fast thawing means immersing the container in a 37 °—42 °C water bath until the valve is thawed. This may be as short as 2 min ($\sim$ 98 °C/min) (2) for aortic valves in 20 ml of medium or, in our experience, 12—14 min ($\sim$ 15 °C/min) for aortic and pulmonary valved conduits with a total combined volume of 100 ml for valve and medium. In cryobiological terms, these extremes would both fall in the range of an intermediate thawing rate. This difference in thaw rate may be insignificant if the corresponding cooling rate was near the tissue optimum: slow warming of tissues exposes the cells to less osmotic shock because smaller temporal osmotic gradients are experienced during warming, resulting in better tissue viability (8). We are not aware of any studies in which the effects of changes in warming rate on allograft viability have been tested.

The dilution of cryoprotectant from the allograft tissue should be done in a stepwise manner. This will tend to reduce the osmotic stress. However, due to the fact that most cryoprotectants exhibit cellular toxicity, the dilution should be carried out in an expedient manner.

Conclusion

Cryopreserved allograft heart valves have a number of advantages over non-viable allografts and alternate valves. The major factors influencing the viability of cryopreserved heart valves are: (1) the duration of warm and cold ischaemia experienced during procurement and transportation of the tissue; (2) use of sterilisation procedures which optimise both tissue sterility and cell viability; (3) selection of appropriate cryoprotectants and cooling rates; (4) storage below $-$ 135 °C; (5) rapid thawing and gradual dilution of cryoprotectants.

Although cryopreserved heart valves have been used clinically for nearly 25 years, very few in-depth studies have been undertaken to evaluate and understand this method of heart valve preservation. Several investigators have used a variety of freezing protocols, which appear to be acceptable, but which have not been evaluated for tissue viability. Consequently, methods of cryopreservation are being used which in essence are poorly understood. We propose, that if the variables discussed in this paper are properly evaluated, this method of preservation will yield even better results for tissue viability and longevity which will ultimately benefit the patient.

References

1. Al-Janabi N, Gibson K, Rose J, Ross DN (1973) Protein synthesis in fresh aortic and pulmonary valve allografts as an additional test for viability. Cardiovasc Res 7: 247
2. Armiger LC, Gavin JB, Barratt-Boyes BG (1983) Histological assessment of orthotopic aortic valve leaflet allografts: Its role in selecting graft pre-treatment. Pathology 15: 67
3. Bank HL, Schmehl MK, Brockbank KGM (1988) Endothelial and fibroblast viability assays for tissue allografts. In: Yankah C A et al. (eds) Current concepts on the use of aortic and pulmonary allografts for heart valve substitutes, Berlin 7—9 September 1987. Steinkopff, Darmstadt
4. Barratt-Boyes BG, Roche AHG (1969) A review of aortic valve homografts over a six and one-half year period. Ann Surg 170: 483

5. Brockbank KGM, Bank HL (1987) Measurement of postcryopreservation viability. J Card Surg 2 (Suppl): 145
6. Frim J, Mazur P (1983) Interaction of cooling rate, warming rate glycerol concentration and dilution procedure on the viability of frozen-thawed human granulocytes. Cryobiology 20: 657
7. Henney AM, Parker DJ, Davies MJ (1980) Estimation of protein and DNA synthesis in allograft organ culture as a measure of cell viability. Cardiovasc Res 14: 154
8. Leibo SP, Farrant J, Mazur P, et al (1970) Effects of freezing on marrow stem cell suspensions: Interactions of cooling and warming rates in the presence of PVP, sucrose, or glycerol. Cryobiology 6: 315
9. Leibo SP, Mazur P, Jackowski SC (1974) Factors affecting survival of mouse embryos during freezing and thawing. Exp Cell Res 89: 79
10. Lockey E, Al-Janabi N, Gonzalez-Lavin L, Ross DN (1972) A method of sterilizing and preserving fresh allograft heart valves. Thorax 27: 398
11. LoGrippo GA, Overhulse PR, Szilagyi DC, Hartman FW (1955) Procedure for the sterilization of arterial homografts with beta-propiolactone. Lab Invest 4: 217
12. Mazur P (1965) Causes of injury in frozen and thawed cells. Fed Proc 24 (Suppl 15): 175
13. Mazur P, Schmidt J (1968) Interactions of cooling velocity, temperature, and warming velocity on the survival and frozen and thawed yeast. Cryobiology 5: 1
14. McGregor CGA, Bradley JF, McGee JO'D, et al. (1976) Tissue culture, protein and collagen synthesis in antibiotic sterilized canine heart valves. Cardiovasc Res 10: 389
15. Meeker IA Jr, Gross RE (1951) Sterilization of frozen arterial grafts by high voltage cathode-ray irradiation. Surgery 63: 45
16. Mochtar B, van der Kamp AWM, Roza-DeJongh EJM, Nauta J (1974) Cell survival in canine aortic heart valves stored in nutrient medium. Cardiovasc Res 18: 497
17. O'Brien MF, Stafford G, Gardner M, Pohlner P, McGiffin D, Johnston N, Brosnan A, Duffy P (1987) The viable cryopreserved allograft aortic valve. J Cardiac Surg 2 (Suppl): 153—167
18. van der Kamp AWM, Nauta J (1979) Fibroblast function and the maintenance of the aortic valve matrix. Cardiovasc Res 13: 167
19. van der Kamp AWM, Visser WJ, van Dongen JM, et al (1981) Preservation of aortic heart valves with maintenance of cell viability. J Surg Res 30: 47
20. Wallace RB, Giuliani ER, Titus JL (1971) Use of aortic valve homografts for aortic valve replacement. Circulation 43: 365
21. Watts LK, Duffy P, Field B, et al (1976) Establishment of a viable homograft cardiac valve bank: 1. A rapid method of determining homograft viability. Ann Thorac Surg 21: 230
22. Wilson AT, Bruno P (1950) The sterilization of bacteriological media and other fluids with ethylene oxide. J Exp Med 91: 449
23. Yankah AC, Sievers HH, Bursch JH, et al (1984) Orthotopic transplantation of aortic valve allografts. Early hemodynamic results. Thorac Cardiovasc Surg 32: 92
24. Bank HL, Brockbank KGM (1987) Basic principles of cryobiology. J Cardiac Surg 2 (Suppl): 137

Authors' address:
Albert E. Heacox, Ph.D.
CryoLife, Inc.
Suite 142, 2211 New Market Parkway
Marietta, Georgia 30067
U.S.A.

Endothelial and fibroblast viability assays for tissue allografts

H. L. Bank, M. K. Schmehl, K. G. M. Brockbank*

Department of Pathology and Laboratory Medicine, Medical University of South Carolina, Charleston, South Carolina, U.S.A., and * CryoLife Inc., Marietta U.S.A.

Introduction

To perfect methods for the freezing, storage and subsequent transplantation of cells and tissues, it is important to set the criteria for success at the outset. Therefore one or more criteria should be defined which accurately maintain the ability of the system to carry on its physiological function. For example, a frozen-thawed vein should be capable of performing as a conduit after implantation. The vein should not be prone to stenosis, aneurysms, or leakage around the suture lines, and should ideally be non-thrombogenic. Since thrombosis and vascular tone is dependent upon the presence of an intact endothelial lining, a viable cryopreserved allograft should have an intact endothelial lining. For heart valves, the presence of a high percentage of the fibroblasts which are capable of resynthesizing the collagenous matrix of the valve, as well as maintaining the mechanical integrity, is the primary consideration. The viability of any tissue after cryopreservation is dependent in part upon handling during procurement and prefreezing storage. Any exposure to non-physiological conditions, such as ischemia, hypoxia, or anoxia causes direct toxicity to most cell types or sensitizes the cells to the subsequent stresses of freezing and thawing. Careful selection of the cryobiological variables can minimize but not eliminate the loss in viability. Major considerations include the type of cryoprotective agent used, the concentration of that agent, the temperature of exposure, cooling rate, warming rate, osmotic effects, media effects, and dilution scheme. If the goal is to optimize survival of an organ or a specific cell type, then each of the major cryobiological variables must be optimized individually and all the component steps must be optimized with respect to each other, since all of the variables interact in determining the ultimate survival of the cells. In vitro assays are useful to reduce the huge number of variables and to establish tentative optimal conditions prior to time consuming in vivo testing.

In this manuscript several viability assays are described for the assessment of heart valve and vein viability. The vein and heart valve cryopreservation procedures used protocols developed for the CryoLife, Inc.

Viability assays

A variety of assays (Table 1) are used to optimize tissue procurement, transport and cryopreservation. These assays can be classified in five principle groups: (1) Mor-

Table 1. Commonly used heart valve viability assays.

Component tested	Analytical method	References
Fibroblasts	Proliferation in situ	5, 9
	Proliferation in vitro	5, 10
	Protein synthesis	1, 5, 7, 8, 10
	Collagen synthesis	7, 10
	Glucose uptake	11
Endothelial cells	Viability dye test	15
	Protein synthesis	8
Valve integrity	Mechanical testing	8, 12
Valve morphology	Microscopy (LM & TEM)	3, 4, 8, 11, 13

phological procedures, including routine histology, surface antigen localization, and transmission electron or scanning microscopy are used for rapid selection of the most promising experimental procedures, (2) proliferation studies, (3) metabolic assays, (4) implantation or (5) mechanical assays. The appropriateness of a given assay depends on the specific tissue and the function which is being optimized. In this paper we have focused on the use of the first three assays.

Morphological procedures are currently used in our laboratory to evaluate heart valves and venous tissue. To quantitate the morphological integrity of endothelial cells, we use morphometric analysis. 1-μm sections are scored using an optical grid and the viability expressed as $(100 - \%$ loss of cells$) - (\#$ of hypertrophic nuclei $*$ $(100 - \%$ loss $/ \#$ of nuclei$))$.

By the use of this index, much of the subjective aspects of comparing different treatments can be eliminated. Figures 1—4 are light micrographs of unfrozen canine saphenous veins, illustrating the typical morphology encountered. All key observations are subsequently verified by electron microscopy.

A rapid fluorometric method has been developed to evaluate the cellular viability of heart valves. The assay differentiates between viable and nonviable cells by the simultaneous use of the inclusion and exclusion dyes, acridine orange (AO) and propidium iodide (PI). When viewed by fluorescent microscopy, viable cells fluoresce green, while nonviable cells fluoresce bright red. The green fluorescence is due to the binding of the membrane permeable AO to the nucleic acids, acid mucopolysaccharides and polyphosphates. The red fluorescence is due to the entry of PI into dead cells where it forms a complex with the nucleic acids. When live and dead cells are superimposed, a yellow color is observed. This yellow color is due to the combination of red and green fluorescence. Although the AO and PI assay measures membrane integrity, the results of this assay correlates with other measures of cell viability. The AO/PI assay is capable of simultaneously visualizing live and dead cells in intact valves and is sensitive enough to detect individual dead cells within a valve composed of thousands of living cells.

Proliferation studies are most useful when the tissue or organ can be dissociated into an isolated population of cells. Such assays measure the reproductive potential of the cells. For these assays to be quantified, the number of cells and their functional

44

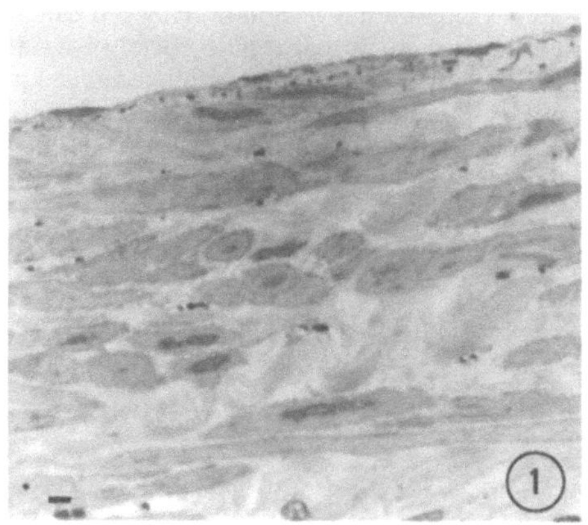

Fig. 1. Longitudinal section of normal canine saphenous vein. Elongated endothelial cells containing flattened nuclei line the intimal surface. Smooth muscle cells embedded in a collagen matrix can be seen in the media. The adventitial layer consists of loose connective tissue composed primarily of collageneous bundles and elastic network. Original magnifications, 250X, from 1-μm plastic sections stained with Toluidine Blue (bar = 2.5 μm).

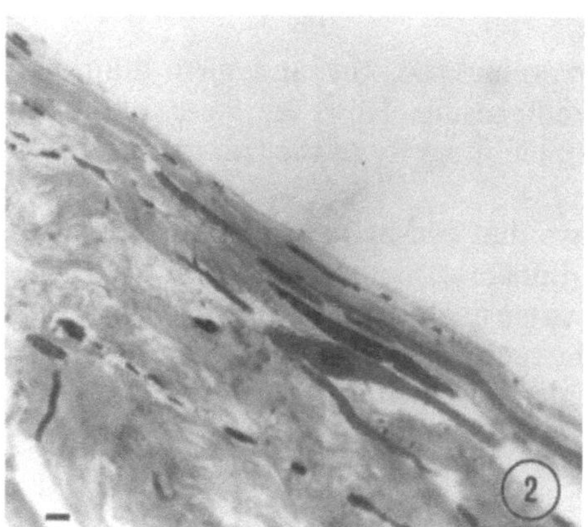

Fig. 2. Longitudinal section of saphenous vein after the endothelium was removed by collagenase digestion showing remnants of the intima on the surface. Some disorganization is apparent in the medial and adventitial layers (bar = 2.5 μm).

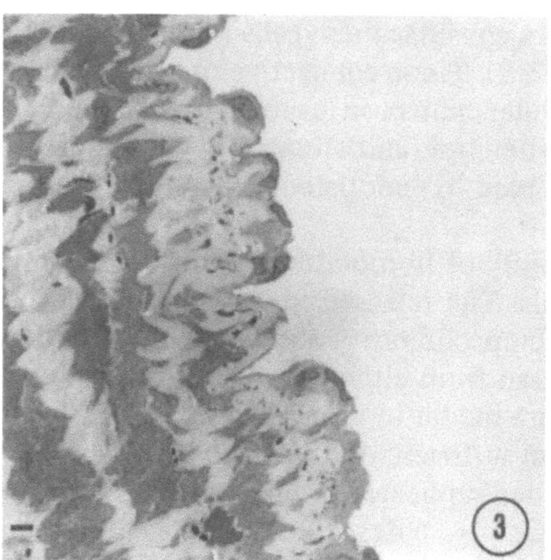

Fig. 3. Longitudinal section of canine saphenous vein in venospasm. The ruffled luminal surface is lined by irregularly shaped endothelial and smooth muscle cells. The endothelial cells appear to have contracted, resulting in irregularly shaped nuclear profiles. The underlying layer appears as a complex pattern created by the contraction of muscle (bar = 2.5 μm).

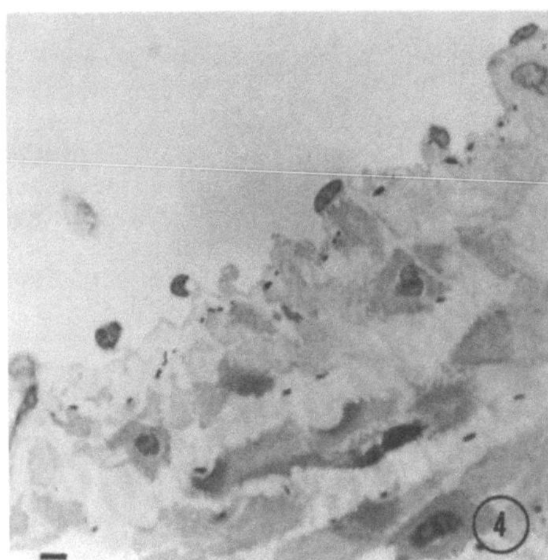

Fig. 4. Longitudinal section of damaged canine saphenous vein. Hypertrophic nuclei protrude into the lumen or are being exfoliated. The underlying tissue is disorganized, appears to have lost its vascular tone and the cells are degenerating (bar = 2.5 µm).

capacity must be related back to the control values, i.e.: the equivalent dilution of the starting population which yields comparable results. However, these studies provide little information on the three-dimensional integrity of the frozen and thawed tissue or organ.

There are a wide variety of metabolic assays that can be used to indirectly assess the viability of the tissues. Radioisotopic uptake of compounds such as labelled proline, glucose or deoxyglucose are used extensively with excellent results. Such assays can be used either for the uptake of the radioisotopes or the release of labelled radioisotopes from cells as a result of freezing and thawing.

Heart valve viability

Heart valves are composed of fibroblasts and endothelial cells in addition to the extracellular matrix. Most studies on heart valve viability focus on aortic valve fibroblasts (Table 1) because several authors consider these cells a prerequisite for long-term function of transplanted valves (2, 9). These connective tissue fibroblasts are responsible for production of intercellular matrix in heart valves (7) and are considered to be crucial for the long-term function and strength of the implanted tissue. There has been much less attention paid to endothelial cell viability during procurement and preservation of valves.

One excellent method of assaying the viability of fibroblasts is to digest the valve matrix using collagenase to release the cells. The released fibroblasts can then be plated in tissue culture media to measure their proliferative abilities, using a limiting dilution assay. In this assay, the cells released from either the matrix of the valve, or the intima of veins, are diluted in culture media in a series of microtiter wells. Typically, we use two-fold dilution steps and sufficient dilution steps to obtain both positive and negative cultures. Three to four replicates of eight culture wells are used per dilution step. After growth at 37 °C for ~ 6 days, the replicate cultures are scored for viable cells. The expected frequency of proliferating fibroblasts can be

46

calculated by the Poisson distribution. Wells are scored as positive if a clonal unit of four or more cells are identified. Typically, the plot of the number of positive cultures gives a sigmoid response when a number of replicates are averaged. Replotting the data as a negative logarithm of a fraction of negative cultures versus dilution yields a linear relationship. Although most investigators use a regression analysis to estimate the number of viable cells, we have shown through Monte Carlo simulations, that a chi-squared analysis is preferable. The regression analysis yields a very high variance while a weighted t-test typically produces values 10 % lower than expected.

A number of studies have estimated the function of fibroblasts by analysis of protein synthesis (1, 5, 7, 8, 10). Total activity is assessed by the incorporation of radioactivity into tissue before homogenization and counting (6, 8, 15). Autoradiography can be used not only to assess cell protein synthesis but to distinguish between cell death and impaired protein synthesis of each cell (5, 7, 8). For example, Van der Kamp and Nauta (7) compared the in vivo uptake for ^{3}H-methionine, which was predominantly incorporated in non-collagenous proteins, and ^{3}H-proline for collagen synthesis is aortic valves. Thus, autoradiography can indicate which cells have the potential of regaining their normal activity. Unfortunately, autoradiography is relatively expensive and time consuming compared with liquid scintillation or gamma counting of the homogenized tissue. An effective way to study protein synthesis in tissues is to use isotopic uptake coupled with autoradiography. This combination of methods determines whether there are any significant changes in protein synthesis per cell or changes due to cell death.

Most studies (8) show that when heart valves obtained from experimental animals are properly handled, they retain viable endothelial cells. However, the endothelium is destroyed within 24 to 48 h post mortem. Using a different approach, Yankah (14) reported that the rat valve endothelium appeared to be viable for at least 40 h post mortem, as determined by the alcian blue dye exclusion technique.

It is not clear how important the survival of heart valve endothelial cells is in the survival of transplanted tissue. The absence of endothelium may lead to insufficient fibroblast nutrition, the formation of thrombi and calcification. Unfortunately most techniques for harvesting the cells cause extensive mechanical abrasion of the endothelial lining cells. In addition, the handling of the valve at the surgical implantation serves to further damage the surface of these cells. Several studies address the viability of endothelial cells using techniques such as silver staining of endothelial cell cement (6), alcian blue exclusion (14), autoradiography (8) and quantitative morphology, which has been used in our laboratory. In general, those assays which measure functional attributes of endothelial cells yield far lower estimates of viability than silver or vital staining.

In summary, we find that the endothelial cells from human heart valves are often damaged during procurement or subsequent processing. Further experimentation is required to develop procurement and preservation techniques for these cells.

References

1. Al-Janabi N, Gibson K, Rose J, Ross DN (1973) Protein synthesis in fresh aortic and pulmonary valve allografts as an additional test for viability. Cardiovasc Res 7: 247

2. Angell WW, Lanerolle P de, Shumway NE (1973) Valve Replacement: present status of homograft valves. Prog Cardiovasc Dis 15: 589
3. Gavin JB, Barratt-Boyes BG, Hitchcock GC, Herdson PB (1973) Histopathology of "fresh" human aortic valve allografts. Thorax 28: 482
4. Gavin JB, Monro JL, Wall FM, Chalcroft SCW (1973) Fine structural changes in the fibroblasts of canine heart valves prepared for grafting. Thorax 28: 748
5. Henney AM, Parker DJ, Davies MJ (1980) Estimation of protein and DNA synthesis in allograft organ cultures as a measure of cell viability. Cardiovasc Res 14: 154
6. Innes BJ, Thomson NB, Aywers W (1969) Postmortem changes in endothelial cells of aortic valve homografts. J Thorac Cardiovasc Surg 58: 416
7. Kamp AWM van der, Nauta J (1979) Fibroblast function and the maintenance of the aortic-valve matrix. Cardiovasc Res 13: 167
8. Kamp AWM van der, Visser WJ, Dongen JM van, Nauta J, Galjaard H (1981) Preservation of aortic heart valves with maintenance of cell viability. J Surg Res 30: 47
9. Lockey E, Al-Janabi N, Gonzalez-Lavin L, Ross DN (1972) A method of sterilizing and preserving fresh allograft heart valves. Thorax 27: 398
10. McGregor CGA, Bradley JF, McGee J O'D, Wheatley DJ (1976) Tissue culture, protein and collagen synthesis in antibiotic sterilized canine heart valves. Cardiovasc Res 10: 389
11. O'Brien M (1987) The viable cryopreserved allograph aortic valve. J Cardiac Surg: 2 (Suppl): 153—167
12. Parker R, Randev R, Wain WH, Ross DN (1978) Storage of heart valve allografts in glycerol with subsequent antibiotic sterilization. Thorax 33: 638
13. Rajotte RV, Shnitka TK, Liburd EM, Dossetor JB, Voss WAG (1977) Histological studies on cultured canine heart valves recovered from — 196 °C. Cryobiology 14: 15
14. Yankah AC, Randzio G, Wottge HU, Bernard A (1985) Factors influencing endothelial cell viability during procurement and preservation of valve allografts. In: Thiede A, Deltz E, Engemann R, Hamelmann H (eds) Microsurgical models in rats for transplantation research. Springer-Verlag, Berlin, p 107

Authors' address:
Harvey L. Bank
Department of Pathology and
Laboratory Medicine
Medical University of South Carolina
Charleston, SC 29425
U.S.A.

Discussion

Chaired by: D. Behrendt, USA

GUNNING:

The idea of grafting parts of the body from one person to another has inspired a number of legends and myths. The use of the aortic valve homograft, however, is of recent origin, dating from the experiments of Lam, Heimbecker, Murray, Gunning and Duran in the 1950s and 1960s. As a result of their work, the aortic homograft has become established as an accepted replacement for the diseased aortic valve and has now become an important part of the cardiac surgeon's armamentarium. Difficulties of harvesting, preservation and surgical technique have been largely overcome. Cryopreservation seems to represent a distinct advance in preservation.

KUMPER:

I would like to describe a new method of measuring the integrity of endothelial cells of the aortic valve of the rat. It is known that endothelial cells take up alcian blue into their cytoplasm when the cell membrane is altered. The ratio of viable to nonviable cells can be estimated by counting the light and dark cells manually through a microscope. Mr. Yankah improved this technique by using a photometer microscope to measure objectively the transmission of light through individual cells. A reference point is placed next to the endothelial cell and the transmission is set to 100%. Then the measuring point is placed on an endothelial cell and its transmission is measured. With this technique we have found that there was no great difference between using DMSO and using nutrient medium for storage. Even at − 80 °C storage temperature, an increasing loss of cell integrity occurs during the first 80 days of storage.

Thus, we hope we have found a method to test the influence of cryopreservation techniques on endothelial cells.

BEHRENDT:

Mr. Ross, if I understood your opening remarks correctly, you indicated that structural integrity, not cell viability, is the essential factor. But many of the other speakers focused on viability and methods to preserve and measure it, indicating a belief that cell viability is crucial. Would you please comment on this apparent difference of opinion?

ROSS:

The importance of cell viability and preservation techniques lies in their influence on structural integrity in the long-term.

BANK:

I think we understand your concept of structural integrity. However, long term maintenance of structural integrity may depend on preservation of fibroblasts and endothelial cells. That this may be the case is suggested by the fact that your results show a fall off in valve integrity at 8 or 9 years, whereas Dr. O'Brien is reporting much longer survival.

ROSS:

I cannot explain the difference. I do not think that cells are remaining viable in our allografts. They may be remaining viable in the grafts of others, but I doubt whether the maintenance of viability for the length of time that the homograft survives.

BANK:

One of the problems we may be dealing with here relates to the definition of terms. When the term "fresh allografts" is used, this has a certain connotation that the valve is not dead. Perhaps we should be using the terms "allografts" as opposed to "denatured allografts" in order to avoid any type of confusion. The term "fresh" would indicate "alive" to most people; yet you were not using it in that context. Perhaps rethinking some of the terminology might avoid problems in the future.

BODNAR:

Dr. O'Brien, in the next session of the conference, I will compare two groups of viable valves. One will be fresh nutrient viable, the other frozen viable. But both were viable. Therefore, one cannot compare his two groups to draw conclusions on the importance of viability, both groups being "viable".
What I find to be the largest problem is that in manufacturing these valves there cannot be strict quality assurance at every single step of preparation. Nobody is checking on the true viability of these valves at their origin. Therefore, I am not sure we know that those valves we have been calling "viable", were viable at all. If we could implement the sort of research methodology which has been described in this symposium in clinical practice and get this sort of information on all valves, we could decide in 10 years' time if viability is important.

O'BRIEN:

The two series referred to by Dr. Bodnar were totally different from one another. The first series employed absolutely nonviable valves which were kept in nutrient medium antibiotic solution for up to 70 days. Their nonviability has been borne out in various tests. This type of valve, before implantation, is nonviable and certainly every valve we have explanted in the long-term is nonviable. The second series is totally different, as we will present later. With these valves which are viable, sterile procurement is fairly essential. Surprisingly, sterile valves can be procured from the autopsy room with a surgeon or attendant scrubbing up and removing the valve. We do this fairly soon after death. The mean time after death for procurement in our cryopreserved group in 15 h. We have been doing this now for the cryopreserved clinical implants for 12 1/2 years. Initially, we took bacteriological cultures from the pericardium, blood, myocardial tissue and, of course, from the valve once it was put in its nutrient medium. All valves have been taken within 24 h of death. So, we think that sterility is essential because it can allow the use of low-dose antibiotics for a short time.
Thus, as we look back now on our two series, we can readily answer the question of the importance of viability to which Dr. Bodnar has referred.
Minimum handling of the tissues is essential and it is surprising how much damage the surgeon does to the valve. We have always checked our viability in an esoteric way. We have taken the pulmonary valve as well from the same donor and done a simple glucose metabolic uptake on a leaflet from that valve in tissue culture. At the same time we have cryopreserved a pulmonary valve leaflet and then at the time of using the aortic valve, we have examined the viability of that remaining pulmonary leaflet. The actual aortic valve that is implanted is also examined for glucose metabolism before it is cryopreserved. We were doing this in our experimental work for more than 3 years before we began clinical application. So, in conclusion, we are very keen on demonstrating that the tissue we use is viable. Any criticism we would make would have to do with the fact that we have not got a quantitative measurement of viability.

50

BEHRENDT:

Dr. O'Brien, do you believe that cryopreservation confers some special advantage over the technique of fresh antibiotic preservation in regards to cell viability?

O'BRIEN:

The "fresh" antibiotic preserved valve becomes progressively nonviable the longer it is kept. Cryopreservation is simply a method of storage. We would actually prefer to implant any valve within 24 h of donor death and, if we cannot do that, then we would cryopreserve it. So, in either situation, we would put in a viable valve. We would not use a nonviable valve, i.e. one stored in antibiotics for a long time without cryopreservation. If fact, we discontinued that technique in 1975.

ROSS:

Dr. O'Brien has convinced us that he is putting in valves which are initially viable. In my view, that maintains tissue integrity. The evidence he has produced that these valves are viable 5—10 years later indicates that he has put in nondamaged valves, which is a good thing. Viability is a good indication that you have not damaged the valve. But what is the evidence that they are still viable later?

BARRATT-BOYES:

There are three points I would like to address:
The first is that all the previous discussion about viability of the cells ignores what is happening to the ground substance. It would be our impression that anything happening to the collagen in the ground substance of the leaflet is probably more important, in fact, than the viability of the cells. This can occur with antibiotics of certain types and there is no question that you may alter in a very dramatic way the behavior of the so-called "viable" leaflet.
The second point is that all of our evidence in animal experiments involving transplanted leaflets in dogs indicates that, while a leaflet implanted within 2 h of collection is quite clearly viable, the cells gradually disappear if you follow those animals serially. Now, one could question whether this data can be actually transferred to the human model. I believe we can, because our only human data also support this. So, viability at the time of implantation, does not mean, necessarily, that these valves are going to remain viable. Nor does subsequent culture of that valve at removal, because a host reaction over the cells can give a positive culture.
The third point I would like to make is that I do not agree that you cannot use an antibiotic solution of low concentration and still obtain valves cleanly, but not sterilely. We do not believe that sterile collection is important. While it is important that the valve be sterile and not damaged by the procurement process, if you would limit your collection to sterile techniques, the number of valves available will be greatly reduced. I think it is a very important point that if we are to use this device in a realistic way and in a reasonable number of people, we will have to look beyond obtaining all of these valves sterilely, particularly in the brain dead donor.

Contribution for discussion:
Problems of homograft procurement

A. L. Moulton

Section of Thoracic and Cardiovascular Surgery, University of Nebraska,
Omaha, Nebraska, USA

Prior to commercial availability of glutaraldehyde-preserved heterograft valves and conduits (mostly porcine) in the early 1970s, cadaver homografts were frequently used in the United States for valve replacement and conduits. As we now know, the methods of preservation for those homografts — quick freeze and gamma ray irradiation — potentiated early degeneration and calcification. Thus disappointing clinical results, combined with the ready availability of commercially prepared porcine heterografts in a wide range of sizes (so each institution could maintain a full inventory) led to the dismantling of most institutions' tissue banks.

More recently, as this symposium attests, the early- and long-term advantages of homografts which have been preserved by less deleterious methods have again become recognized. Unfortunately, general availability is a genuine problem.

My comments are intended to examine some of the difficulties encountered in the procurement of these homografts. I will concentrate on several areas: (1) the availability of suitable tissue for donation, where there may be legal, emotional as well as logistical problems; (2) difficulties in the *timely* procurement of available tissues without damage or contamination; (3) the problems in getting tissue from the site of procurement to the preservation area; (4) the surgical preparation of the tissue; and (5) potential difficulties in the actual preservation of the homografts.

To emphasize these difficulties, I have obtained data from the Nebraska Organ Retrieval System. In addition, the CryoLife corporation has kindly provided me with data based on approximately 3,000 homografts sent to them for processing from 1984 up to and including 1987.

Since potential homograft donors are restricted to damaged, beating hearts, many may be patients who have received fatal trauma. In cases of homicide or industrial or auto accidents, the cause of death may be an important legal issue. Obtaining coroner's consent is a necessary, often difficult and time consuming, and sometimes impossible task.

Notification of the next of kin, and obtaining the necessary permission, may require time that threatens the viability of the donor tissue.

Particularly in potential paediatric donors, establishment of custodial (and therefore permission) rights may be difficult. When the potential donor is a possible victim of child abuse, the legal need to determine the cause of death, as well as the moral implications of having a parent who possibly killed the child also give consent for organ donation, may make donation difficult or impossible.

Even when there are no legal difficulties, emotional factors may predominate. There is emotional significance attached to the heart as the "seat of the soul", so that families who may be willing to donate other tissue for transplantation frequently are reluctant to donate cardiac tissue. In Nebraska in 1986, only 46% of multi-organ donors were heart donors. In 1987, it was 52%. For the donor who has suffered a sudden and unexpected event, the family may have greater difficulty overcoming their sudden grief than a family who have had hours or days to adjust to the possibility of neurological death, and have probably been preliminarly contacted about the possibility or organ donation. For the tissue donor with a non-beating heart, this time factor may be more critical; the combined time for notification of death, adjustment and obtaining consent may exceed the safe limits for tissue viability. For the grieving family who donates a heart for whole organ transplantation, there can be some consolation that the heart is keeping some other patient alive and in some sense their loved one still lives as long as the heart is beating. Though homografts may also save a patient's life, there is not the same immediate emotional gratification for the donor family to serve as an impetus for donation. Similarly, if the potential donor is not going to provide multiple organs for transplantation, many organ procurement agencies are not motivated to approach families about tissue donation for implantation at an indefinite future date. The director of one large procurement agency has been quoted as saying he felt procurement of non-beating hearts was "vulturistic". Unfortunately, some of the procurement agencies' lack of enthusiasm may be financial, since the fee for procurement, at least in the CryoLife system, is only $ 100.00, as opposed to several thousand dollars for a heart for transplantation.

As a result of these multiple factors, the homograft tissue being sent to CryoLife for cryopreservation comes almost exclusively from multi-organ donors. Other procurement groups have noted similar trends, so the huge source of potential homograft donors with non-beating hearts is presently virtually untapped.

Once the legal and emotional aspects have been overcome, tissue is procured and transported to the preservation site. As already noted, with the exception of a few institutions such as the University of Alabama, most centres in the U.S. have not re-established their tissue banks after dissembling them in the 1970s. Most, therefore, have chosen to transport the tissue to the CryoLife Laboratories just outside Atlanta, Georgia. Though most come from damaged beating heart donors, with an effective transport system, less than 1% of tissue arrives outside the 24-h period acceptable for transplantation and most arrive within 16 h of procurement. Tissue cryopreserved more than 24 h after procurement has a higher incidence of cusp degeneration, calcification, and suture line dehiscence. Despite the impressive potential for logistic problems, less than 1% of the tissue arriving at CryoLife has to be discarded because of inadequate cooling, packaging, and insulation or excessive transport time.

Infection results in discarding 7—8% of tissues sent for cryopreservation, but each homograft is cultured at four different stages during the processing. Since the number of homografts from non-beating heart donors is so small, it is impossible to tell whether there is a difference between beating heart donors (usually multiple organs obtained in the operating room) and cadaver donors (which are frequently procured in the morgue).

When a heart is procured for homograft preservation, it is important to obtain as adequate length of aorta (distal to, and including, the arch vessels) and the pulmonary arteries (PAs) (including the confluence plus the proximal portions of left and right PAs). In the material being sent to CryoLife, damage to the aorta at the time of procurement is rare; but in approximately 40%, the PAs have been damaged, usually with inadequate length of the left and right PAs. Since, as Dr. Clark has shown us, one of the main indications for use of a PA homograft is to simultaneously replace the main PA and its proximal branches which may have been damaged by prior banding or shunts, failure to obtain adequate length severely limits the use of the PA homografts.

During the dissection of the aorta from the PA and the heart (with its attached mitral leaflet), the aorta is still damaged only rarely. But the thin-walled and friable PA is damaged in another 10% of cases during this dissection.

I will not dwell on cryopreservation techniques, but this multi-staged procedure must be performed properly to ensure that all available tissue is procured for possible future use. By concentrating on some of these problem areas, hopefully we can increase the quantity of homograft tissue which reaches this stage.

Author's address:
A. L. Moulton MD
Professor of Surgery
Section of Thoracic and Cardiovascular Surgery
42nd and Dewey Avenue
Omaha
NE 68105-1065
USA

Contribution for discussion:
Heart valve procurement in Berlin

F. Keller*, A. C. Yankah, S. Schüler, R. Klän*, G. Offermann*,
H. Warnecke, R. Hetzer

* Klinikum Steglitz, Free University Berlin. German Heart Center, Berlin
(West), Germany

Introduction

Theoretically, every patient who dies in a hospital can be considered a heart valve
donor. Practically, this is impossible because of logistic and moral reasons. In December 1986, the Berlin Heart Valve Procurement Program was initiated by the
German Heart Center (2). Since then, two main sources for heart valve procurement
have been established: (1) heart transplant recipients and (2) multi-organ donors.

Organisation and methods

The failing hearts of heart transplant recipients are suitable for heart valve procurement. All serological and immunological data are available. Organisation and surgery are done by the surgeons of the German Heart Center, Berlin. The valves are
dissected and prepared for cryopreservation immediately after heart explant.
Multi-organ donors are the second source for heart valve procurement. There are,
however, several requirements for heart valve procurement from organ donors.
Namely, the permission for multi-organ donation must be obtained from the relatives of the donor and secondly, the serological and immunological data of the donor
must be available. Heart valve procurement is part of the task work of the transplant-
coordinator.
The following criteria and protocol apply to heart valve donors: diagnosis of dissociated brain death is required; relatives of the donor should be asked for an explicit
permission for heart valve procurement; the donor age should be less than 55 years;
sepsis, HIV-infection or previous contact with HIV risk groups must be excluded.
For each heart valve donor, the following data are recorded (Eurotransplant Nec-
roheart Report): name, age, diagnosis of underlying and other diseases, cause of
brain death, date and time of organ donation, blood group (O, A, B, AB), HLA class
I (A, B) and class II (DR) antigens, HIV Elisa (if positive: Western blotting), HBs
antigen, cytomegalovirus titer (unspecific IgG and IgM).
Initially, donor hearts were explanted by the heart surgeon. Recently, explantation
was done by the operating urologist. For heart valve procurement the pericardium
is opened through median sternotomy or left lateral thoracotomy and the heart is
explanted at the transsection of the vena cava inferior/superior and from pulmonary
arteries at the hili. Transsection at the aortic arch close to the carotid artery interna

sinistra is made to produce a long aortic conduit. The explanted heart is rinsed in Eurocollins solution and packed in sterile plastic bags comparable to kidney organ donation. The plastic baggage with the donor's heart is placed in an ice box (+ 4 °C). The ice box is transferred within 6 h to the German Heart Center, where dissection of the aortic and pulmonary valve conduit is performed. The valves are cryopreserved in nutrient medium (human serum albumin and RPMI 1640).

Results

Within 9 months, 95 heart valves from 58 heart transplant recipients were procured (1). Within the same period, only 16 heart valves were procured from eight multiorgan donors (Fig. 1). Heart valve procurement was restricted to those multiorgan donors whose hearts were not suitable for cardiac transplantation (Table 1). The mean age of heart valve donors was 40 years (± 14 years). The heart of the donor was not suitable for transplantation, mainly because of circulatory instability requiring high catecholamine dosage. Only in one case was the permission by the relatives of the donor restricted to heart valve donation and no heart transplantation could be performed.

Conclusions

The failing heart of cardiac transplant recipients is suitable for valve procurement in 82% of cases (1). The disadvantage of obtaining heart valves from transplant recipients is the short ascending aorta conduit. A long aortic conduit is only available from organ donors. For heart valve procurement from organ donors the relatives of the donor must be explicitly asked for permission for heart or heart valve donation.

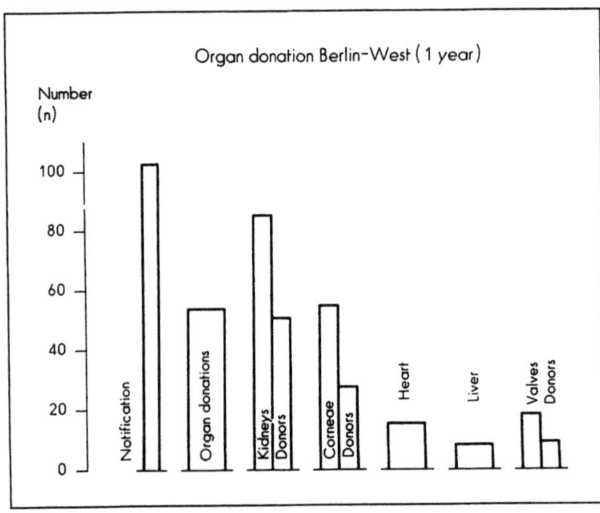

Fig. 1. Heart valve procurement as a part of multi-organ donation program.

Table 1. Heart valve procurement from multi-organ donors in Berlin (West) between December 1986 and September 1987.

Donor age (years)	Unsuitable hearts for heart transplantation (reasons)
28	circulatory instability
51	no permission
46	cardiomyopathy
29	circulatory instability
15	cardiomyopathy
44	circulatory arrest
53	coronary heart disease
54	complex arrhythmias

Additionally, serological and immunological data are required. These criteria are met only in the case of multi-organ donation. Heart transplantation has a clear priority over heart valve procurement. Procurement of heart valves from multi-organ donors, therefore, is restricted to those conditions where the heart is not suitable for transplantation. The donor heart was unsuitable for transplantation mainly because of circulatory instability and intrinsic heart disease of the donor.

References

1. Schüler, S, Yankah C, Zhang B, Warnecke H, Hetzer R. Allogenic valve procurement in cardiac transplantation. This volume, p 13—16
2. Yankah AC, Hetzer R (1987). Derzeitige und zukünftige Trends bei der Transplantation allogener Herzklappen. Z Herz Thorax Gefäßchir 1: 12—19

Authors' address:
F. Keller, M.D.
Klinikum Steglitz
Free University Berlin
1000 Berlin (West)
Germany

Basic principles of transplantation immunology

W. Müller-Ruchholtz

Department of Immunology, University of Kiel, F.R.G.

Transplantation means surmounting the biological barrier between individuals. To achieve this has been one of the dreams of mankind for thousands of years as, for example, expressed in former centuries by paintings and sculptures showing the saints Cosmas and Damian — rather than devils — grafting a deceased black man's leg onto a white patient, whose own leg had to be amputated.

Today the scientifically established basic fact is that reactions against foreign cells are governed by immunological mechanisms. This had to be made clear, and it did not become so until the research by P. B. Medawar. His pioneering animal experiments were performed in 1943 in London and consisted of skin grafts between rabbits. A second graft from the same source of origin was rejected specifically in an accelerated fashion. Medawar won the Nobel Prize in 1960.

The *basic biological problem in transplantation* may be characterized as follows: The function of the immune system consists in recognizing and maintaining the biological individuality and integrity of the organism. This is a vital function. Its definition implies the definition of immunology as the science of self-non-self discrimination. Thus, as already mentioned, the transplantation of cells, tisues and organs signifies the crossing of the biological barrier between individuals and therefore represents a basic challenge to the above function. This indicates that the transplantation surgeon challenges the immunologist fundamentally and vice versa.

However, much depends on the *type* of graft, as shown in Table 1. Avital implants, be they of tissue origin, otherwise derived or synthetic, should not be called transplants. For the sake of clarity, the latter term should be reserved for living cells, since only they can truly replace a lost cell function. The degree of histoincompatibility, which clearly differs between non-MHC (major histocompatibility complex)-determined allogeneic, MHC-determined allogeneic and xenogeneic grafts, may also vary remarkably within each of these three types of grafts. The terms

Table 1. Types of grafts.

Term	Features	Immune reactions
autologous	intra-individual	none
syngeneic	id. twins, inbreds	none
allogeneic, non-MHC	intra-species, weak incomp.	weak-moderate
allogeneic, MHC	intra-species, strong incomp.	strong-very strong
xenogeneic	inter-species, very str. incomp. broad range	often hyperacute
tissue implant,	nonvital	
allogeneic	intra-species	none
xenogeneic	inter-species	perhaps some

homograft instead of allograft and heterograft instead of xenograft have been obsolete for many years. It may be pointed out that the immunological analysis of transplantation, i.e., animal experimentation, requires grafting between inbred strains. (This is the reason why we in Kiel have established so many models in inbred rats, from cornea grafting and transplantation of a large variety of parenchymal organs to bone marrow transplantation.)

The *immunogenicity* of a graft, i.e., its capacity to elicit an immune response, is determined by the following parameters:

1. The degree of histoincompatibility, as governed by the number and strength of cell surface antigens that differ between donor and recipient. It should be mentioned that an increasing body of experimental data indicates that even the so-called strong, MHC-determined transplantation antigens appear to be remarkably weak per se, i.e., when taken out of the context of a living, metabolically active cell.

2. Certain characteristic features of the grafted cells. The most prominent features are viability, extent of surface antigen expression, metabolic activity (enabling the cell to release socalled second signals, such as interleukin 1, see below) and, naturally, the number of cells. Each of these features may vary over a broad range.

3. The localization of the cells within the graft. Immunologically privileged, "inaccessible" sites have been described in the cornea, cartilage, central nervous tissue, etc. However, this kind of immunological privilege has been shown to be no all-or-none phenomenon. In the context of the present topic, namely heart valve transplantation, it may suffice to mention that the endothelial cells are accessible primarily, whereas the fibroblasts are not, as long as the endothelial layer is intact.

The *most important molecules* in transplantation immunology are the so-called strong, MHC-determined transplantation antigens and those molecules that effect the specific immune reactivity against certain accessible epitopes of the antigens. These are the immunoglobulins (antibodies) and the T-cell receptors on the surface of specifically reactive T-lymphocytes. Strikingly, all of these molecules are composed of polypeptide chains of remarkable structural homology, as outlined in Fig. 1. Therefore they are considered to be members of the same "gene superfamily", which are evolutionarily derived from one primordial cell surface structure gene. The non-constant domains of the molecules determine both the reaction specificity of the immunoglobulins and T cells and the biological individuality of an organism in terms of its MHC structures (which are common to the genome though not necessarily to the surface expression of all nucleated cells of a given organism). It is only a limited number, of the order of a few to a few hundred, of different genes (gene segments) that determine the fascinating diversity of all these molecules by making use of the combinatorial possibilities following from the variety of compositions of the non-constant parts of the molecules.

To better understand this highly important issue with regard to man's MHC transplantation antigens, we may briefly look at the present understanding of the *immunogenetics of HLA*. This is outlined in Fig. 2. In contrast to the genetic determination of the ABO blood group system (one gene locus with three alleles), we know of a whole region composed of many loci. Among loci that appear to carry silent genes there are several loci which are occupied by one of many alleles that determine many different antigenic specifities. The fascinating polymorphism, to say it again, derives from the large number of combinations that are possible because

60

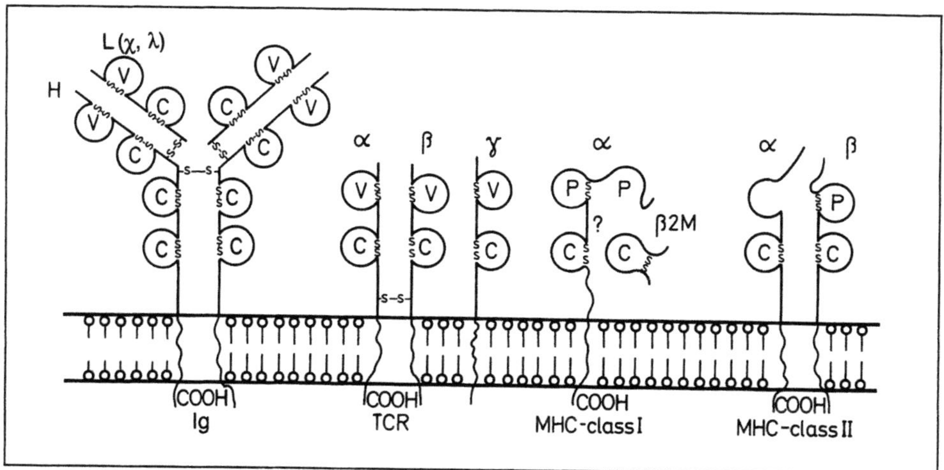

Fig. 1. Immunoglobulin gene superfamily. A group of molecules appears to be evolutionarily derived from a primordial cell surface receptor. Depicted are only those members that are involved in immune reactions, i.e., antigen handling. Note the composition of polypeptide domains (homology units), a number of which are rather constant (c). Immunoglobulin (Ig) and T-cell receptor (TCR) contain variable domains (v) the structures of which are encoded by genes resulting from gene rearrangement in ontogeny. MHC class I and II molecules contain polymorphic domains (p) whose structures are constant in the individual but have emerged from remarkable variations in phylogeny.

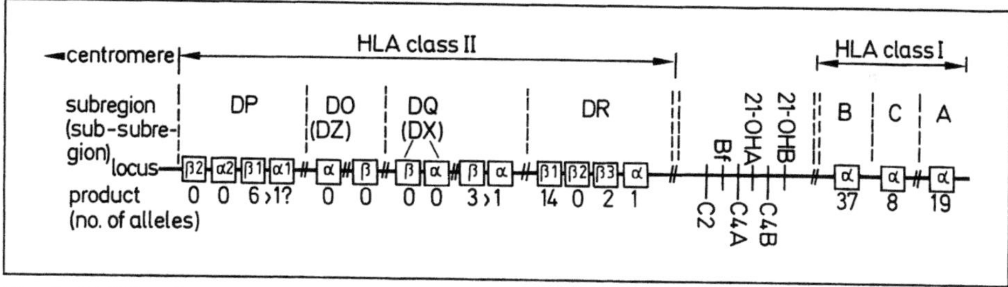

Fig. 2. MHC region of human chromosome 6. A schematic map of the gene loci and cell surface products, as presently understood. The number and order of the loci remain to be confirmed. Some genes do not appear to be expressed. Some loci demonstrate a genetic polymorphism which is not detectable, as yet, at the cell surface expression level. The total number of allelic products is almost certainly not yet known.

an individual's HLA pattern is composed of the various alleles of the various loci. The MHC class I and class II cell surface expression, whether constitutive or induced by a large variety of immunological or nonimmunological stimuli, varies on the different cells of the organism. Until recently it was thought that class I molecules are ubiquitously found whereas class II molecules were constitutively expressed on cells that are immunoreactive, such as antigen-presenting macrophages and dendritic cells, B lymphocytes and activated T lymphocytes. But this simplistic view could not be upheld; it may suffice here to state that we are presently collecting much more data which will hopefully allow us to better understand the pertinent rules of

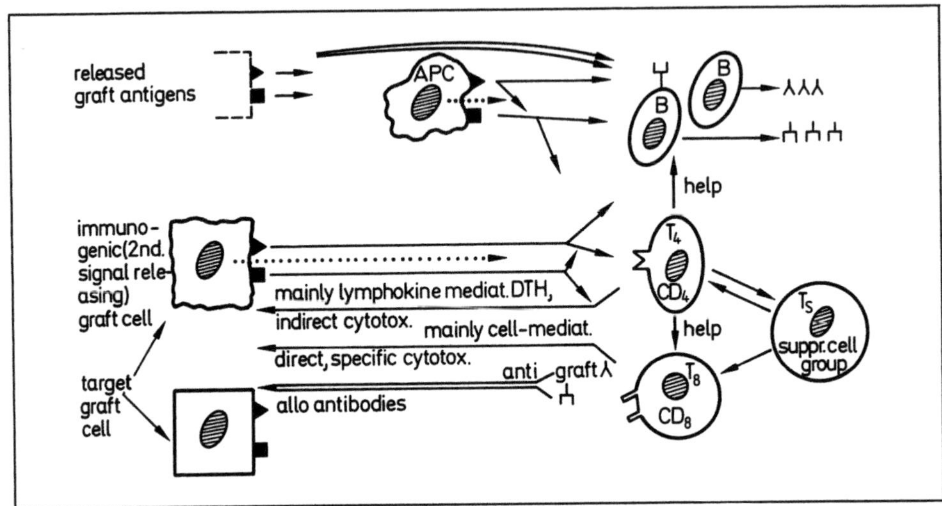

Fig. 3. Cell interactions for immunological recognition of and attack against grafts (simplified outline). (▲) MHC class II antigen; (■) MHC class I antigen. (·····>) 2nd signal, such as Il-1. (APC) antigen presenting cell of the recipient. Lymphokine effects: B help (Il-4) and T8 help (Il-2), increase of graft MHC expression (γ IFN), macrophage activation (γIFN). Non-MHC antigens are not indicated; they are recognized and targeted with the help of MHC molecules.

nature in the near future. Also, I shall restrict myself here by only hinting at the fact that the biological role of MHC cell surface structures is certainly not to serve as transplantation antigens but to act as cell interaction molecules. Again, we are only at the beginning of our understanding in that we are only describing the essential role of MHC molecules for the interaction of T-lymphocytes with antigens.

The main events of *immune recognition and immune destruction* of a graft are outlined in Fig. 3 and may be divided into three aspects.

1. Grafted cells are immunogenic not just by virtue of their foreign cell surface structures which may act as transplantation antigens. Second signals have to be provided, the best presently known, but certainly not the only one, being interleukin 1. A nonviable cell or a metabolically incompetent cell is not immunogenic but may, nonetheless, become the target of an immune reaction initiated otherwise. On the other side, antigen presenting cells (APC) of the recipient, such as macrophages and dendritic cells, may handle released transplantation antigens and thus "restore" graft immunogenicity. We are still in the process of trying to understand under what circumstances these APC do or do not become active.

2. A number of different lymphocyte subsets become activated. Firstly, the CD4+ T cells (synonyms: T4 cells, inducer/helper lymphocytes) may be described as the MHC class II molecule-handling cells. Secondly, the CD8+ T cells act as MHC class I molecule-restricted cells. Thirdly, a group of regulator T cells with specifically suppressive potential become activated. (Most of these cells also carry the CD8 marker.) And fourthly, B lymphocytes differentiate into antibody-producing plasma cells.

3. The graft destruction may be initiated by one or several of three immunologically specific trigger events, which in general are followed by unspecific but biologically

62

Table 2. Immunological manipulation of rejection.

---

(1) **Reduction of immunogenicity of the graft**
    degree of histoincompatibility: tissue typing
    features of graft cells:
        selective elimination of cells, downregulation of cells
    privileged localiz. of the cells:
        consideration of variables

(2) **Reduction of reactivity of the recipient**
    nonspecific long-term immunosuppression:
        management of effects vs. side-effects
    ⇓ the ultimate modulation
    graft-specific immunotolerance:
        reprogramming of immune reactivity

---

highly efficient sequential events. Firstly, upon specifid interaction with their target antigen, T lymphocytes release a umber of lymphokines which indirectly mediate cytotoxicity. This has been referred to as delayed type of hypersensitivity (DTH) reaction, effected by CD4$^+$ cells. However, CD8$^+$ cells may also become capable of releasing lymphokines. Secondly, cytotoxic T effector cells may directly effect the destruction of graft cells. This has been observed mainly (but again not only) with T cells carrying the CD8 marker. Thirdly, antibodies may initiate graft damage. However, it must be added that, functionally similary to T suppressor cells, destruction-blocking antibodies may be observed (so-called graft-facilitating or graft-enhancing antibodies).

The *prevention of graft rejection* by immunological manipulation is at the centre of our interest. It is based on what has been outlined above. The two principal approaches, namely reduction of immunogenicity of the graft and reduction of reactivity of the recipient, are outlined roughly in Table 2. The concern about limitation of the degree of histoincompatibility has maintained its great value, wherever tissue typing is possible — as to be expected from the systematic animal experimentation data. It may be pointed out that two approaches toward reduction of immunogenicity will increasingly become research "hot spots": (1) The selective elimination of those cells from a graft that represent strong immunogenicity carriers but are not required for the function of the graft. In this context, Lafferty's concept of passenger cells is to be broadened, because a number of residential cells need to be considered as well. (2) Downregulation of either MHC antigen expression or second signal production. Certain drugs, such as corticosteroids or cyclosporine A, appear to be useful, but only as long as they continue to be given. The regulation of MHC expression at the genetic level, as it occurs naturally in a number of cells, will hopefully open new doors of research. Finally, it must be repeated again and again that on the side of the graft recipient, the ultimate goal remains induction and maintenance of immunotolerance rather than immunosuppression. There is good reason to expect that this can be achieved in the human, too, and that the lower the graft's immunogenicity is, the easier it will be in the human. At present we know of many impressive animal models of immunotolerance, but we know terribly little with regard to man. To a large extent, I believe, this is so because of poor cooperation between surgeons and immunologists.

The *application* of the above outlined basic principles of transplantation immunology to heart valve transplantation should be the major concern of the subsequent session. Let me therefore finish with some introductory questions and remarks: (1) What is really known about endothelial cell and fibroblast viability of a valve, of their metabolic activity and immunogenicity (as they can be studied in established in vitro tests before the valve is grafted)? (2) Only when that is known, can the question as to the role of the degree of histoincompatibility be studied conclusively. It certainly needs to be studied, not just in one centre but in as many places as possible. (3) What is really known about MHC antigen expression on human valve endothelial cells (rather than other species or other endothelial cells) and fibroblasts? There were claims that they do not express MHC class II antigens; however, we have seen some 10—20% of valve endothelial cells constitutively expressing these antigens. Does this vary under certain circumstances and/or under certain genetic conditions? (4) How do we get information about the potential of the recipient's immune system to recognize transplantation antigens at the particular position of a functioning heart valve? (5) If sensitization takes place, how accessible are the graft's target cells for immune effector cells and/or antibodies? (6) What about the recipient potential and the biological requirement to replace endothelial cells and/or fibroblasts following their immune destruction, if that takes place? (This question clearly differs from that relating to cell repopulation following some kind of devitalizing treatment before the valve is grafted.)

References

1. Müller-Ruchholtz W, Müller-Hermelink HK (1988) Introduction to Transplantation Immunology. In: Sale GE (ed) The Pathology of Transplanted Organs. Butterworths.

Author's address:
Prof. Dr. Dr. W. Müller-Ruchholtz
Abteilung Immunologie
der Universität Kiel
Brunswiker Str. 4
D-2300 Kiel
F.R.G.

Cryopreserved and fresh valved aortic homograft conduits in a chronic sheep model: Haemodynamic, angiographic and histological comparisons

R. A. Jonas, G. Ziemer, L. Armiger, L. Britton, A. R. Castaneda

Department of Cardiac Surgery, Children's Hospital and the Department of Surgery, Harvard Medical School, Boston, U.S.A., and the Department of Pathology, Auckland University, New Zealand

Introduction

In 1949, Gross (1) demonstrated that simple freezing to − 72 °C of the canine aortic homograft, followed by subsequent implantation, resulted in a high rate of failure due to aneurysm and rupture. Since that time there have been major advances in preservation methods. We thought that it was important to repeat the large animal experimental model studies performed by Gross in order to compare storage of aortic homografts using current techniques of cryopreservation relative to simple storage in a nutrient medium at 4 °C.

Materials and Methods

15 aortic homografts were harvested immediately after death of donor sheep with a mean weight of 23 kg at approximately 4 months of age. Eight homografts were immersed for 48 h at 4 °C in an antibiotic solution composed of cefoxitin 240 mg/ ml, lincomycin, 120 mg/ml, polymyxin B, 100 mg/ml, vancomycin, 50 mg/ml, and amphotericin, 25 mg/ml, in Eagle's cell culture medium. The homografts were then stored for 1—4 days in plain Eagle's culture medium at 4 °C prior to implantation (Group A). Seven homografts were placed in ice-cold normal saline in a sterile container and were shipped to the CryoLife procurement plant. Following immersion for 48 h at 4 °C in the same antibiotic solution as Group A, these homografts were frozen in a controlled rate liquid nitrogen freezer (− 196 °C) with 10 % DMSO as cryoprotectant (Group B).

The homografts were inserted into recipient sheep of similar size and weight as the donor sheep, between the right ventricle and pulmonary artery bifurcation without the use of cardiopulmonary bypass. The main pulmonary artery was divided and oversewn. Right heart catheterisation studies were performed at 6 weeks, 4 months, and 9 months. A pullback gradient was obtained between the pulmonary artery and right ventricle. Cardiac output was calculated using thermodilution and right ventricular and pulmonary artery angiograms were performed. 50 % of the animals were sacrificed at 4 months and the remainder at 9 months. Histological analyses were performed in New Zealand.

Results

There were three early deaths. Two of these animals were from the fresh group. One animal had an unrecognized right haemothorax and one remained in persistent congestive failure following prolonged intraoperative resuscitation. One animal from the cryopreserved group died suddenly 11 weeks after surgery. At post mortem examination, the homograft was found to have ruptured. Histologically, there was evidence of infection.

The weight gain of the animals (51 %) was similar between the two groups. There was an increase (73 %) in transconduit gradient with time, starting with a gradient of between 20—30 mm at 6 weeks after surgery, increasing to approximately 40—50 mm at 4 months with a further slightly increase by 9 months. There was no significant difference (p = 0.67) between the gradients in the cryopreserved group and the fresh group.

Figure 1 illustrates the typical angiographic appearance of the homografts. There was frequently a gradient at the point of take-off of the large single first branch trunk, arising from the aorta. Anastomotic gradients were also found, as in the proximal anastomotic stenosis shown in Fig. 2. Fig. 3 is the angiogram taken 6 weeks after surgery in the animal from the cryopreserved group that died 11 weeks after surgery. There is a kink at the midpoint of the homograft with a filling defect which may be an infected thrombus. There is also a proximal bulge in the posterior wall of the homograft where the rupture subsequently occurred. All homograft conduits were found to be heavily calcified by 4 months from the time of surgery. This was verified both by X-ray and histologically.

The homograft conduits were examined histologically from two points of view, namely, as a conduit looking at the aortic wall and as a valve looking at the valve

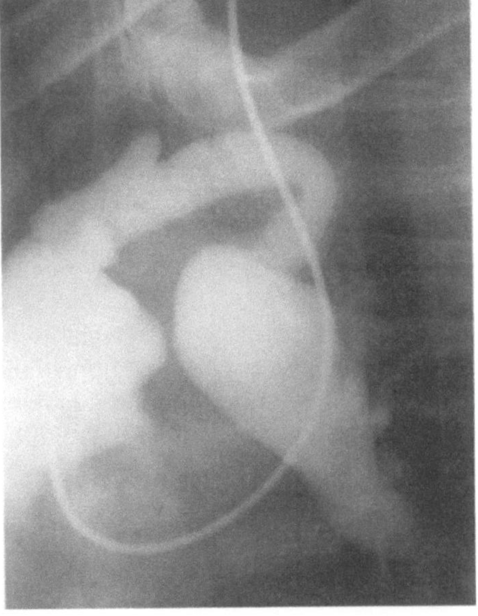

Fig. 1. Typical angiographic appearance of sheep homograft placed between the right ventricle and pulmonary artery. Prominent calcification of the homograft wall is visible.

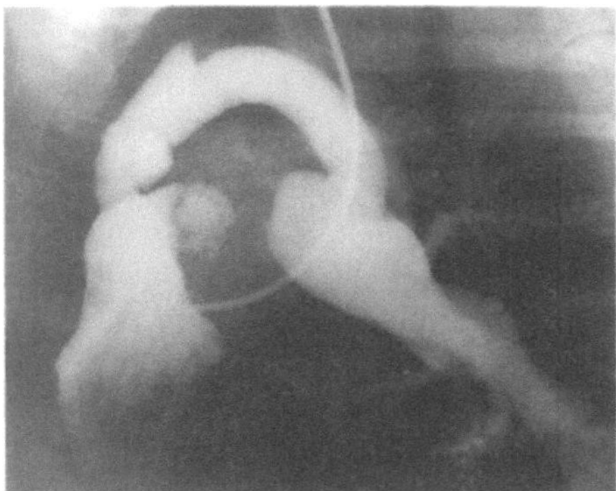

Fig. 2. Proximal anastomotic stenosis between the right ventricle and aortic homograft.

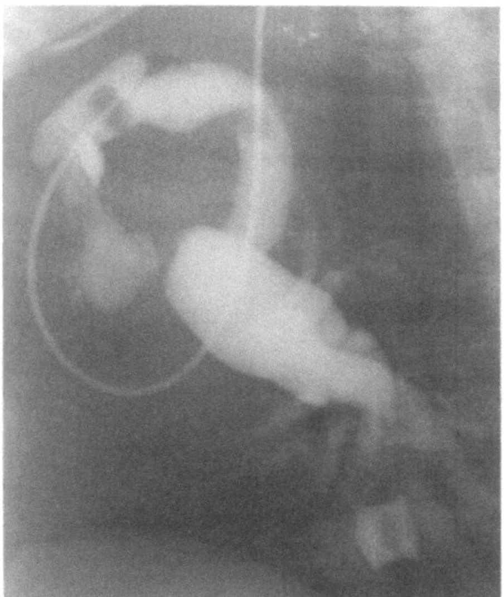

Fig. 3. Pulmonary angiogram 6 weeks following surgery in an animal which received a cryopreserved homograft. A filling defect distal to the midpoint kink is noted, together with a bulge in the posterior wall proximally, which was the site of subsequent rupture.

leaflets. The normal sheep aortic wall has particularly prominent smooth muscle within the media. Islands of smooth muscle are surrounded by elastic fibres. After 9 months of implantation, the most dramatic finding in the aortic wall was the disappearance of smooth muscle, often with persistence of spaces which had been occupied by these muscle islands. There was frequently some fibrosis within the adventitia and often red blood cell infiltrates within the adventitia. Calcification was always present. Often there were areas of separation between calcified plates and the remainder of the aortic wall. Some conduits showed relatively heavy lymphocytic infiltration in the adventitia. This may represent an immune phenomenon. Careful comparison of the fresh and cryopreserved groups failed to reveal any significant difference from the point of view of conduit calcification, loss of muscle cells, or intimal proliferation. There was a suggestion that lymphocytic infiltration within the adventitia was more prominent in the cryopreserved group than in the fresh group.

There was a variable loss of cellularity from valve leaflets following either method of donor treatment. However, intracuspal thrombus of unknown significance appeared more prominent in the cryopreserved group relative to the fresh group. There was a surprising persistence of endothelium on the valve cusps with both methods of preservation. However, factor VIII immunofluorescence was not used to positively identify the cells which were morphologically indistinguishable from endothelial cells.

Conclusions

This study demonstrates that in the sheep model, cryopreservation with current techniques does not significantly alter the functional integrity of aortic homograft conduits placed between the right ventricle and pulmonary artery relative to antibiotic treated aortic homografts stored in nutrient medium for up to 4 days. There are some minor differences in histological appearance with a suggestion of greater immune reactivity of the cryopreserved homografts. The significance of intracuspal thrombus, seen within the valve leaflets of the cryopreserved homografts but not in antibiotic treated homografts stored at 4 °C, is not known.

References

1. Gross RE, Bill AH, Peirce EC (1949) Methods for preservation and transplantation of arterial grafts. Surg Gyn Obstet 88: 689—701

Authors' address:
Richard Jonas, M.D.
Department of Cardiac Surgery
Children's Hospital
300 Longwood Avenue
Boston, MA 02115
U.S.A.

Homograft valve calcification: Evidence for an immunological influence

L. Gonzalez-Lavin, J. Bianchi, D. Graf, S. Amini, C. I. Gordon

Deborah Research Institute, Deborah Heart and Lung Center, Browns Mills, New Jersey and Robert Wood Johnson School — UMDNJ, New Brunswick, New Jersey, U.S.A.

Introduction

Long-term function of valved conduits used in the correction of congenital heart malformations are of utmost importance since these procedures are usually performed in children. Many conduits have been utilised for this purpose; however, fresh antibiotic sterilised aortic homografts have yielded the best long-term results (1—2). These results are suboptimal due to unpredictable calcification of the conduit which occurs at various intervals, and to various degrees of severity. We, along with others, have questioned the possible relationship between immunogenicity and these degenerative changes (3—6). The results of our investigation are the basis of this report.

Materials and Methods

31 pairs of mongrel puppies, 6 months old and weighing 10—15 kg, were divided into two groups: Group A consisted of 11 dogs receiving homografts from related donors (donor and recipient from the same litter); Group B consisted of 20 dogs receiving homografts from unrelated donors. Animals were cared for according to the guidelines set forth in the "Guide for the care and use of laboratory animals", published by the National Institute of Health (1978).

Conduit preparation

The homografts were procured within 48 h of donor death and dissection was performed with clean but nonsterile technique. The conduits were sterilised and stored in an antibiotic nutrient medium at 4 °C (Table I) for 2—21 days.

Implantation

Under general endotracheal anaesthesia, the aortic homograft was implanted between the right ventricular outflow tract (RVOT) and the main pulmonary artery (MPA) without the aid of cardiopulmonary bypass. After completion of both suture lines, the native MPA was ligated at its base, so all blood flow was directed through the conduit.

Table 1. Antibiotic nutrient medium.

RPMI # 1640 with L-glutamine	
10% fetal calf serum	
Cefoxitin	240 µg/ml
Ticarcillin	2.5 mg/ml
Neomycin	250 µg/ml
Polymixin	100 µg/ml
Mycostatin	500 U/ml

Explantation

The animals were maintained for a mean of 117 days, ranging from 12 to 174 days (Group A, 105 $\pm$ 12; Group B, 123.5 $\pm$ 7.9; p = 0.11), at which time the homografts were excised. The specimens were divided longitudinally through the midportion of the graft to make two equal halves of the specimen. One half was submitted for tissue calcium determination and the other half for histological examination.
Tissue calcium determinations were performed by colorimetric analysis with ortho-cresolphthalein complexone. Histological examination was performed utilising von-kossa, gomori trichrome, and haematoxylin eosin.

Statistical analysis

Results were analysed using the t-test and F-test.

Results

Histology

Each specimen was divided into four sections of interest: the leaflets (when they were identifiable), the proximal third, the middle third, and distal third of the aortic root. Histological findings between the two study groups were significantly different: in Group A (donor related), specimens disclosed significantly less calcification than those in Group B. Where severe calcification was present, both groups demonstrated calcification in proximal, mid and distal sections without any apparent area being predominant. All sections in both groups demonstrated a sequential pattern leading to calcification. The pattern apparently commenced with initial elastosis, that is, reduplication and splitting of elastic fibre so as to widen the wall. These spaces, which were more prominent in Group B, contained a mucinous substance which, under haematoxylin and eosin sections, is consistent with an acid mucopolysac-charide (Fig. 1). These changes appeared to be followed by both an acute and a chronic inflammatory infiltrate of polymorphonuclear leukocytes, plasma cells and lymphocytes and then by calcific deposition, together with thrombosis and bone formation (Fig. 2). The bulk of this lesion was in the inner third of the aortic wall, suggesting a protective mechanism relating to the vasa vasorum. The exact nature

70

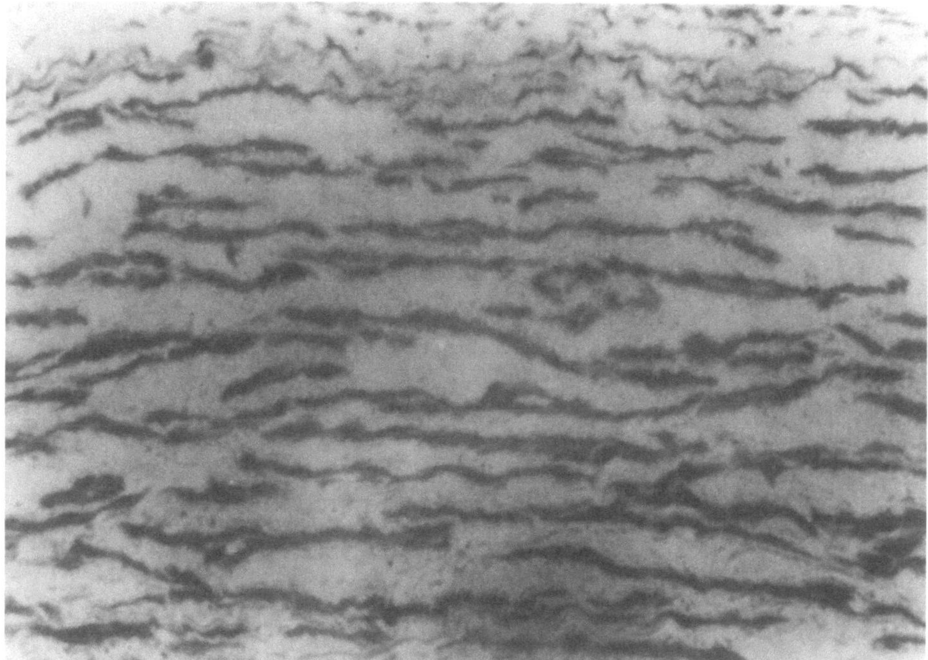

Fig. 1. Wall of homograft from Group A demonstrating elastosis with depositions of acid mucopolysaccharide material between elastic fibres (haematoxylin and eosin; original magnification x40).

of the acid mucopolysaccharide could not be determined, but appeared to be the precursor of calcification. As in the clinical setting, calcification was significantly greater in the aortic wall than in the valve leaflets. In summary, histological sections depicted that in genetically-related animals there was minimal elastosis, myxoid deposition, and significantly less calcification.

Calcium determination

The calcium (Ca^{++}) tissue determinations were expressed as milligrams of calcium per gram of dry tissue (mg calcium/g dt). Where discernible, the valve leaflets were removed from the rest of the specimen and subjected to the same analysis (Table 2).

Discussion

A fresh aortic-valve bearing homograft is the conduit of choice when repairing severe congenital heart malformations in children and young adults (1, 7–9); consequently, their long-term function is of utmost importance. Previous studies concerning host tissue invasion of homograft valves have identified a host-graft inter-

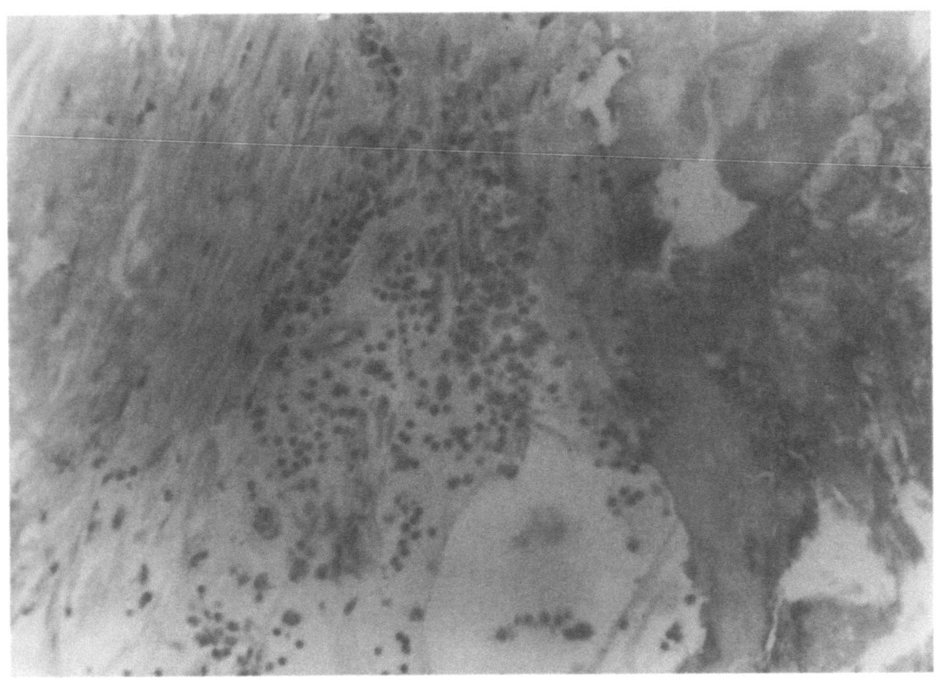

Fig. 2. Wall of homograft from Group B demonstrating elastosis with subsequent calcification and granulation tissue reaction (haematoxylin and eosin; original magnification x40).

Table 2. Calcium determinations (mg/g dry tissue).

	Group A (Related)	Group B (Nonrelated)	p-value
Leaflet	7.89	14.4	0.14
(± SEM)	± 1.68	± 4.07	0.03
Aorta	24.89	56.75	0.02
(± SEM)	± 7.6	±10.9	0.04

face, characterized by infiltrates of macrophages, lymphocytes and a smaller number of plasma cells (10–12). All this work has been done in adult dogs or with adult human homograft valves.

Most of the recent studies attempting to assess the influence of host cellular and immunological effects on degenerative changes of valves have been performed in heterograft valve materials, with disagreement regarding the immunological evidence. Some authors have shown evidence of hypergammaglobulinemia, plasmacytosis and immune complex deposition in calcified cusps (13). Talbert et al. (14) reported microscopy evidence of an immune-mediated host response in a case of bioprosthetic valve failure. On the other hand, some investigators have reported that neither immune nor nonspecific inflammatory cell contact is necessary for bioprosthetic heart valve calcification (15).

72

To assess more carefully the immunological influence on homograft aortic valve conduits, the present study was designed to mimic conditions seen in the clinical setting, i.e., the grafts were implanted orthotopically, haemodynamic parameters were stable and similar to those seen after repair of RVOT in humans, and the animal model was metabolically similar to children in need of these procedures.

Perhaps the most important aspect of this study was observing a genetically related group which demonstrated a significantly lower degree of degenerative changes, suggesting a protective mechanism that is lacking in the other group. As in the clinical setting, calcification was significantly greater in the conduit wall than in the valve leaflets.

The higher calcium content in both tissues in the unrelated group, as well as the significantly higher variance in the unrelated group, suggest a relationship between degeneration and an immunological influence.

These findings are relevant to the current methods of homograft valve procurement and preservation, since one would expect a higher immunological reaction when the implanted tissue retains viability on a larger scale. The current tendency in this field, based on previous experience (1, 10, 16) is to procure grafts as early as possible after death and attempt to preserve their viability as highly as possible. Our current policy is to obtain homovital homografts from brain dead, heart beating donors, where the viability of the graft should be optimal (17). It is important then to consider the possibility of a significantly higher immunological response to the homovital grafts. Our experimental study has also allowed us to detect differences in the origin and progression of the degenerative changes between the two groups. Based on these results, a consideration of immunosuppression, may be suggested, at least temporarily, after implantation of homovital grafts in growing individuals.

References

1. Kay PH, Ross DN (1985) Fifteen years' experience with the aortic homograft: The conduit of choice for right ventricular outflow tract reconstruction. Ann Thorac Surg 40: 360
2. diCarlo D, DeLeval MR, Stark J (1984) "Fresh", antibiotic sterilized aortic homografts in extracardiac valved conduits. Long-term results. Thorac Cardiovasc Surg 32: 10
3. Ross DN (1982) The evolution of the biologic valve. In: Cohn LH, Gallucci V (eds) Cardiac Bioprostheses, Proceedings of the Second International Symposium. Yorke Medical Books, New York, p 1—8
4. Mohri H, Reichenback DD, Barnes RW, Nelson RJ, Merendino KA (1967) Studies of antigenicity of the homologous aortic valve. J Thorac Cardiovasc Surg 54: 564
5. Tector AJ, Boyd WC, Korns ME (1971) Aortic valve allograft rejection. J Thorac Cardiovasc Surg 62: 592
6. Buch WS, Kosek JC, Angell WW (1971) The role of rejection and mechanical trauma on valve graft viability. J Thorac Cardiovasc Surg 62: 696
7. Stark J (1983) Concordant transposition and left ventricular outflow tract obstruction. In: Stark J, deLeval M (eds) Surgery for Congenital Heart Defects. Grune and Stratton, London, p 363
8. Fontan F, Choussat A, Deville C, Doutremepuich C, Coupillaud J, Vosa C (1984) Aortic valve homografts in the surgical treatment of complex cardiac malformations. J Thorac Cardiovasc Surg 87: 649
9. Kirklin JW, Barratt-Boyes BG (1986) Ventricular septal defect and pulmonary stenosis. In: Kirklin JW, Barratt-Boyes, BG (eds) Cardiac Surgery. John Wiley and Sons, New York, p 749—758
10. Gavin JB, Herdson PB, Monro JL, Barratt-Boyes BG (1973) Pathology of antibiotic-treated human heart valve allografts. Thorax 28: 473

11. Gavin JB, Barratt-Boyes BG, Hitchcock GC, Herdson PB (1973) Histopathology of "fresh" human aortic valve allografts. Thorax 28: 482
12. Armiger LC, Gavin JB, Barratt-Boyes BG (1983) Histological assessment of orthotopic aortic valve leaflets allografts: Its role in selecting graft pre-treatment. Pathology 15: 67
13. Rochini AP, Weesner KM, Heidelberger K, Keren D, Behrendt D, Rosenthal A (1981) Porcine xenograft valve failure in children: An immunologic response. Circulation 64: II-162
14. Talbert W Jr, Wright P (1982) Acute aortic stenosis of a porcine valve heterograft apparently caused by graft rejection: Case report with discussion of immune mediated host response: J Texas Heart Inst 9: 225
15. Levy RJ, Schoen FJ, Golomb G (1986) Bioprosthetic heart valve calcification. Clinical features, pathobiology, and prospects for prevention. CRC Critical Reviews in Biocompatibility 2: 147
16. Gonzalez-Lavin L, Al-Janabi N, Ross DN (1972) Long-term results after aortic valve replacement with preserved aortic homografts. Ann Thorac Surg 13: 594
17. Gonzalez-Lavin L, McGrath L, Graf D (1987) A homograft bank. New Jersey Medicine 84: 109

Authors' address:
Lorenzo Gonzalez-Lavin, M.D.
Chairman, Department of Surgery
Deborah Heart and Lung Center
Browns Mills, New Jersey 08015
U.S.A.

Pathology of human explanted aortic valve homografts: A comparative morphological study with porcine aortic valve explants

Y. A. Goffin, L. M. Gerlis, W. M. Jones

Cardiac Research Unit, Killingbeck Hospital, Leeds, U.K.

Aortic valve homografts and porcine aortic valve bioprostheses differ mainly in two aspects: a slightly different anatomy — particularly at the commissures — and different methods of preservation, namely, antibiotic sterilisation in the former, and glutaraldehyde fixation in the latter.

The aim of this study is to compare the alterations in explants of these two different types of biological valves after medium to long-term implantation in patients.

A full morphological study (Table 1) compares six aortic valve homografts (AVH), all antibiotically treated, with six glutaraldehyde-fixed porcine aortic valves (PAV). The valves had been implanted for between 37 and 152 months; eight in mitral and four in aortic position; all but two valves were mounted on a stent.

Table 1. Methods of comparing homograft and PAV explants.

Routine macroscopy and microscopy (paraffin: HE, elastin)
XR (low KVP)
Polarizing light
Frozen sections
Special stains: fat, fibrin(ogen), amyloid, glycogen (aortic wall)
                RNA (immunocytes and other active cells)

Typical mode of failure for AVH was cusp rupture at the commissure (unmounted valves) or detachment of the aortic wall from the stent (mounted valves); for PAV, paracommissural calcifications with radial tears (Ishihara 1 type).

Histological differences observed between the two valve types were (Table 2): (a) Under ordinary light: in AVH, homogenization of collageneous structures with loss of fibroblast staining and exceptional calcifications in leaflets; in PAV: spongy degradation with accumulation of insudated plasma constituents and frequent calcific nodules of extrinsic intramural form in PAV cusps; (b) Under polarized light: in AVH, better preservation of collagen birefringence and density, absence of secondary lipid crystal (cholesterol) formation in any of the explants; in PAV, marked evidence of collagen fibre rupture and frequent cholesterol crystal deposition in the cusps.

Both series of biological valves were made of dead tissue and colonized only by host leucocytes and histiocytes.

It is concluded that the relatively better clinical behaviour and less morphological degradation of long-term aortic valve homografts do not result from the preservation

Table 2. Comparative study of homograft and PAV explants.

Histological observations	Antibiotically treated aortic valve homografts	Glutaraldehyde-treated porcine aortic valves
Nucleus staining	↙	↙
Desquam. endothelium	+ + +	+ + +
Collagen bundles	fragmentation	fragmentation
Basal substance	extracted	extracted (progressive)
Calcification	few small in cusp	frequent in collageneous cord of commissural area and spongiosa body of leaflets
Infiltration of plasma constituents	0 − + + in wall (flowing)	+ −+ + + (accumulation in masses)
Cholesterol crystals	0	+ −+ + + in 4/6
Amyloid deposits	1/6	2/6
Lymphocyte infiltration endothelization (partial)	rare 1/6	rare 2/6

of living fibroblasts, but rather from the differences in the anatomical structures of the commissural areas and/or the mode of preservation. In other words, it seems that the prominence of the collageneous cords and the glutaraldehyde fixation both favour the calcification of porcine aortic valve bioprostheses.

Authors' address:
Y. A. Goffin
Cardiac Research Unit
Killingbeck Hospital
Leeds
U.K.

Antigenicity and fate of cellular components of heart valve allografts

A. C. Yankah*, H.-U. Wottge**, W. Müller-Ruchholtz**

German Heart Center Berlin, Berlin (West), Germany, and Dept. of Immunology of the University of Kiel, FRG**

Introduction

Although the allograft aortic valve is celebrating 25 years of clinical use, very few of the normally asked clinical questions have actually been resolved.

Fresh, viable (allovital) and freshly preserved viable and nonviable aortic valve allografts have been found clinically to be eminently satisfactory and will function for a certain reasonable period due to their excellent haemodynamic and physiological functions in the absence of postoperative thrombosis and thromboembolism without any anticoagulant therapy.

At the stage of precision and perfection in valve surgery, maximum longevity and reduced patient morbidity are to be desired and these can only be achieved through combined clinical and laboratory studies on the fate of cellular components in vivo. The purpose of the experimental work therefore is to study the fate of the cellular components of aortic allografts in a rat model. An attempt will be made to answer the following questions:

1. Do the fibroblasts persist or die or are they replaced by host cells?
2. Is re-endothelisation of heart valves possible?

Material and Methods

Animals

Young inbred male rats of the strains (RT), AS (RT1^l). (CAP × LEW)F1 hybrid, CAP (RT1^c), weighing 230—300 g, maintained in the Department of Immunology of the University of Kiel, FRG, were used throughout this study. Recipients were LEW, and donors were LEW (syngeneic), AS (weakly allogeneic, MHC identical, non-MHC different), (CAP × LEW)F1 (MHC semiallogeneic) and CAP (strongly allogeneic, MHC and non-MHC different). The strains used in this study were selected on the basis of the rejection times of skin transplants as an indicator of histoincompatibility differences.

---

* Research supported by the University of Kiel, Dept. of Cardiovascular Surgery, F.R.G.

Preparation of donor aortic valve allografts

Under ether anaesthesia and sterile conditions, the heart was explanted via median sternotomy. The valve graft, containing the myocardium and approximately 8 mm of the ascending aorta, was dissected and the coronary ostia closed with sutures. The graft was rinsed in isotonic saline and either freshly transplanted heterotopically in the infrarenal aorta or preserved in nutrient medium containing 20% fetal calf serum and antibiotic solutions and stored at 4 °C for 14 days.

Heterotopic transplantation

Using microsurgical techniques (Zeiss operating microscope, × 10 magnification or operating telescopic eye glasses, × 4 magnification) the infrarenal abdominal aorta was exposed by midline laparatomy. The aorta was mobilised from the inferior vena cava, occluded and divided between the two clamps. The allograft was interposed between the stumps of the aorta by proximal and distal anastomosis using continuous 8-0 prolene sutures (Fig. 1a, b). The anterior valve leaflet was partly incorporated into the proximal anastomosis, causing the trileaflet valve to become incompetent. Valve incompetence was desirable to ensure complete blood washout in the sinus valsalva during systole and diastole and therefore prevent thrombosis in the aortic root. This model can be used ideally for immunological studies.

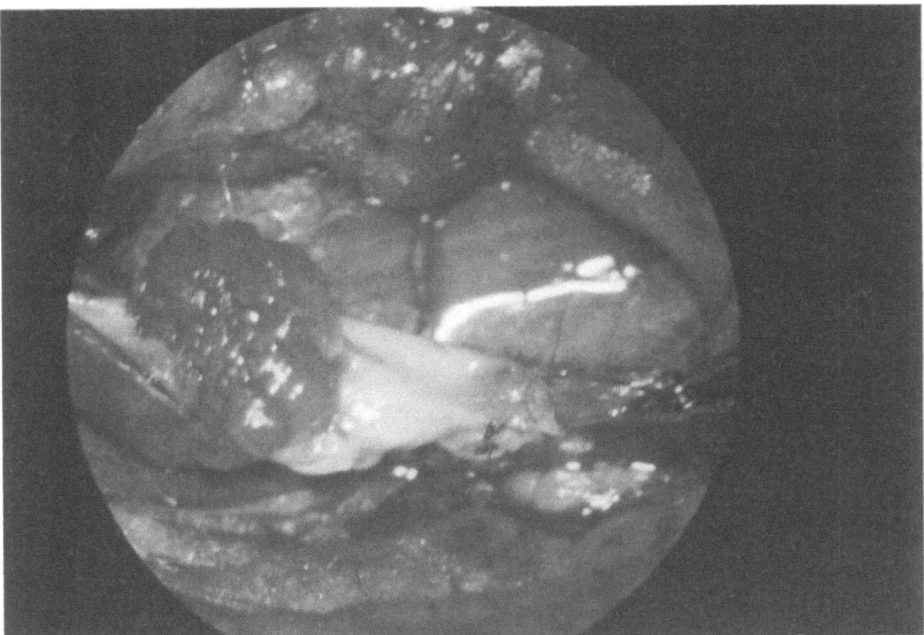

Fig. 1a. Heterotopic transplantation of aortic valve allografts in rats. Interposition of the allograft in the infrarenal aorta by proximal and distal anastomosis using 8-0 prolene continuous suturing technique for the posterior and anterior line (× 10).

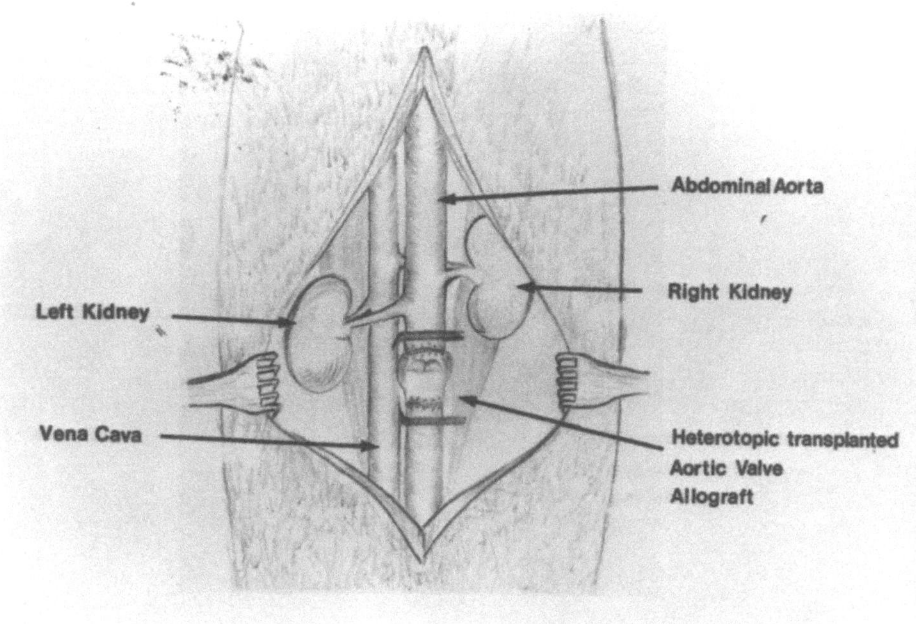

Fig. 1b. Illustration of heterotopic transplantation of aortic valve allograft conduit in the infrarenal aorta.

Skin grafting

3 weeks after heterotopic valve allograft transplantation, recipients were challenged with 1 cm full thickness skin grafts syngeneic to the donor aortic allografts. Skin graft rejection or survival was diagnosed macroscopically and confirmed by intravenous injection of 0.2 ml disulphine blue dye (0.62%) to demarcate avascularised rejected skin grafts (10). There was no prompt dye uptake in the skin grafts after intravenous injection of dye on the day of rejection. Daily visits were made 2 days after skin transplantation. The 95% confidence limit (CL) was established from the mean values of the rejection times and the standard deviations (×).

Histological preparations for immunofluorescence, light and scanning electron microscopy (SEM) studies

Animals were sacrificed 20, 50, 100 or 150 days after heterotopic aortic valve allograft transplantation. The valve and the aorta were dissected and prepared for the following examinations: The antigenicity of allografts and the antibody formation against valve surface antigens were demonstrated by indirect and direct immunofluorescence techniques. The technique is described elsewhere (13). For light microscopy, the valves were embedded in paraffin and sections were stained with hae-

79

matoxylin and eosin (Ladewig, Gemsa, von Kossa) to evaluate rejections, the structural integrity of the tissues and degenerative processes. For scanning electron microscopy (SEM), the valves were fixed in 4% glutaraldehyde in 0.05 M cacodylate buffer (pH 7.4). The technique of preparation has already been described (14).

Results

Light microscopy

Synergeneic strain combination (LLEW → LEW): In the viable grafts, the endothelium of the valve leaflets was preserved and hypercellular. There were no identifiable mononuclear cell infiltrates besides foreign body giant cells which were recognized around the suture lines on day 20. The media was normocellular with regularly organized collagen fibres and structures on days 50, 100 and 150.

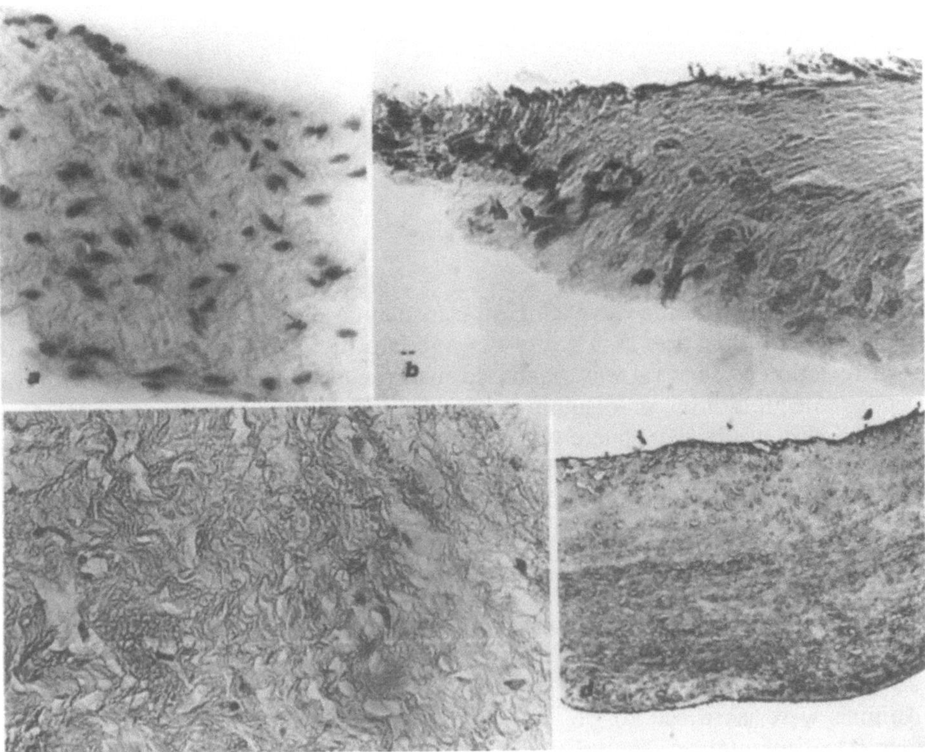

Fig. 2. Histological findings of aortic valve allograft. (a) 50th postoperative day. Normal cellularity syngeneic strain combination, LEW-LEW; (b) 50th postop. day. Prominent loss of endothelial cells and focal mononuclear cell infiltrations and reduced cellarity; AS-LEW (c) 100th postop. day. Valve stroma almost acellular with a few fibroblast-like cells and macrophages. Irregular collagen fibres; (d) 250th postop. day. The valve is acellular with destroyed ground substance, AS-LEW.

80

Weakly allogeneic (AS → LEW) and MHC semiallogeneic strain combinations (CAP × LEW)F1- > LEW:
The endothelia of the viable valves were preserved and showed intense nuclear staining from days 20 to 100. The media showed focal mononuclear cell infiltrations on day 20, which had resolved partially but with regular collagen fibres and persistent fibroblasts and macrophages by day 50. The graft was completely acellular, the collagen fibres were disorganized in some areas with macrophages around them (Fig. 2) on days 100 and 150.
Strongly allogeneic strain combination (CAP → LEW): The endothelia of the viable grafts were cellular with pyknotic cells that showed weak nuclear staining on day 20. At this time there were already diffused infiltrations of mononuclear cells in the subendothelial tissues and media. On day 50, the endothelial cells were destroyed and the collagen fibres appeared disorganized with abnormal structures. There were areas of fibroblast necrosis surrounded by round cell infiltrates in the media. On day 100 there were no recognizable endothelial cells, but rather a thick neointimal matrix of fibrin. The media contained few round cell infiltrates and the collagen fibres were disorganized with breaks in their structures.

Nonviable grafts:

Syngeneic strain combination (LEW → LEW): The nonviable allografts showed unstained pyknotic endothelial cells and a denuded endothelia on day 20 and a thin neointima on days 50 and 100. There were few mononuclear cells and fibroblasts in the media on days 20 and 50. The media contained organized collagen fibres and structures on days 20, 50 and 100.
Grafts from the weakly allogeneic (AS → LEW) strain combinations: On day 20 the endothelia contained a few recognizable, unstained, abnormal, and pyknotic cells with areas of fibrous dysplasia, and the media showed a few mononuclear cell infiltrations. On day 50 the grafts displayed an endothelium denuded of cells, characterized by fibrous dysplasia and the formation of a thin neointimal matrix of fibrin. Partial resolution of the focal mononuclear cell infiltrates and a few areas of disorganized collagen fibres with abnormal structures were observed at this time. On day 100 the grafts were covered with a thick neointimal matrix of fibrin. The media was acellular and the collagen fibres were disorganized in some areas with breaks in their structures.

Scanning electron microscopy (SEM)

Syngeneic strain combinations (LEW → LEW): The endothelial of the viable grafts appeared normal and preserved without intercellular gaps on days 50 and 100.
Weakly allogeneic (AS → LEW) and MHC semiallogeneic (CAP × LEW)F1 → LEW strain combinations. The endothelia of the viable grafts appeared normal but with areas of wide intercellular junctions on day 50. On day 100 the endothelia were partly denuded and on day 150 completely denuded (Fig. 3a, b).
Strongly allogeneic strain combination (CAP → LEW): The endothelial cells of the viable grafts were detached and destroyed on day 50 and the underlying tissues were characterized by fibrous dysplasia. The remaining endothelial cells appeared ab-

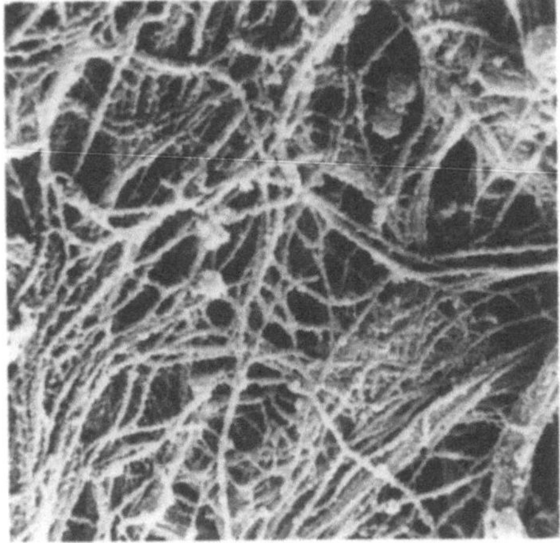

Fig. 3a. Transplanted allograft with denuded endothelium showing collagen fibres and cellular infiltrates. Non-MHC, different weakly allogeneic, AS → LEW 150 postoperative day (SEM × 2000).

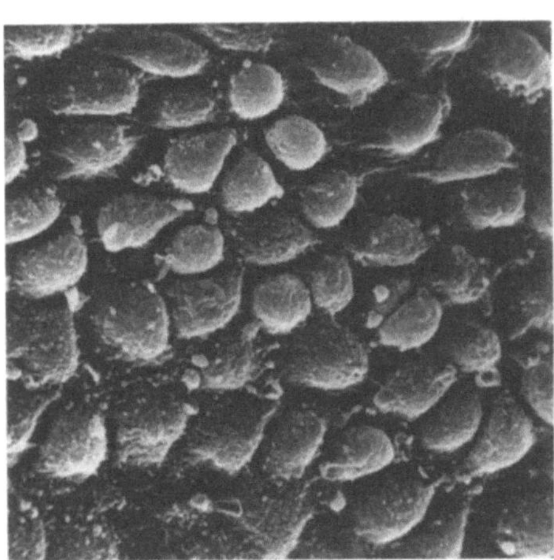

Fig. 3b. Fresh allograft with intact endothelium (SEM × 2000).

Table 1. Scanning electron microscopy (SEM) of aortic allograft: Influence of the degree of histoincompatibility on endothelial degeneration.

Strain combinations	Fresh viable graft	
	50 days	100 days
LEW → LEW (syngeneic)	O	O
AS → LEW (weakly allogeneic)	+ + +	+ +
(CAP × LEW) F1 → LEW (MHC-semiallogeneic)	+ + +	+ +
CAP → LEW (strongly allogeneic)	+ +	−

Symbols: O = Tight intercellular junctions, normal-looking cells; + + + = Partly tight and partly loosed intercellular junctions; + + = Loose and detached, destroyed irregular abnormal cells. Fibrous dysplasia of endothelium. − = No recognizable endothelial cells. Neointimal matrix of fibrin layer.

normal, detached and disorganized. On day 100 a thick neointimal matrix of fibrin
with discrete calcific deposits had formed after detachment of the endothelial cells.

Nonviable grafts:
Synergeneic strain combination (LEW → LEW): The nonviable allografts displayed
a denuded endothelium with fibrous dyplasia on days 50 and 100.
Weakly allogeneic (AS → LEW) strain combinations: The allografts in the three
strain combinations showed similar morphological changes in the endothelial surface. The grafts were denuded of endothelial cells on day 50 and a thin neointimal
matrix of fibrin had formed. On day 100 the endothelia were covered with a thick
neointimal matrix of fibrin (Table 1).

Antigenicity and immunogenicity

Indirect immunofluorescence following treatment with anti-LEW and anti-CAP was
used to identify antigen on donor or recipient endothelial cells (Fig. 4). To investigate their immunogenic potential to induce specific antidonor-MHC antibodies, the
allografts were used as targets in direct immunofluorescence studies on days 20 and
50. The cells of the LEW strain could not be identified on the AS and CAP grafts
on days 20 and 50. The endothelial cells of the donor allografts (AS or CAP) reacted
positively with the FITC labelled anti-rat Ig on days 20 and 50. However, there was
a decrease in the intensity of immunofluorescence on day 50 in the strongly allogeneic system which was in accordance with the destruction of the endothelial cells
shown by SEM (Tables 1 and 3).
Donor strain skin grafts were used to challenge the allograft recipients 3 weeks postoperatively. The results of donor-specific skin transplantation are summarized in
Table 2. Weakly allogeneic strain combination (AS → LEW): The rejection of the
skin graft was accelerated (9.2 ± 0.77 days; Control AS → LEW, 11.87 ± 0.77
days). Third strain grafts (CAP) were rejected normally (CAP → LEW): 7.3 ± 0.8
days, n = 15,95% CL). MHC semiallogeneic strain combination (CAP × LEW)F1 →

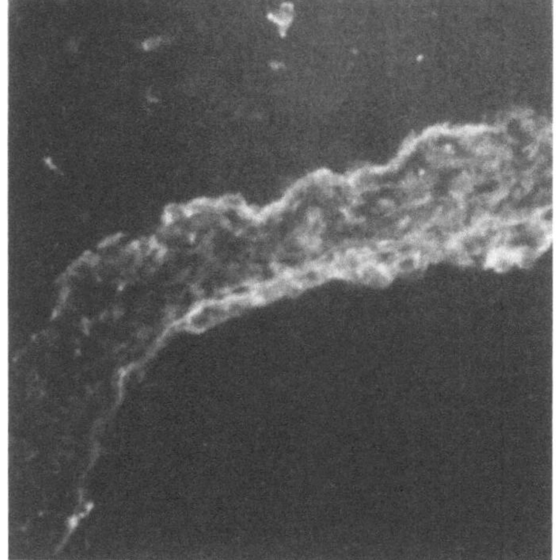

Fig. 4. Expression of endothelial surface antigens by indirect immunofluoresence technique.

Table 2. Sensitizing potential of viable aortic valve allografts investigated by survival of indicator skin grafts.

Strain combination of aortic valve allografts	Survival time (± SD) of donor strain skin grafts			
	Valve recipient n		Normal control n	
LEW → LEW (syngeneic)	20	no rejection	20	no rejection
AS → LEW (weakly allogeneic)	15	9.20±0.77	15	11.89±0.74
(CAP × LEW) F1 → LEW (MHC semiallogenic)	13	5.69±0.86	15	8.15±0.86
CAP → LEW (strongly allogeneic)	15	3.80±0.80	15	7.30± 80

SD = Standard Deviation

Table 3. Results of immunofluorescence study of endothelial cells of transplanted allografts.

Antiserum	Transplanted allografts					
	LEW postoperative days		AS		CAP	
	20	50	20	50	20	50
FITC labelled anti-rat Ig	−	−	+ +	+ +	+ +	+
Anti-LEW (CAP × LEW)	+ +	+ +	−	−	−	−
Anti-CAP (LEW × CAP)	−	−	−	−	+ +	−

Symbols: − = no reaction; + = weak positive reaction; + + = strong positive reaction.

LEW: Skin grafts syngeneic to the donor strains were rejected 5.69 ± 0.86 days postoperatively (Control: (CAP × LEW(F1 → LEW 8.15 ± 0.86 days). Control grafts (AS) from a third strain were rejected normally (AS → LEW; 11.9 ± 0.74 days, n = 15,95% CL). Strongly allogeneic skin combination (CAP- > LEW): The skin grafts syngeneic to the donor strain were rejected in an accelerated manner 3.8 ± 0.8 days). The third party control strain skin grafts (BD) were rejected normally (BD → LEW, 95% CL; 7.15 ± 0.98 days; n = 13).

Because of the destruction of the endothelia of allografts in the MHC fully allogeneic combination at day 50, further investigation was no longer necessary. The non-MHC, weakly allogeneic allografts (AS) were used to observe the possibility of re-endothelialisation after rejection of their endothelia cells at 100 days. Observations made at 150 days postoperatively, using indirect immunofluorescence, revealed no identifiable host-specific endothelial cells, which was confirmed by endothelial cell markers using anti-Factor VIII and Lectine Ulex europaeus I (Fig. 5).

Discussion

Histologically, the collagen fibres of fresh viable grafts were regular on day 50 and disorganized with macrophages around them in some areas on day 100. On day 100

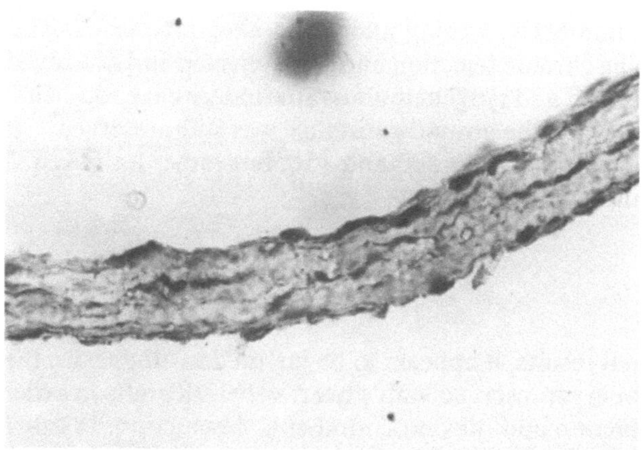

there were still a few recognizable focal macrophage cell infiltrates. The ongoing degenerative changes led to the formation of a thick neointimal matrix of fibrin by day 100.

The nonviable grafts showed regular collagen fibres and persistent fibroblasts and macrophages on day 50. The collagen fibres appeared disorganized on day 100 with macrophages identifiable around them and no fibroblasts.

The SEM findings of destruction and the loss of endothelial cells in viable grafts in the allogeneic donor-recipient combinations were primarily caused by immunological reactions, as shown by accelerated rejection of subsequent valve donor strain skin grafts (second set reaction) and by specific antibody production, demonstrated by the direct immunofluorescence.

The main immunogenic strength of the valve has been attributed to the endothelial cells of the valve leaflets (13), which thus presumably form the primary target for immunological attacks. This is particulary likely, since endothelial cells are known to express histocompatibility antigens as part of their cell membrane (9, 13). Thus the rejection of heart valve allografts differs from the "classical" graft rejection because they heal in place and cause no immediate haemodynamic disturbances. The presence of antibodies reacting against the surface antigens of the endothelial cells of the transplanted valve allografts indicates that the allografts are immunogenic. Although the immunological attack against aortic valves and corneas depends on the degree of histoincompatibility, corneal grafts are not destroyed in their "privileged" position even in the strongly allogeneic system (4).

Since the viability of the endothelial cells and their physiologic and metabolic functions are a prerequisite for the long-term survival of heart valve grafts (3, 11) it was important to investigate the possibility of re-endothelization of denuded donor valve grafts by the host. Indirect immunofluorescence with anti-LEW showed negative reactions with the donor strain target endothelial cells of viable non-MHC weakly allogeneic AS and MHC fully allogeneic CAP, nonviable non-MHC AS and syngeneic LEW allografts at days 50, 100 and 150. The results demonstrated no evidence of migration of host specific endothelial cells to the donor grafts irrespective of histocompatibility and viability. The findings were confirmed by endothelial cell markers using antifactor VIII (6, 8) and Lectine Ulex europaeus I (2, 7). The endothelial cells of the viable non-MHC weakly allogeneic allografts were maintained at day 50 while undergoing chronic rejection and were rejected and destroyed at day 100. The nonviable non-MHC and syngeneic allografts underwent endothelial degeneration already at day 50, while the ground substance was still preserved. Re-endothelization was not observed on days 100 and 150, but rather a thickened neointima as shown by SEM and light microscopy.

Conclusions

In the light of these experimental results, it appears to be justified to emphasize the need for tissue typing of fresh or cryopreserved viable heart valve allografts in order to minimize immunological reaction and prevent endothelial destruction. In other words, the possibility that the cellular components of incompatible aortic valve used clinically will be destroyed should be stressed.
The cellular components of the incompatible valve allografts disappear without replacement by host cells.
Monoclonal antibodies can be useful tools for identifying the cellular components of allografts.
It might not be necessary to cross match for nonviable heart valves, however, unspecific cellular reactions should be expected.
Degeneration of the allografts was characterized by macrophage infiltrations around the degenerated collagenous matrix.

Acknowledgement

The authors are grateful to Prof. A. Bernhard, Head of Dept. of Cardiovasclar Surgery, University of Kiel; Prof. Müller-Hermelink, formerly in the Dept. of Pathology, University of Kiel, now the Head of the Dept. of Pathology in Würzburg University; Prof. Thiede, Kidney Transplant Unit; Prof. Seifert, Head of the Dept. of Experimental Surgery in the Dept. of General Surgery, for their interest, advice and support; Dr. Saß for his assistance in the immunofluorescence work; Miss Liborius, Miss Nicklisch and Mr. Kümper for their laboratory support in the viability studies and Mrs. Lee for her technical assistance in the preparation of the manuscript.

References

1. Bodnar E, Wain WH, Martelli V, Ross DN (1979) Long-term performance of 580 homograft and autograft valves used for aortic valve replacement. Thorac Cardiovasc Surg 27: 31
2. Borisch B, Möller P, Harms D (1983) Lektin Ulex Europaeus I als Marker in der Differentialdiagnose Gefäßtumoren. Pathologe 4: 241—243
3. Freudenberg N, Riese KH, Freudenberg MA (1983) Well-established functions of endothelium. Gustav Fischer Verlag Stuttgart, New York, p 16
4. Gronemeyer U, Müller-Ruchhotz W (1974) Allogene Hornhauttransplantation bei Inzuchtratten. Albrecht von Graefes Arch Exp Ophthal 190: 319
5. Hammon JW, O'Sullivan MJ, Oury J, et al (1974) Allograft cardiac valves. A view through the scanning electron microscope. J Thorac Cardiovasc Surg 68: 352
6. Hoyer LM, de los Santos RP, Hoyer JR (1973) Antihemophilic factor antigen. Localization in endothelial cells by immunofluorescence microscopy. J Clin Invest 52: 2737

7. Holthöfer H, Virtanen I, Karieniemi AL, Hormia M, Linder E, Mielttinen A (1982) Ulex europaeus I lectin as a marker for vascular endothelium in human tissues. Lab Invest 47: 60
8. Jaffe EA (1984) Culture and identification of large vessel endothelial cells. In: Jaffe EA (ed) Biology of endothelial cells, Martinus Nijhoff, p 1—13
9. Moraes JR, Stastny P (1977) A new antigen system expressed in human endothelial cells. J Clin Invest 60: 449
10. Müller-Ruchholtz W, Gundermann KD (1964) Ein einfacher Farbtest zur Erkennung der Durchblutung von Hauttransplantation in vivo. Z Immun Forsch 127: 450
11. Ryan US, Ryan JW (1984) Cell biology of pulmonary endothelium. Circulation 70 (Suppl III), III: 46
12. Penta A, Quereshi E, Yacoub MH et al (1984) Patient status 10 or more years after "fresh" homograft replacement of the aortic valve. Circulation 70 (Suppl I), I: 182
13. Yankah AC, Feller AC, Thiede A, Westphal E, Bernhard A (1986) Identification of surface antigens of endothelial cells of fresh preserved heart allografts. Thorac Cardiovasc Surg 34: (special issue) 1—108
14. Yankah AC, Dreyer W, Wottge H-U, Müller-Ruchholtz W, et al (1986) Kinetics of endothelial cells of preserved aortic valve allografts used for heterotopic transplantation in inbred rat strains. In: Bodnar E, Yacoub M (eds) Biologic and Bioprosthetic Valves. Yorke Medical Books, p 73—84

Authors' address:
A. C. Yankah, M.D.
German Heart Center
Augustenburger Platz 1
1000 Berlin (West) 65
Germany

Immunohistopathology of cardiac valve allograft explants

H. K. Müller-Hermelink, A. C. Yankah*

Institute of Pathology, University of Würzburg and *German Heart Center, Berlin (West), Germany

Introduction

There is renewed interest in the use of fresh and cryopreserved cardiac valve allografts in view of good functional results avoiding the use of anticoagulants thromboembolism, haemorrhage and usually sudden death as complications seen with mechanical valves. However, some doubts remained on cellular viability of allografted valve endothelial cells and fibroblasts as well as the possibility of immunological mediated allograft rejection. We investigated, therefore, those cases with acute valve insufficiency after relatively short periods after transplantation. It will be shown that after short periods of implantation the usual cryopreserved cadaver heart valves are completely, or at least almost, devoid of viable donor cells and that viable cells within the transplant to a major extent represent inflammatory cells, in particular macrophages of probable host origin.

Materials and Methods

Between 1982 and 1986, 65 cryopreserved heart valve allograft transplants have been performed at the centre of cardiac surgery at the University of Kiel. 41 were in aortic, 24 in pulmonary position. Four valves, all in aortic position, had to be replaced by synthetic valves for acute valve insufficiency (Table 1).
There were three adult patients and one child. The time of explantation ranged from 9 days to 4 months (Table 2). No infection was found by microbiological and microscopic monitoring. The explantation and preservation of donor valves was similar to other cases. Interestingly, in three cases, ABO-incompatibility was noted retrospectively.
The tissue of explanted valves was investigated by routine histology and paraffin sections. In addition, a detailed immunohistological analysis in situ was performed on paraffin sections (Table 3) and on snap-frozen fresh tissue (Table 4) in order to look for immunological mechanisms. The most important reactions were the following: (1) identification of macrophages, (2) demonstration of lymphoid cells and subsets, (3) demonstration of endothelial cells and (4) identification of possible serological immune mechanisms.

---

* Formerly Dept. of Cardiovasc. Surgery, University of Kiel.
The study was supported by the Institute of Pathology, University of Kiel.

Table 1. Heart valve allografts (Kiel, 1982–1986).

Localization	Total #	Donor		Recipient		Explanted #
		P	A	Child	Adult	
Aortic valve	41	2	39	7	34	4
Pulmonary valve	24	9	15	21	3	—
Total	65	11	54	28	37	4

Table 2. Characteristics of explanted heart valve allografts.

Recipient	TPTX	Preparation time after death of donor	Preservation temperature and time °C/d	ABO
CR (47 yrs)	9 d	23 h	+ 4 °C/12 d	incomp.
HD (15 yrs)	14 d	18 h	−30 °C/20 d	comp.
SW (59 yrs)	4 wk	1 h	−30 °C/82 d	incomp.
TW (59 yrs)	16 wk	1 h	+ 4 °C/ 8 d	incomp.

Legend: TPTX = Time Posttransplant.

Table 3. Immunohistochemical investigation of paraffin sections.

Antibody	Specificity	References
Moab:		
HAM 56	macrophages	Gown et al. Am. J. Pathol. 125 (1986): 191
UCHL 1	T-lymphocytes	Smith et al. Immunol. 58 (1986): 63
Ki B3	B-Lymphocytes (similar to CD45R)	Feller, Kiel
Polyclonal antisera (rabbit):		
anti-IgM		
anti-IgG		
anti-IgA	Immunoglobulins	Dakopatts, Denmark
anti-K		
anti-L		
anti-C3c	Human C3c	dto.
anti-UEA I	endothelial cells	Ey-Laboratories, San Mateo, USA

Results

As a consistent finding in all explanted valves most of the valve tissue was acellular.
No endothelial cell coat could be found at the surface. Mainly in the earlier explantation times the fibrous valve stroma showed some dissociation by oedematous fluid
at the sides that were facing the arterial blood stream in situ. In the vicinity of valve
ruptures, interstitial haemorrhages were seen too. The fibrous strands of stromal

Table 4. Immunohistochemical investigation of cryostat sections.

Antigen	Moab	Specificity
CD3	Leu4	T-cell receptor associated Pan-T reagent
CD22	To15	Pan B
Ki M1	Ki M1	Macrophages and dendritic cells (APC for T-cell responses)
Ki M6	Ki M6	Macrophages
others:		
UEA	—	Terminal L-fucose: endothelial cells

tissue were dissociated by oedematous fluid, seen at its maximum in a valve 2 weeks after transplantation and much less prominent in a valve 4 weeks after transplantation (Fig. 1). The birefringence of collagen was altered at that time, pointing to an early degenerative change. On this background of acellular stroma collagenous tissue, some foci of viable cells with moderate to high cellularity are found. These are localized in the vicinity of valve ruptures or tissue irregularities at the surface of the leaflets (Fig. 2) at the base of the valve, a loose pannus-like granulation tissue was seen growing over the surface of the acellular valve transplant. These characteristics have already been noticed in early studies of homograft histology(2, 3).

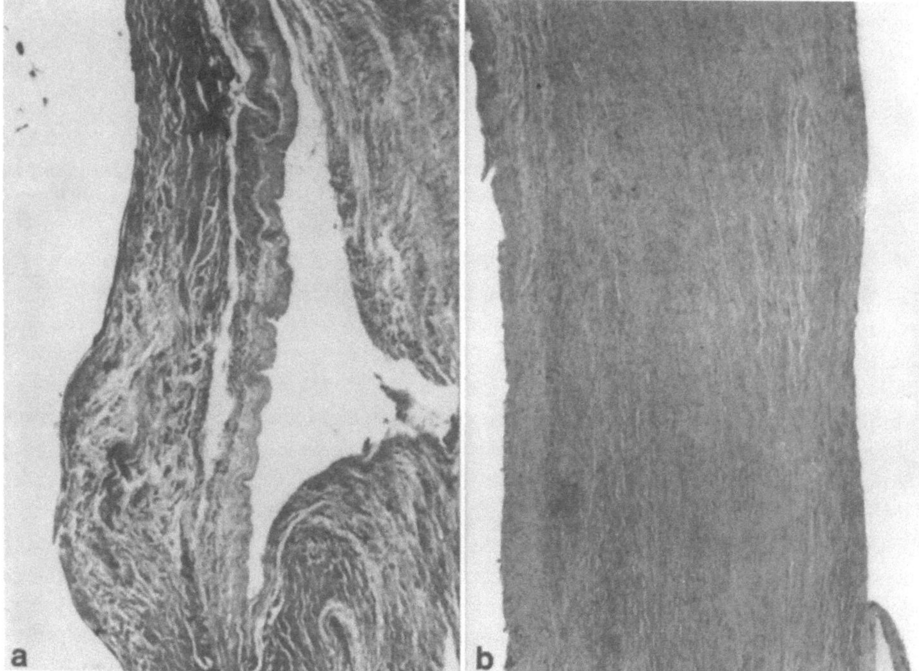

Fig. 1. Acellularity and early degeneration with oedema in explanted heart valve at (a) 2 weeks after transplantation (b) 4 weeks after transplantation. HE; × 80 magnification.

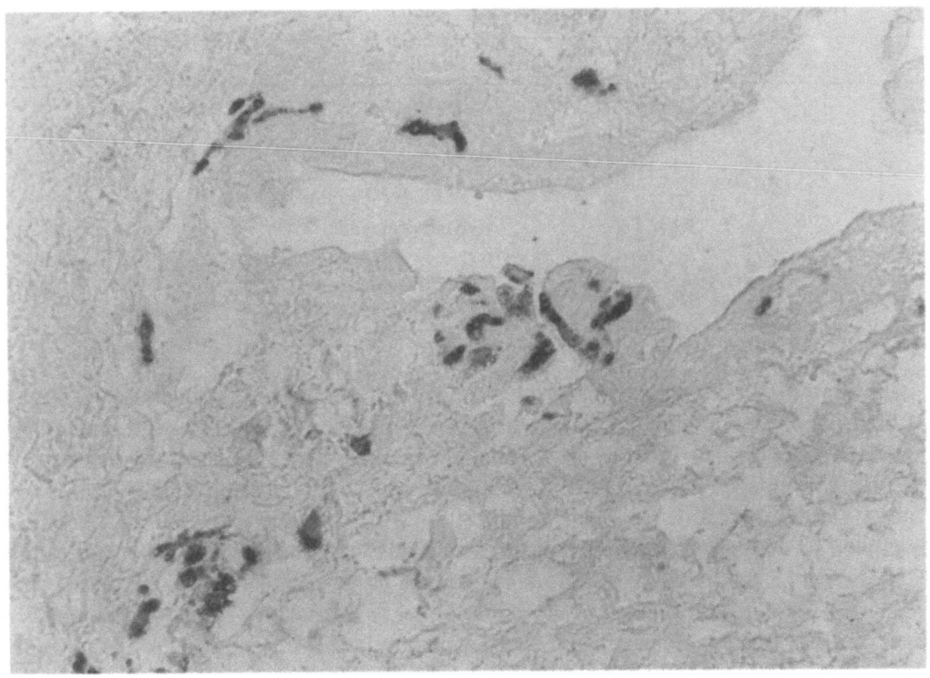

Fig. 2. Immunohistological demonstration of macrophages at the surface and the deeper stromal part of explanted heart valve tissue 4 weeks after transplantation (HAM 56; indirect immuno peroxidase reaction; × 200).

Immunohistochemical studies

Monoclonal antibody immunohistochemistry revealed that almost all viable cells in the transplant were macrophages. Individual cells in the fibrous stroma with well staining nuclear structure, as well as flat cells at the valve surface and a collection of rounded, foam-like cells in the stroma, showed a definite positive reaction for the macrophage-specific monoclonal antibody HAM 56 (4). In some areas (Fig. 2) it can be shown that monocytes/macrophages attach to the surface in the region of clefts and irregular surface structures. They migrate to the central parts where the cells are larger and represent mature macrophages with vacuolated cytoplasm. No viable endothelial cells or fibroblasts were found by immunohistochemistry nor lymphocytes of T or B subset in three of the four cases.. Two valves showed reactivity with antibodies to IgM at the valve surface, as well as a spot-like reactivity with antibodies to activated complement component C3C in areas which may have been originally occupied by stromal fibroblasts. This creates the possibility for an antibody-mediated immune mechanism, especially in cases of ABO-incompatibility.
A mitral valve explanted at 8 weeks after transplantation was heavily destroyed (Fig. 3). Histologically, it showed the strongest infiltration of host cells which accumumulated in a granuloma-like fashion around degenerated collagenous tissue. This aspect resembled the structure of rheumatoid necrosis. Immunohistologically there was a very strong infiltration of macrophages reacting with the monoclonal antibody

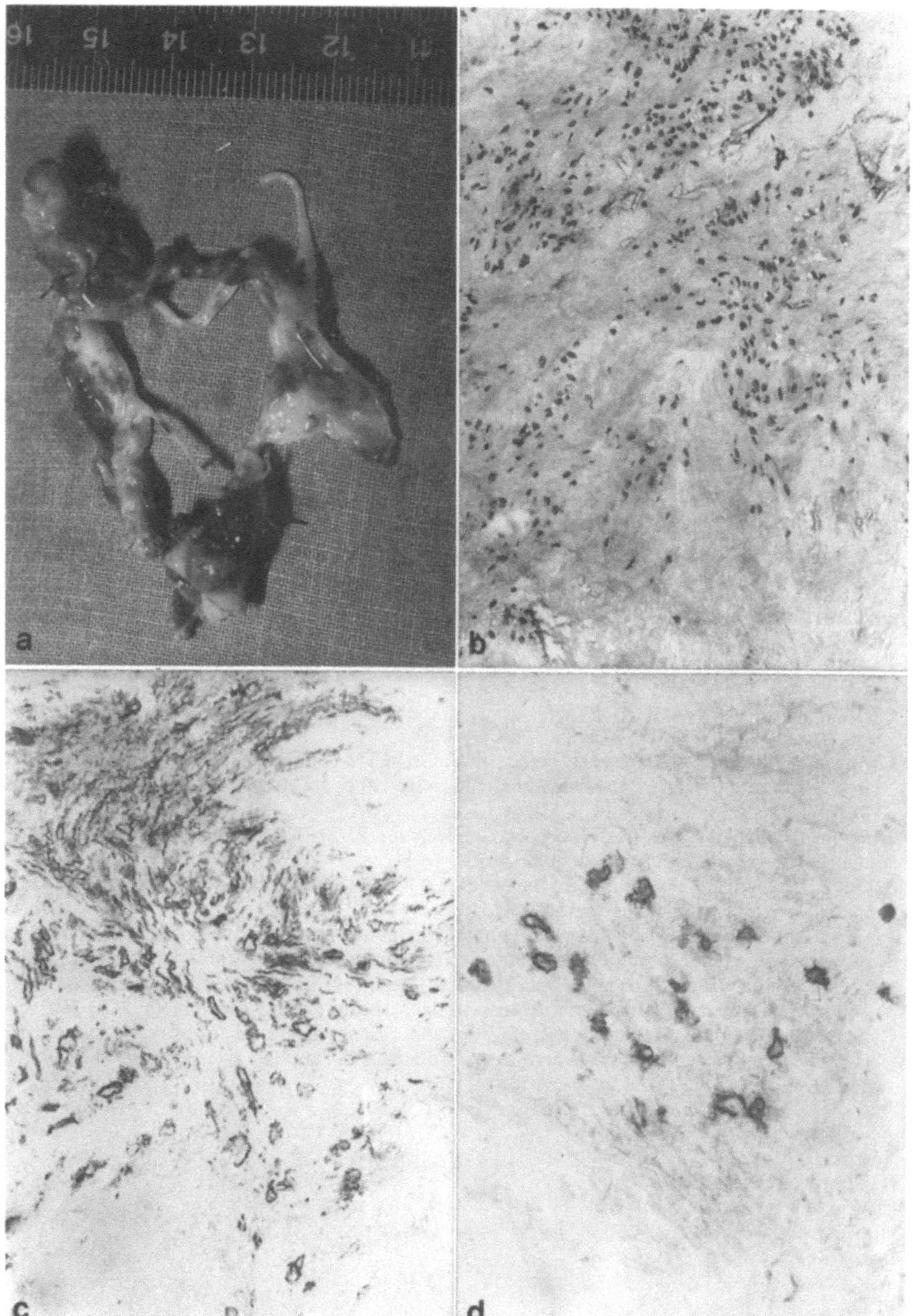

Fig. 3. Mitral allograft explant at 8 weeks after transplantation. (a) Macroscopical aspect. (b) Granuloma-like dense infiltration of valve tissue with focal collections of inflammatory cells and collagen degeneration (HE, × 130). (c) Demonstration of macrophages with monoclonal antibody Ki M1 (indirect immunoperoxidase, × 200). (d) Demonstration of Pan T-cell antigen CD 3, showing a minority of T-lymphocytes (indirect immunoperoxidase, × 200).

Ki M1 on cryostat-sections (Fig. 3c) and also other macrophage-specific antigens (Ki M6, Ki M8). In addition, this case was the only one showing a minority of T-lymphocytes mainly of the CD-4 subtype. This cellular component may represent a concomitant inflammatory infiltration which is seen in many types of chronic inflammation.

Conclusions

Heart valve allografts explanted early after transplantation were almost completely acellular, which is in contrast to reports suggesting viability of fibroblasts after cryo-preservation of cadaver heart valves (1, 5) but confirms earlier results (2, 3). Mucoid oedema and collagen matrix degeneration, seen early after transplantation, are less prominent in a later transplant. Viable cells in the valve stroma are of recipient origin, consisting mainly of macrophages: macrophages attach at the surface and migrate to the stroma of the transplant. Increasing numbers are found with time after transplantation. Macrophage infiltration is increased in the foci of degeneration. Two valves show deposition of immunoglobulins and of activated complement (C3C) at the valve surface, suggesting that antibody-mediated mechanisms may be of relevance in accelerating the degeneration process. There is no clear evidence of a cellular immunological allograft rejection.

References

1. Angell WW, Angell JD, Oury JH, Lamberti JJ, Grehl TM (1987) Long-term follow-up of viable frozen aortic homografts. A viable homograft valve bank. J Thorac Cardiovasc Surg 93: 815—822
2. Gavin JB, Barratt-Boyes BG, Hitchcock GC, Herdson PB (1973) Histopathology of "fresh" human aortic valve allografts. Thorax 28: 482
3. Gavin JB, Herdson PB, Monro JL, Barratt-Boyes BG (1973) Pathology of antibiotic-treated human heart valve allografts. Thorax 28: 473
4. Gown AM, Tsukada T, Ross R (1986) Human atherosclerosis. II. Immunocytochemical analysis of the cellular composition of human atherosclerotic lesions. Am J Pathol 125: 191—207
5. Livi U, Abdulla A-K, Parker R, Olsen EJ, Ross DN (1987) Viability and morphology of aortic and pulmonary homografts. A comparative study. J Thorac Cardiovasc Surg 93: 755—760
6. Norton AJ, Ramsay AD, Smith SH, Beverley PCL, Isaacson PG (1986) Monoclonal antibody (UCHL1) that recognises normal and neoplastic T cells in routinely fixed tissues. J Clin Pathol 39: 399—405

Authors' address:
H. K. Müller-Hermelink MD.
Chairman, Professor of Pathology
University of Würzburg
Institute of Pathology
Würzburg
FRG

Applications and limitations of histocompatibility in clinical cardiac valve allograft surgery

M. H. Yacoub

Harefield Hospital, Harefield, National Heart and Brompton Hospital, London, U.K.

During the last few years there has been a vast accumulation of knowledge with regard to allograft rejection mechanisms accompanied with development of powerful tools for studying this problem. In addition there has been an accumulation of data specifically related to the homograft valve. The question, therefore, is: Do we know enough to-day to make firm recommendations with regard to clinical practice? In this chapter I shall try and review some of the evidence in an attempt to answer the following questions:
1. Does rejection play a role in determining the fate of aortic valve homografts?
2. If so, is it cell- or antibody-mediated?
3. Can we modify the process of rejection?
4. Are we really justified to use immune suppression on the current evidence we have?
Current knowledge indicates that allograft rejection depends on antigen presentation which involves Class-2 major histocompatibility (MHC) antigens (DR, DP or DQ) which is expressed by specific cells; this activates T-helper cells which then secrete lymphokines which enhance Class-2 antigen expression and activate cytotoxic T-cells which then attack the target organ. For the target organ to be attacked it has to express Class-1 MHC antigen. That was the knowledge until very recently when, through a very elegant experiment, a group of researchers have genetically modified cells to delete the DNA which encodes for Class-1 antigen and showed that Class-2 antigen can function not only as an antigen presenter, but also as a target for cytotoxic T-cells in the absence of Class-1 antigen. We do know the major histocompatibility Class-1 antigen structure which is formed of five domains (Fig. 1), three extra-cellular, one in the bilipid layer and one intracellular. We know the sequence of these polypeptides, and their genetic coding. Similar knowledge has accumulated in relation to Class-2 antigen which is very similar to Class-1 antigen molecule, the T-cell receptor and to the molecule of antibodies, showing that they probably all evolved from the same gene family several million years ago. The gene encoding the MHC antigens is located on the short arm of chromosome 6 (Fig. 2), and is closely related to the gene encoding the compliment system. The DNA is encoding Class-1 and Class-2 through a process of transcription and translation can then be expressed on the cell surface. This is important, because we now have tools to study the major histocompatability antigens not just on the surface of the cell, but through the use of molecular probes specific for MHC antigens either polymorphically or monomorphically. We can look at the messenger RNA encoding them regardless of whether the antigen is expressed on the cell or not. Through the

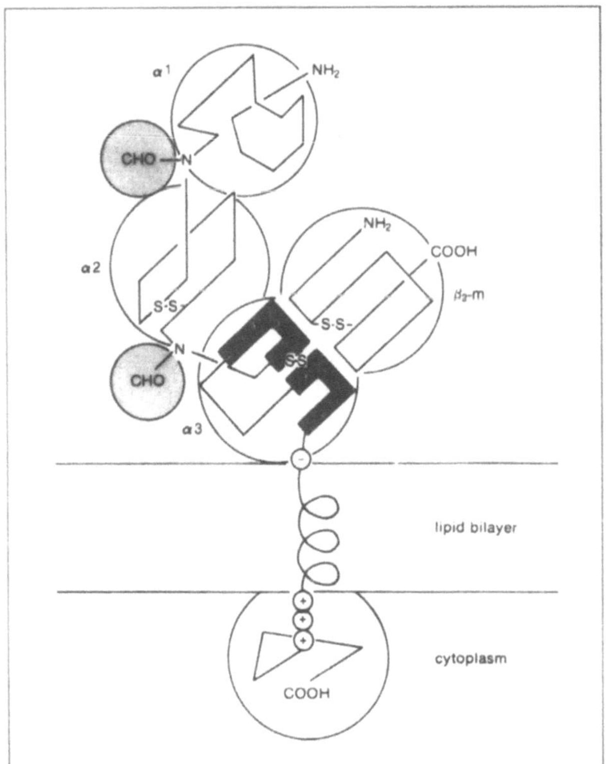

Fig. 1. Diagnostic representation of the molecular structure of Class-1 MHC antigen.

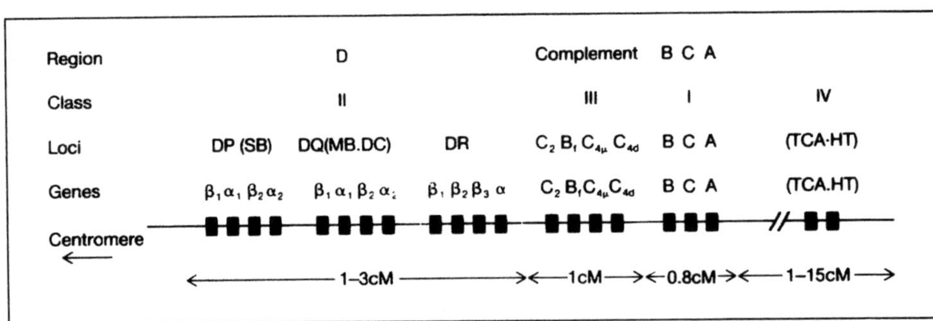

Region		D			Complement	B C A	
Class		II			III	I	IV
Loci	DP (SB)	DQ(MB.DC)	DR		C_2 B_1 $C_{4\mu}$ C_{4d}	B C A	(TCA·HT)
Genes	$\beta_1 \alpha_1 \beta_2 \alpha_2$	$\beta_1 \alpha_1 \beta_2 \alpha_2$	$\beta_1 \beta_2 \beta_3 \alpha$		$C_2 B_1 C_{4\mu} C_{4d}$	B C A	(TCA.HT)
Centromere ←							

$\leftarrow$ — 1–3cM — $\rightarrow$ $\leftarrow$ 1cM $\rightarrow$ $\leftarrow$ 0.8cM $\rightarrow$ $\leftarrow$ — 1–15cM — $\rightarrow$

Fig. 2. Genetic loci encoding MHC antigens.

use of monoclonal antibodies we now have a relatively straightforward methodology for looking at the antigen expression by immunocyto-chemistry. Using this technique Dr. Marlene Rose has shown in our laboratory that, contrary to the prevailing dogma which states that all somatic cells should express Class-1 antigens on the cell — this is not so in the case of the heart (Fig. 3a). Under normal conditions the myocytes do not express any Class-1 antigen which implies that they cannot act as targets to immunological damage. Further work has shown that, just prior to or

96

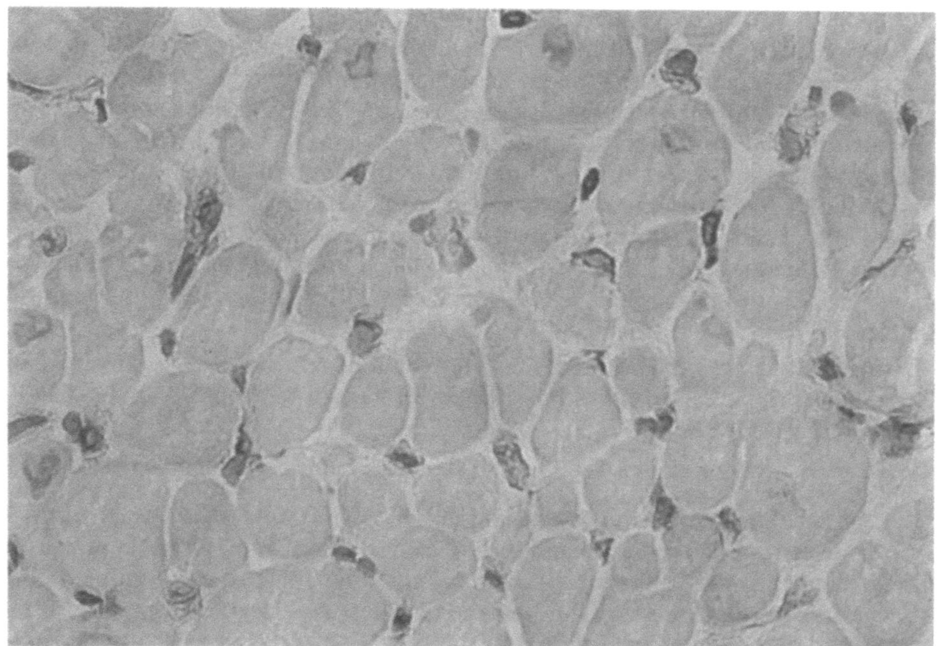

Fig. 3a. A section of a normal heart stained by immunocytochemistry using W6/32 monoclonal antibody showing no Class-1 antigen expression by myocardial cells.

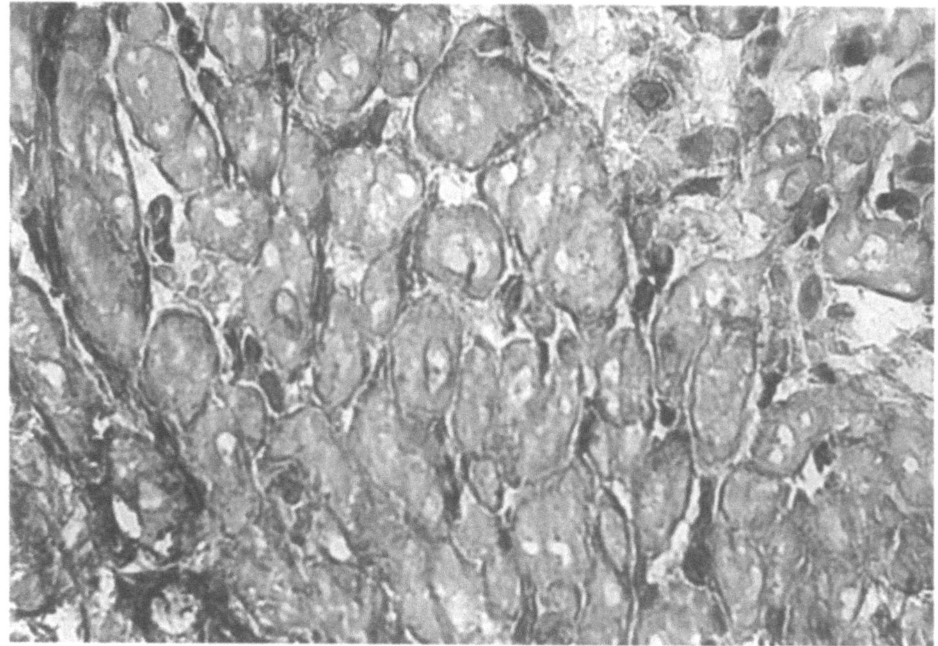

Fig. 3b. Section of the heart during acute allograft rejection stained as in Fig. 3a, showing induction of strong Class-1 MHC antigen expression by the myocardial cells.

during acute rejection episodes, there is induction of very strong Class-1 antigen expression on the myocytes (Fig. 3b) (1, 2). Although our knowledge of how the cells are attacked is relatively good it is by no means complete and, up to recently, it was thought that the mechanism by which the cytotoxic T-cells attack the target cells are through the secretion of specific proteins which actually have been isolated and termed perforins, because they perforate the cell membrane which causes cell destruction. More recently another mechanism has been suggested (Fig. 4), this involves a receptor mediated mechanism which enables the cytotoxic T-cell to induce a series of chemical reactions inside the cell which produces cell destruction — so, in effect, rather than murder the cell, the T-cells induce the target cell to commit suicide.

Further research into the basic mechanisms could be relevant because if we do understand those, perhaps we could modify the process of rejection.

Does rejection play a role in determining the fate of aortic valve homografts?

This can be addressed in a variety of indirect ways. One of the ways we have utilised was to investigate the presence and localisation of Class-1 and Class-2 antigens in aortic homografts at different times and to study the effect of sterilisation and/or storage on antigen expression. Dr. Amanda Suitters (3), in our laboratory did the following series of experiments:

Valves were obtained within 15 min. of death (generally from cardiac transplant recipients) and examined immediately by immunochemistry. Portions of the same valve were examined 24 h later when kept in a nutrient TC 199 medium at 4 °C.

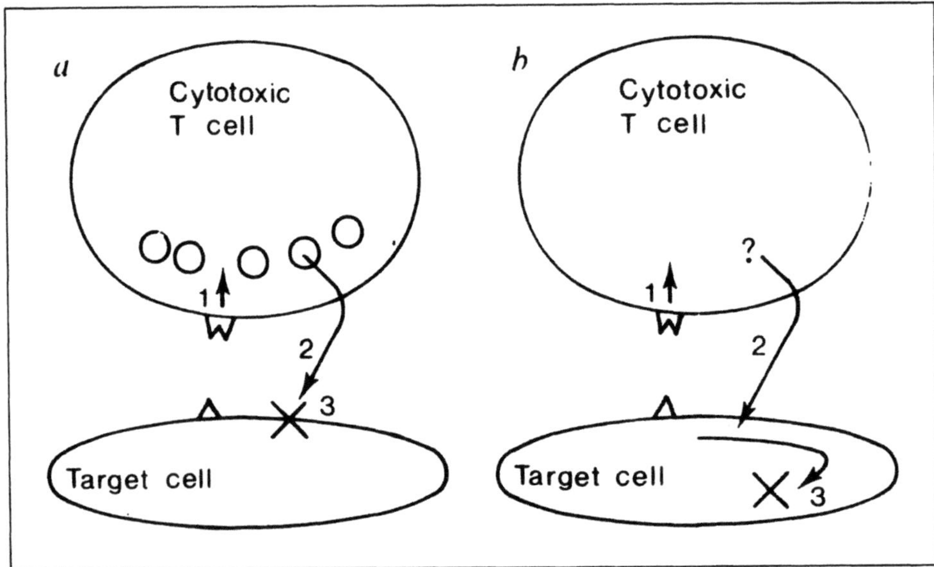

Fig. 4. Diagrammatic representation of the possible mechanisms of destruction of target cells by cytotoxic T-cells.

Valves also were examined from material obtained 1—3 days from routine post mortem and sterilised in antibiotics before and after the sterilisation process and during the period of storage. For this purpose a variety of monoclonal antibodies were used, these included:

1. W6/32, a mouse MAb with specificity against a human nonpolymorphic determinant common to all Class-1 antigens. This antibody was used as a neat tissue culture supernatant and was kindly donated by Dr. C. Navarette and Professor H. Festenstein (London Hospital, London, UK).

2. HLA-DR, a mouse MAb with specificity against Class-2 DR determinant (Becton-Dickinson). This antibody was diluted 1: 10 in PBS.

3. F10-89-4, a mouse MAb that is directed at the common leukocyte antigen. This antibody was diluted 1 : 80 in PBS and was kindly donated by Dr. R. Dalchau and Professor J. Fabre (Blond-McIndoe Centre, East Grinstead, UK.)

4. Factor VIII rabbit heterologous antibody that specifically stains endothelium (Dakopatts Ltd., London, UK). This antibody was diluted 1 : 30 in PBS.

The fresh valve, obtained within 15 min of death and examined immediately did express Class-1 antigen on the endothelial cell quite strongly (Fig. 5). 24 h later, however, there was no Class-1 antigen expression. These cells were shown to be viable and indeed, could be stained by monoclonal antibody specific for endothelial cell, so they just lost MHC Class-1 antigen expression by 24 h. Just what is the relevance of that is still not entirely clear, because — as has been shown with myocytes, lymphokines or other agents could induce Class-1 antigen expression before

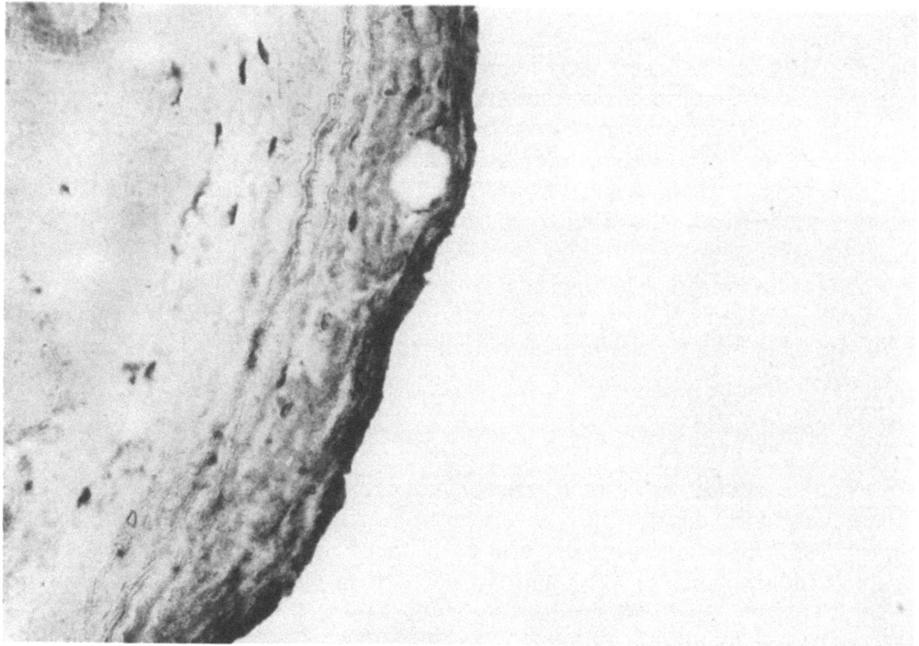

Fig. 5. Photomicrograph of a fresh aortic homograft stained by MAB (W6/32) showing strong Class-1 antigen expression by endothelial cells.

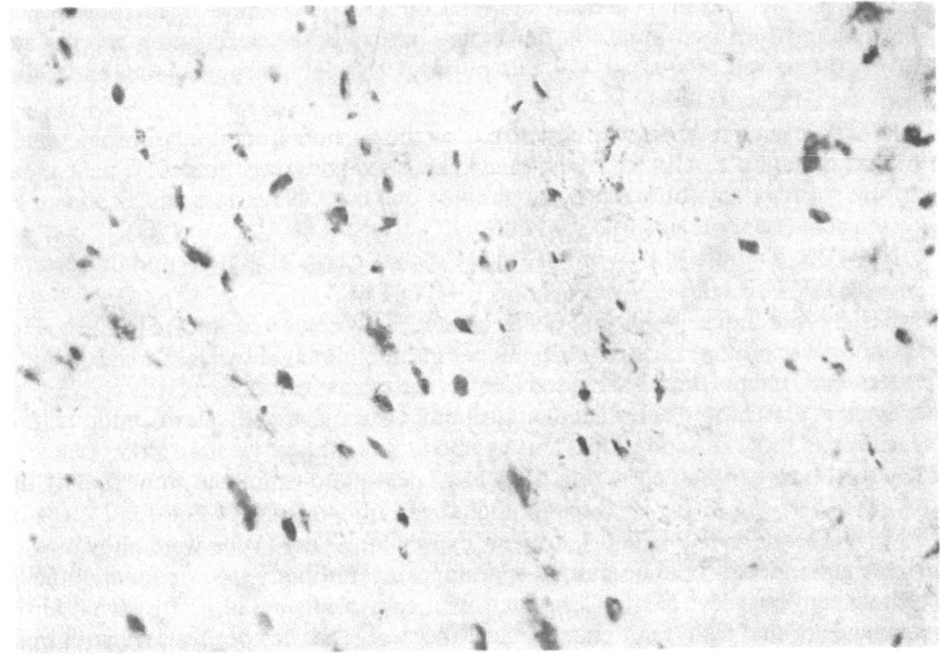

Fig. 6. Stroma of a fresh aortic homograft showing strong Class-2 antigen expression by dendritic cells (see text).

or during rejection. Cells expressing Class-2 antigen were present in the stroma of the valve (Fig. 6). These cells were identified as dendritic cells, in that they did stain with antileucocyte common antigen MAB. They also disappeared after 24 h storage. This indirect study, therefore, shows that fresh homografts immediately after being taken out of the body, without processing, do express Class-1 and Class-2 antigens and that Class-1 antigens are localised to the endothelial cells, and Class-2 are mainly on interstitial cells in the form of dendritic cells. It has also been shown that antibiotic sterilisation and storage produces progressive reduction or disappearance in both types of antigen. The significance of these findings will require further study. We did not either look at these cells with messenger RNA probes, neither did we challenge them with Y interferon or lymphokines.

Can we influence the performance of aortic homografts by immunological means?

For example, should we be matching for ABO compatability? We have attempted to match for ABO compatibility in the group of patients where we obtained homografts from transplant recipients and used them within 24 h and look retrospectively at the influence of ABO matching. But then we have to wait a long time, because we know that homografts do function very well for periods of 7 to 8 years before you start having any number of degenerations to count. What we have shown is that in the medium term, there was no difference between patients who have been matched for ABO compatibility and those who have not, in that specific group of

100

patients receiving very fresh homograft valves. Indeed we have a patient who has had a heart transplant where we crossed the ABO compatibility — a heart from group A donor was transplanted into an O recipient and this patient did not reject and is a "long-term survivor" three year's later. This is, of course, an exception to the rule, because it has been shown that ABO blood groups are expressed on most somatic cells and act as strong transplantation antigens. However, our findings highlight the presence of gaps in our knowledge.

The influence of matching for histocompatibility antigens is also not completely defined. In cardiac transplantation we cross histocompatibility antigens fairly frequently, but are we paying the price? When we looked back at our cardiac transplant recipients who are immunosuppressed, we could not demonstrate an influence of matching for Class-1 MHC antigens on the survival of these patients. However, we could show that there was a significant difference between patients matched for Class-2 specifically DR (Fig. 7) or when we combined matching for DR and HLAB. Patients with two, or more, mismatches had a significantly less favourable survival (4). Currently there are no data relating to the influence of matching for MHC antigens on aortic homograft valve performance.

Are we justified to use immunosuppression for patients receiving homograft valves?

We have limited data on a group of patients who received azathioprine and steroids for 3 months after receiving homovital valves (removed at the time of cardiac trans-

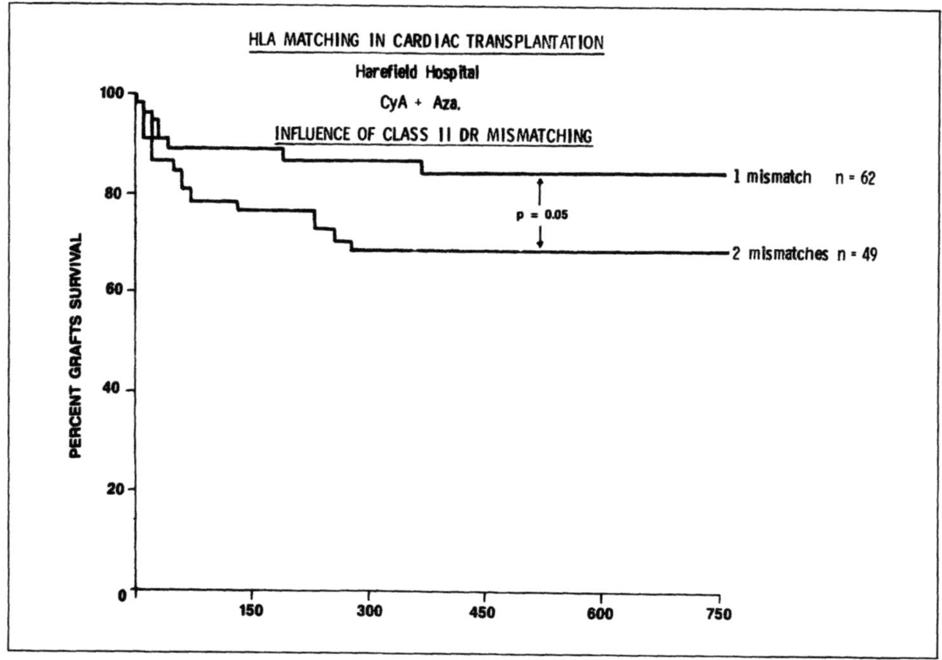

Fig. 7. Actuarial survival curve showing the influence of matching for Class-2 antigens (DR).

101

plantation) and we could not demonstrate any difference in the performance of the valves over a period of 3—4 years, when compared with a historical group of patients who did not receive immunosuppression and we think that the only means of answering this question is through a prospective randomised trial. Current evidence does not provide enough knowledge to subject the patients to the extra hazards of immunosuppression without knowing what benefits they could derive.

Antibody mediated rejection

A positive crossmatch in patients undergoing cardiac transplantation does not always result in hyperacute rejection, however the one year survival of these patients is 55 %. That might not be too bad if you have a very desperate patient where you cannot do anything but transplant him or her, but that shows you that preformed antibodies can have an influence on survival of heart transplants. What is the influence of antibodies on long term results? There is some evidence that accelerated coronary sclerosis in the heart transplant recipient is mediated, either by natural killer cells or antibodies formed de novo.

Similar mechanisms could be operational in the case of homografts, and has to be investigated.

I have to conclude, therefore, that although we know a fair amount about the process of rejection and we have strong tools for studying this, our current knowledge is too patchy to allow us to make firm recommendations. Also, I have to conclude that perhaps there is a very strong need for controlled trials and a lot more research before we can answer the questions posed in this paper.

References

1. Rose ML, Coles MI, Griffin RJ, Pomerance A, Yacoub MH (1986) Expression of Class I and Class II major histocompatibility antigens in normal and transplanted hearts. Transplantation 41, 776—780
2. Suitters A, Rose M, Higgins A, Yacoub MH (1987) MHC antigen expression in segmental biopsies from cardiac transplant patients — correlation with rejection. Clin. Exp. Immunol. 69, 575—583
3. Yacoub M, Suitters A, Khaghani A, Rose M (1986) Localisation of major histocompatibility complex (HLA ABC and DR) antigens in aortic homografts. In: Bodner E, Yacoub M (eds) Biologic and Bioprosthetic Valves. Yorke Medical Books
4. Yacoub MH, Festenstein P, Doyle M, Martin D, McClusky D, Awad J, Gamka A, Khaghani A, Holmes A (1987) The influence of HLA matching in cardiac allograft recipients receiving cyclosporin and azathioprine. Transpl Proc 19, 2487

Author's address:
Magdi Yacoub, M.D.
British Heart Foundation Professor of Cardiac Surgery
Consultant Cardiac Surgeon
Harefield Hospital
Harefield
Uxbridge, Middlesex
U.K.

Discussion

Chaired by: W. Müller-Ruchholtz, FRG, M. H. Yacoub, UK

GONZALEZ-LAVIN:

I would like to present a case that will support some of the data in the discussion already presented by Sir Brian Barratt-Boyes and Mr. Donald Ross, and more recently, by Mr. Yankah. We operated on a 20-year-old lady with a congenital aortic regurgitation. The allograft was taken from a 21-year-old male with a head trauma and was procured under sterile conditions in a vital state 11 hours after death. We put it in a nutrient medium at 4 °C for 11 days, and afterwards the graft was cryopreserved and stored for 208 days. Postoperatively, the recipient developed aortic regurgitation due to sagging of the non-coronary leaflet.
The allograft was explanted 10 months later. At the time of the re-operation we found that the aortic wall of the allograft was adherent to the aorta, so we just excised the leaflets and replaced the valve. In a histological and a cytogenetic analysis we found that the tip of the leaflets was completely acellular, however, the base of the leaflets was cellular, looking pretty much normal. The edge of the base of the leaflet was covered by a single layer of endothelial cells. To examine the integrity of the endothelial cells, immunochemistry was carried out using a polyclonal antibody against factor VIII-related antigens and showing viable and normal looking endothelial cells. The controls for the immunohistochemistry were negative. The tissues for cytogenetic investigations were prepared into single cell suspensions and seeded in tissue culture flasks. The cytogenetic analysis showed no Y-chromosomes in the cultured fibroblasts indicating host origin of those cells. So, I think we have some evidence that one preserves the ground substances Sir Brian Barratt-Boyes and Mr. Donald N. Ross have alluded this morning, that there is some possibility of repopulating these leaflets.

YACOUB:

Were these endothelial cells really repopulating the whole of the leaflets or was it just a little sheet underneath the cusp? We should differentiate between repopulation and that shelf of tissue which comes underneath the valve. And was it on the ventricular aspect or on the aortic aspect?

GONZALEZ-LAVIN:

It was right at the base of the leaflet and in the closer 1/3 of the leaflet towards the base of the leaflet. We analysed it very carefully: it was on the free edge of the leaflet.

MOLINA:

Examination in the long term of our non-viable allograft valves — non-viable when implanted — has led to a consistent concern about acellularity. The valves become thin and perforate any time from 7 years on.
We do not believe that there is host infiltration into the leaflet. We have never seen it and we remain unconvinced by the presentation of others that the host infiltrates into the leaflet tissue itself. We accept sheathing and we also accept, of course, macrophage and lymphocyte infiltration into any type of leaflet. The picture is a little different with the viable valve. A valve at four months shows a central core of cellularity with a surface acellularity appearance. A valve at 2 1/4 years shows, once again, some cellularity in the centre of the leaflet. Altogether, have similar evidence at 2 months, 10 months, 20 months, 2 1/4 years. Another valve at 7 years was, we thought, a viable valve, but there was no cellularity at all; although it was competent, the patient dying of cancer at 7 years, we would have expected this valve to perforate in the near future. The longest was at 9 1/4 years; its cellularity was quite evident. So, we have seen a huge variation in our study: within the same valve, one leaflet has been acellular and the other has been cellular. And then we see differences from patient to patient.

We are actually able to "tissue-culture" these cells. There was a male donor and a female patient and all cells cultured from the leaflet tissue demonstrated donor origin. We are strongly convinced that in some patients, and we do not know how large a group, there will be persistence of donor cells. But there is also a pattern of acellularity and we wonder whether there is a need for refinement of our protocols indicating how we use the valves, collect them, and used them earlier. I would very much value Prof. Yacoub's comments on what we have seen in the long term.

YACOUB:

I really do not know what to say because I agree that there are features which we cannot explain. I am impressed by one of your slides which showed cellularity which could be related to the valve. The rest of the slides seemed again to be showing the type of cells which have been seen in many of the papers we have had this morning. These dark-staining nuclei which could easily be monocytes can now perhaps with the help of the variety of monoclonal antibodies be defined concerning the type of cell they belong to. But the behaviour of valves is certainly inconsistent, as you say, and there are sometimes generalisations without controls, e.g. regarding the age of the donor. We have had a patient with the donor being 74; the valve was performing for 16 years or more and I had the chance to look at it while I was replacing another valve 16 years later from a 74-year-old donor; it was antibiotic-sterilised and is still going. So, there are features which we do not understand, and maybe now we should start to try to understand a bit more about the different determinants. I cannot answer your question very well.

ANGELL:

I want to echo Prof. Yacoub's remarks because our experience with valves at a week, a month, several months, and a few years would suggest exactly what he described. This is, there are cellular components and acellular segments of the valve leaflets and this varies from patient to patient and within the same valve. The fibroblasts can be shown by EM to be producing collagen; this phenomenon persists for at least months to a few years after implantation and drops off progressively. There are 13-year-old frozen valves that are acellular at the time of explantation. This work is also reproducible in experimental animals and we saw no difference between animals and man in the qualitative examinations of the cellular component of the valve leaflet. There is a quantitative difference that is quite striking and probably due to the fact that the dog valves are more cellular and more reactive. I also believe strongly that it is an immunologic phenomenon that we maintain viability at the time the valve is implanted and then reactions are seen post-implantation.

BANK:

One of the problems in any type of transplantation is the presence of immuno-reactive cells, specifically passenger leucocytes and macrophages. Is there any evidence in either the heart valve itself of the surrounding cardiac muscle cells that either of these cell types (a) is present and (b) plays a role in the induction of the immune response?

YACOUB:

Yes, there are definitely a large number of dendritic class II positive cells in the substance of the aortic allograft.

MÜLLER—RUCHHOLZ:

As a transplantation immunologist, I would suggest to you not to restrict the understanding of immunogenic cells to that which Lafferty has introduced as "passenger cell concept". This passenger cell concept should be broadened substantially because we now know of residential cells which are as well MHC class II antigen positive as those passenger cells are. And to those residential cells which are MHC class II positive in the human — but I should stress "in the human" — belong endothelial cells. Not so in the rat, but in the human.

I should add that we do not have extensive studies of how far endothelial cells in the various parts of the vascular network may differ in this respect. Therefore, I would like to see more extensive studies with regard to that tissue you are interested in, namely valves. But, to say it again, expect valve endothelial cells to be potentially good immunogenicity carriers.

YACOUB:

In our study, the endothelium of the valve did not express class II antigens, even in the fresh specimen and unlike what we have seen in the heart where the endothelial cells express both class I and class II quite strongly without challenge. Perhaps if subjected to interleukin-2, for example, they will express and they might have, in the DNA class II antigen, codely like any other endothelium. The worry is that they could express it under challenge.

MÜLLER-RUCHHOLTZ:

Of course, we have to differentiate between the constitutive expression and the induced expression. But you are simply supporting my point, namely that I would suggest more extensive study of when and in which parts of the vascular network the endothelial cells express these antigens.

YACOUB:

But in the allograft valve it seems to be entirely the dendritic cells, the passenger cells, because of double staining data. The cells which express class II antigens were also stained for common leucocyte antigens, so that we thought there is a proof that they were indeed passenger and dendritic.

MÜLLER-RUCHHOLTZ:

In addition to endothelial cells. But they may be MHC antigen negative at the moment when you put them into the recipient and may afterwards become induced to express these antigens a few hours later.

BANK:

We preserved lymphocytes and macrophages under a wide variety of cryobiological techniques and under some conditions it is possible to define cryobiological profiles which apparently destroy the immuno-reactive cells while not adversely affecting the valve tissue.

ROSS:

Could you tell us what the findings are in the ordinary heart transplant recipient who dies for an unrelated course? Those patients have a homovital valve in place, have been under imunosuppression all the time. Do they have a full complement of endothelial cells?

YACOUB:

Yes, they do. If you look at the cells, they look normal to the naked eye and it depends on how the patients died. Whether it was in the hyperacute rejection phase, where you can find some haemorrhages, some infiltration of the valve, or in the long-term ones who died for a variety of reasons where it looked entirely normal. I am aware however, of at least one specimen, in which the valve looked calcified and thickened in a patient who had chronic rejection for 5 years, as if the valve had been attacked. But as you quite rightly say, these patients have been relatively meticulously immunosuppressed.

COHEN:

Not being an immunologist, I would like to confirm Prof. Yacoub's finding in the cornea preservation where we culture corneas for 4 or 6 weeks. After culturing with various techniques we were unable to show any presence of ABO or HLA antigens anymore. Nevertheless, if you transplant these corneas into completely mismatched bad risk, that is, first urgency cornea patients, they do reject. So I think that Dr. Müller-Ruchholtz' suggestion to start further studies is indeed worthwhile.

BODNAR:

I would like to discuss calcification and immunology. Dr. Goffin said first that calcification is exceptional in allografts. That is a wishful thought. We might say that calcification is very rare in allografts inserted into the right side of the heart. But if the allograft is put in the aortic position then calcification will occur.
Gonzales-Lavin presented very impressive series of animal experiments: calcification versus immunology. I have some doubts. There were 3 weeks' time differences between Group A and B in that experiment. Group A, which did not calcify or very little, were killed about 3 weeks earlier than Group B which, among other things, were unrelated donors. If the calcification went along a straight line, it might not be a significant period. But as calcification goes along a logarithmic line, the 3 weeks' difference has to be considered.

GONZALEZ-LAVIN:

First of all we did not attempt to sacrifice Group A before Group B. This was just the normal survival of the animals, so it happened that Group B animals died earlier and this is probably because they have much more calcification than Group A. In answer to Prof. Yacoub we did not do any important identification of immunogenic factors in these groups.

MÜLLER-RUCHHOLTZ:

To make very brief concluding remarks:
1. I would strongly suggest continuing systematic experimental work which should be done in inbred strains, because I am really convinced that from those best-controlled experimental studies you can still learn a lot.
2. Dr. Bank, I am sitting in your boat with regard to the viability problem and I would like to extend this aspect, because viability determines immunogenicity. It is not just the expression or non-expression, the existence or non-existence of transplantation antigens on cell surfaces. I would like to repeat what I said during my lecture, namely that immunogenicity is determined by cell viability plus metabolic activity. So it might be very useful to be more concerned about a standardized definition of viability and to try to define which viability test informs about immunogenicity. We have immunological tools nowadays to study that, MHC-like tests, for example.
3. One question did not come up at all, and I would consider that as an important one: The question of sensitization. In other words, to test whether the recipient of a graft became sensitized. Such has been done in experimental studies and the tools exist. This would be the easiest and most direct approach to answer the question of whether immunological reactions follow allograft transplantation or not.

106

The anatomy of the outflow tracts of the heart and of aortic and pulmonary allografts

S. P. Allwork

Department of Surgery, Royal Postgraduate Medical School, Hammersmith Hospital, London, U.K.

Although the left and right outflow tracts are contiguous they are markedly dissimilar in their morphology. This is due to the striking anatomical differences between the left and right ventricles. The left ventricle is conical in shape and its inflow and outflow tracts are separated only by the anterior leaflet of the mitral valve. The right ventricle is sigmoid in shape and its inlet and outlet valves are separated by a mass of muscle called the crista supraventricularis.

The aortic root and outflow tract of the left ventricle

The aortic root comprises the annulus fibrosus of the aortic valve, its three leaflets and their corresponding sinuses, and the membranous part of the ventricular septum. It is related to both the inflow and outflow portions of the right ventricle via the interventricular and ventriculoatrial components respectively, of the membranous part of the ventricular septum. In addition it is related to the right ventricular outflow by means of the infundibular septum and to the pulmonary artery by the annuli fibrosi of the aortic and pulmonary valves (Fig. 1). The aortic root, which comprises most of the left ventricular outflow tract, is also related to the transverse sinus of the pericardium by means of the left and posterior (noncoronary) sinuses of the aortic valve, and lastly it is related to the left atrium via the apposition of the left aortic sinus and the left atrial wall (1) (Fig. 2).

The left ventricular outflow tract is thus mainly fibrous, but the right aortic sinus and right valve leaflet are bedded in muscle only. This muscle is part of the infundibular septum which separates the left and right outflow tracts.

The aortic valve

The aortic valve consists of both the aortic sinuses and the leaflets as well as the annulus fibrosus (the valve "ring"). The dimension of the annulus determines the size of the valve which in normal adults ranges from 20—30 mm in diameter, the average being 25 mm. In surgical anatomy valve leaflets and their corresponding sinuses are usually designated "left", "right" and "noncoronary": the last is more accurately identified as the posterior sinus and leaflet, while the former are the anterolateral and anteromedial sinuses and leaflets respectively. The three semilunar

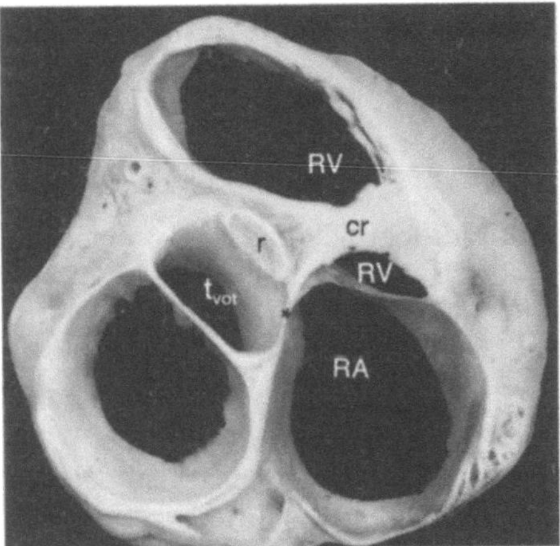

Fig. 1. Transverse section of the outflow tracts of the heart. The membranous septum (*) relates the left ventricular outflow tract (t_{vot}) to both the right atrium (RA) and right ventricle (RV). The right aortic sinus and right leaflet of the aortic valve (r) originate in muscle, they lie a little lower than the other two components of the aortic valve (cr) = crista supraventricularis.

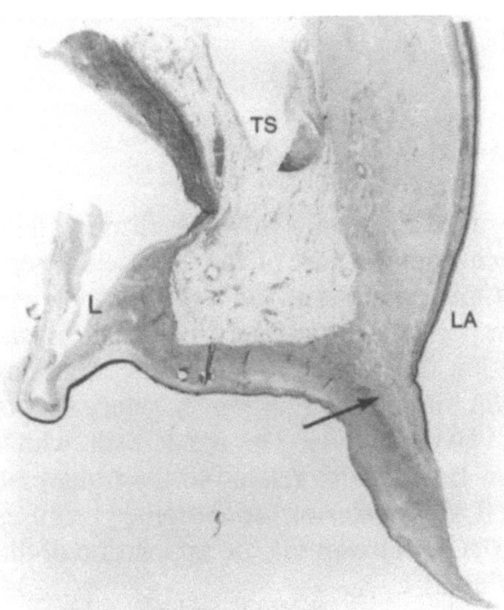

Fig. 2. Histological section through the left aortic sinus and leaflet. The left (L) and posterior (noncoronary) aortic sinuses are related to the left atrium (LA) and to the transverse sinus of the pericardium (TS). The area of aorto-mitral fibrous continuity (arrow) affords additional potential access to the left atrium. Reproduced from ref. (1) with permission.

leaflets of the valve face upwards and each has a small fibrous bleb (the corpus or nodulus Arantii), at the centre of the free edge. Very often there are also fenestrations close to the commissures of the valve, and in babies small blood cysts may be present, although these are commoner on the atrioventricular valves than on the semilunar ones. Neither these nor the fenestrations are of any haemodynamic significance to their original owner, but the fenestrations may become so if such valves are selected as allografts. The noduli Arantii occasionally calcify in old age but as valves are seldom selected from individuals beyond the third, or at the most, the fourth decade of life, this is not likely to be problematical. Histologically the aortic valve is avascular in normal subjects (vascularity in the valve indicates a post inflammatory reaction). The valve consists of fibrous tissue covered with endothelial cells and supported by collagen and an elastic layer on its ventricular aspect. This elastic diminishes with age, contributing to the stiffness sometimes seen in the valves of old people. The aortic sinuses have little elastic tissue, even in young people, as the dense elastic layer of the aorta ceases abruptly at the aortic bar (the beginning of the aortic sinus) (Fig. 2).

Aortic valve allografts

Chemically sterilised aortic valves may last in situ for 18 years or more (2), but deteriorate eventually as the valves become thin and wear into holes, irrespective of either the age of the donor valve or the storage period before implantation.

The outflow tract of the right ventricle

This is structurally much less elaborate than the left as it is entirely muscular. However, the musculature itself is relatively complex.

The outflow tract of the right ventricle consists of the infundibular septum, which separates the left and right channels, the trabecula septomarginalis which demarcates the inlet ond outlet zones of the ventricular septum, and the wedge of muscle between the aorta and the tricuspid valve called the ventriculo-infundibular fold. Together these structures form the crista supraventricularis (Fig. 1). The remaining contributer to the outflow tract is the free wall of the right ventricle which is also muscular.

Although rare in normal hearts, the right coronary artery occasionally passes anterior to the pulmonary valve, thus becoming a part of the outflow tract. This variant of coronary artery disposition occurs with some frequency in cyanotic congenital cardiac malformations, as does anomalous origin of the anterior interventricular (anterior descending) branch from the right coronary artery (3).

Even in the normal heart, the anterior descending branch of the left coronary artery passes close to the lateral margin of the right ventricular outflow tract (Fig. 3), and the first septal branch passes through the infundibular septum.

The pulmonary valve

The pulmonary valve, like the aortic, has a fibrous ring and this ring is attached to that of the aortic valve by a short, inconspicuous fibrous structure, the conus ligament. The pulmonary valve lies superior and a little to the left of the aortic valve so that its most posterior sinus is closest to the right aortic sinus. The sinuses of the pulmonary valve are shallower than those of the aortic valve and do not give origin to coronary arteries.

The pulmonary valve is slightly greater in diameter than the aortic valve, ranging in size from 23—25 mm diameter. The histological structure of the leaflets is the

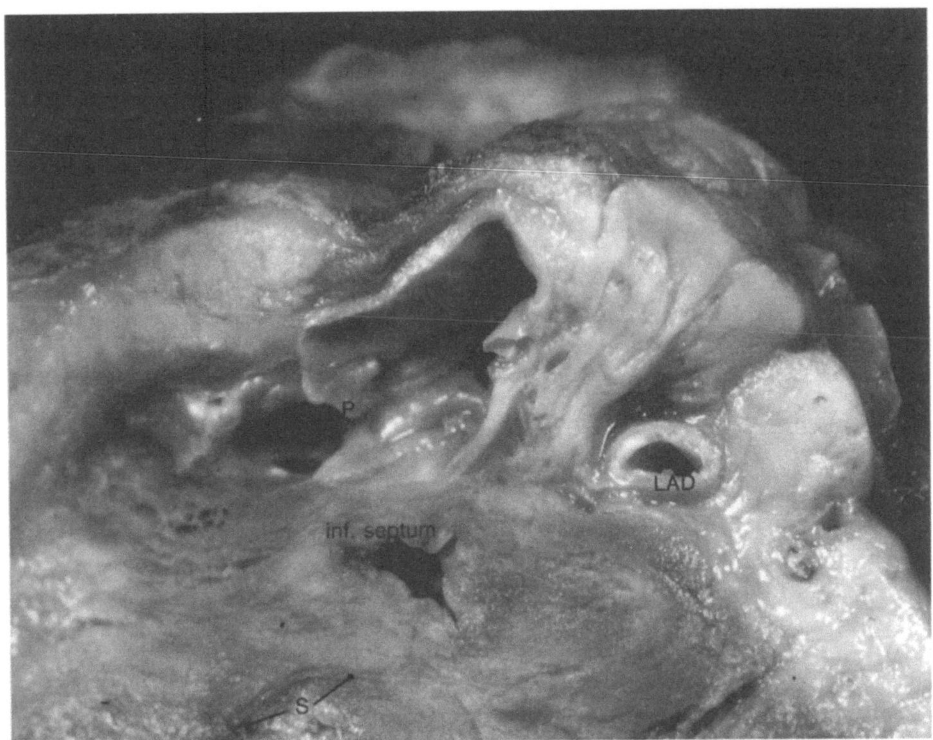

Fig. 3. Transverse section through the right ventricular outflow tract immediately subjacent to the pulmonary valve (P) which originates exclusively from muscle. The anterior descending branch of the left coronary artery (LAD) passes close to the valve. A septal branch (S) passes through the infundibular septum (the infundibular septum is necrotic in this specimen and there is an abcess cavity).

same as that of the aortic valve except that the adventitia of the pulmonary artery is confluent with the epicardium of the right ventricle which is considerably thickened at that point.

Allografts in the pulmonary outflow tract

In a small series of aortic valve grafts implanted in the pulmonary outflow tract (2) the grafts have lasted well: none has required revision up to 20 years later and infective endocarditis has not occurred. There have been no late deaths in this group of patients.

References

1. Allwork SP (1986) The Anatomical Basis of Infection of the Aortic Root. Thorac Cardiovasc Surg 34: 143—148

2. Allwork SP, Pucci JJ, Cleland WP, and Bentall HH (1986) The Longevity of Sterilized Aortic
   Valve Homografts 1967—1972. J Cardiovasc Surg 27: 213—216

Author's address:
Sally P. Allwork
Department of Surgery
Royal Postgraduate Medical School
Hammersmith Hospital
Ducane Road
London W12 OHS
U.K.

Selection of allograft valve size

A. C. Yankah, R. Hetzer

German Heart Center Berlin, Berlin (West), Germany

Introduction

We have perceived the need for a preoperative knowledge of aortic annulus size in individual patients, which will allow proper selection of cryopreserved valve size before cardiopulmonary bypass. The technique of determining valve size from a supravalvular aortic cineangiogram is described.

Materials and Methods

35 patients between 22 and 56 years of age who were undergoing aortic valve replacements were entered in the study. Supravalvular aortic cineangiogram films, taken in the 30° right anterior oblique projection, were used to measure the aortic

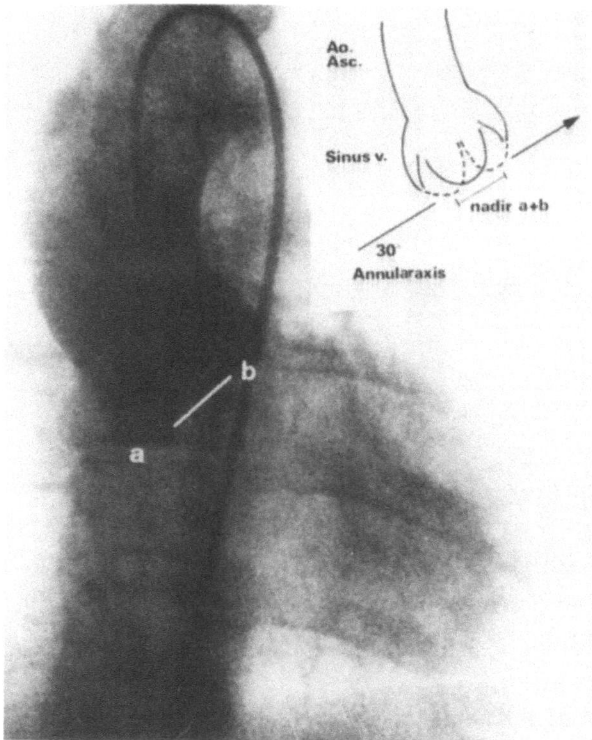

Fig. 1. Supravalvular aortic angiogram in 30° right anterior oblique projection. Nadir a + b = aortic annulus.

annulus. Films with traceable outline of the aortic root and cusps and with projected metal sphere were selected for the study. The true diameter of the metal sphere (TMS ∅) was filmed at each projection to obtain angiographic values of the metal sphere (angiographic metal sphere diameter — AMS ∅) which was used for correction for magnification when converting the angiographic measured external aortic annulus (AEAA ∅) to a true external aortic annulus diameter (TEAA ∅). The measurement of the AEAA was made by joining a transverse line between the two nadirs of the valve cusp (Fig. 1). This method was found on empiric grounds to yield a good in vivo correlation.

Variations of 1—2 mm were found in some patients, especially in those with calcified aortic stenosis; however, the distance between the two nadirs proved to be most reliable and consistent. From the supraaortic cineangiogram, the AEAA ∅ in diastole was measured and the TEAA ∅ was calculated from the following formula:

$$TEAA = \frac{TMS\ \varnothing \times AEAA}{AMS\ \varnothing}$$

The true internal aortic annulus diameter (TIAA ∅) was obtained by subtracting 2 mm from the TEAA.

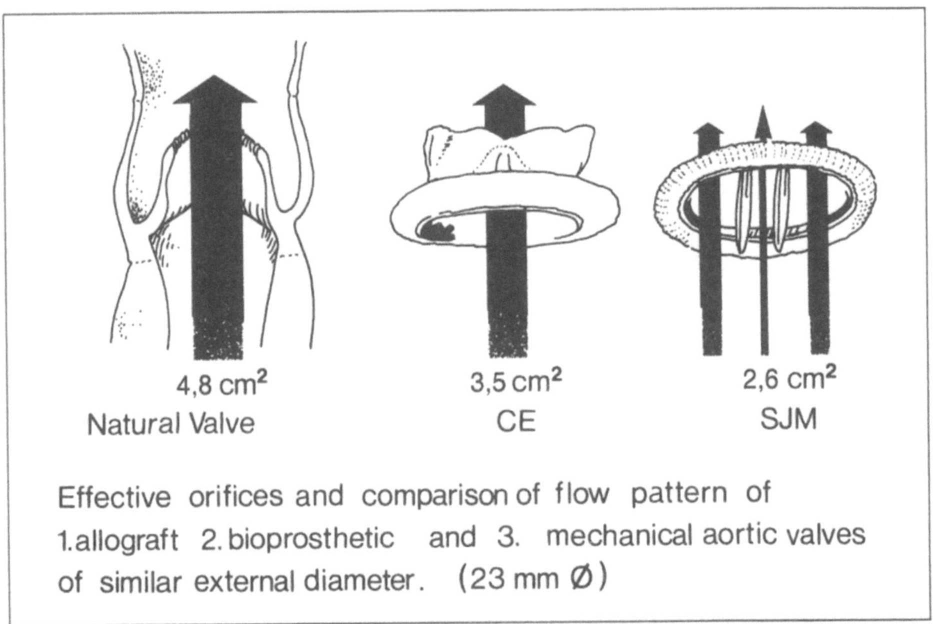

Fig. 2. Effective orifices and comparison of flow pattern of (1) allograft, (2) bioprosthetic and (3) mechanical aortic valves of similar external diameter (23 mm).

Step by step implantation technique of aortic allograft in subcoronary position

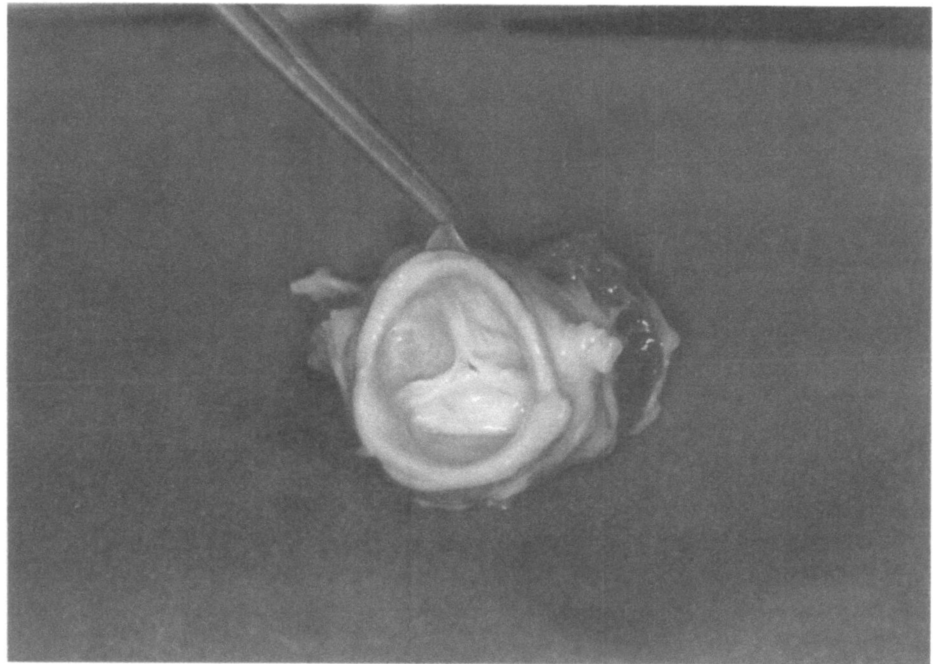

Fig. 3a. Fresh aortic allograft.

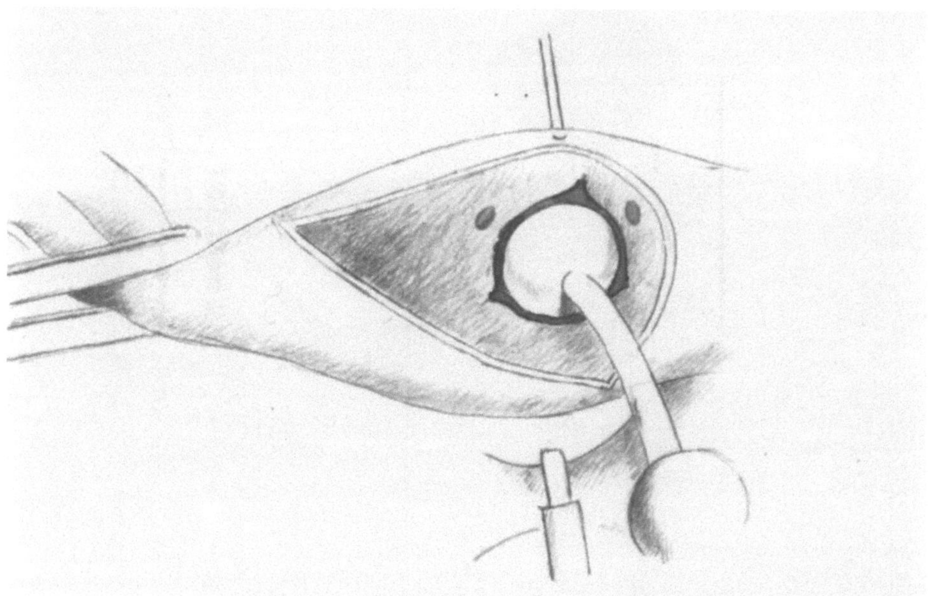

Fig. 3b. Intraoperative invasive measurement of aortic annulus (internal diameter) in an unbeating heart, to compare the preoperative non-invasive measured annulus size.

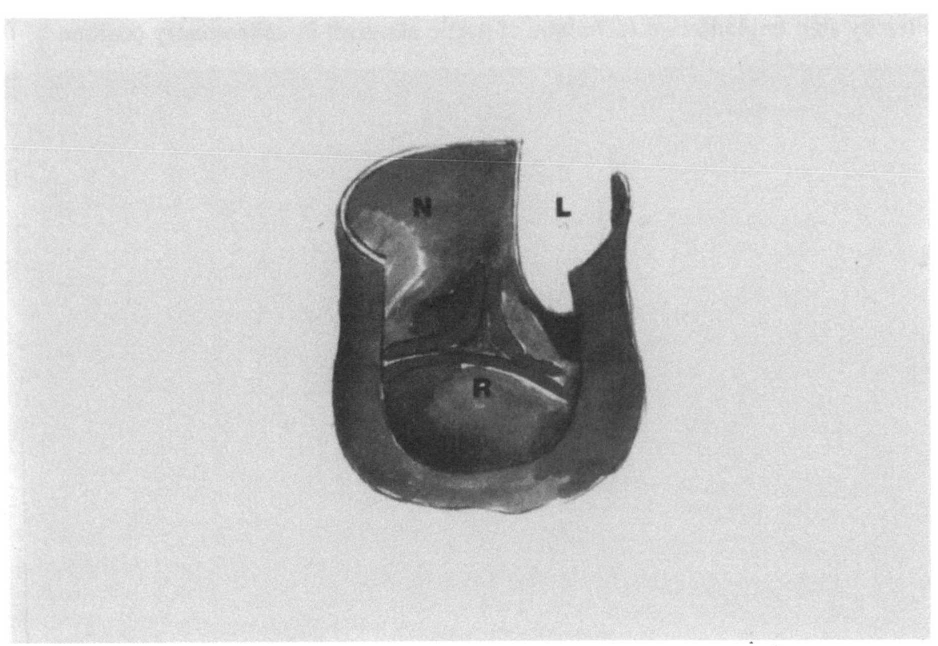

Fig. 4. Trimmed aortic allograft. Scalloped left and right sinus valsalvae, leaving 5—7 mm wall behind for attachment to patient's sinus wall below the coronary ostia.

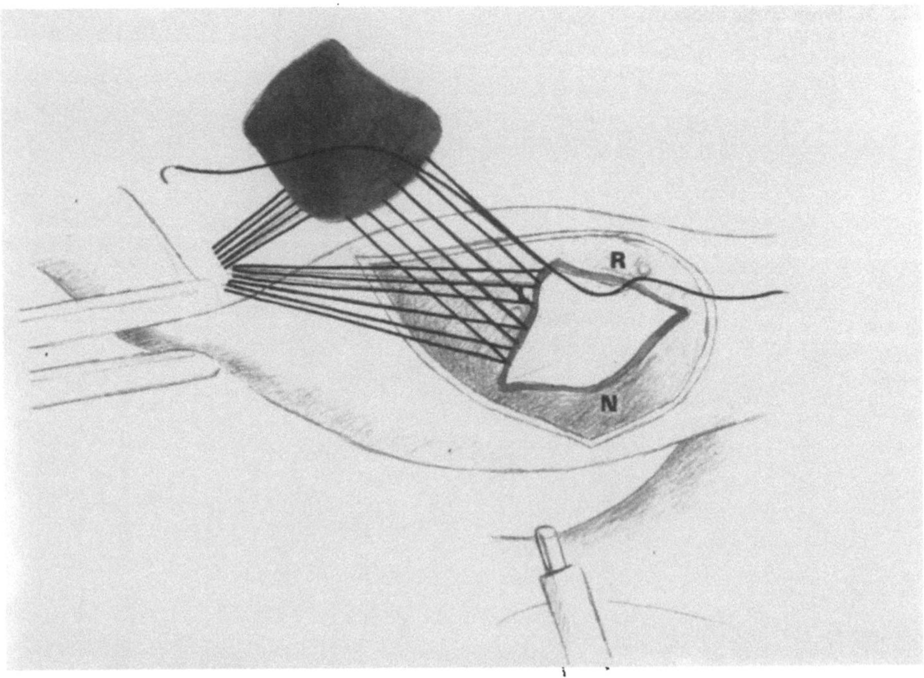

Fig. 5. Multiple interrupted 4—0 prolene sutures are passed through the lower margin of the cusps beginning at the mid point of the left coronary sinus, keeping the allograft at a distance.

116

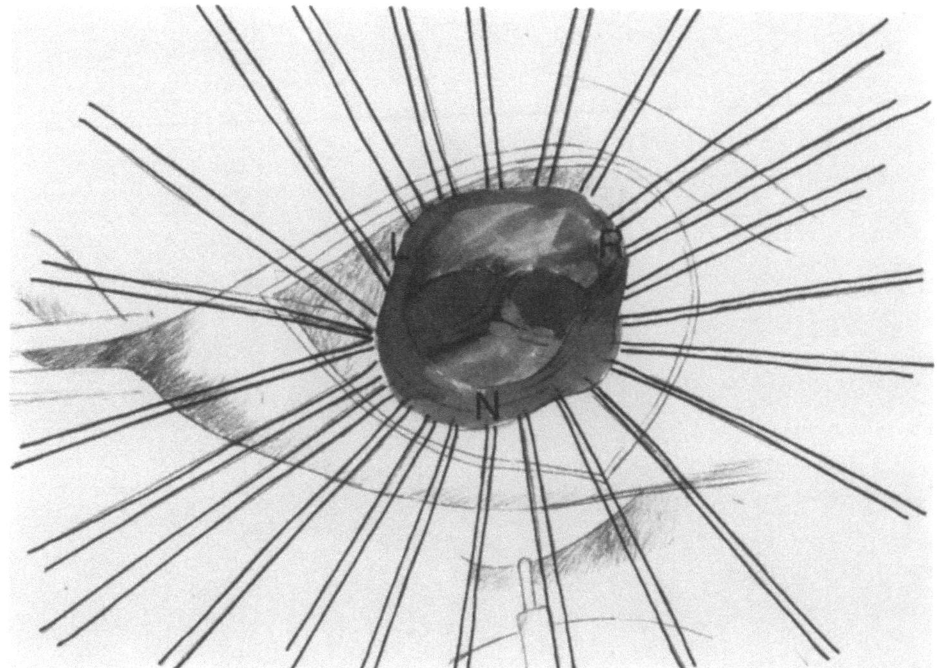

Fig. 6a.

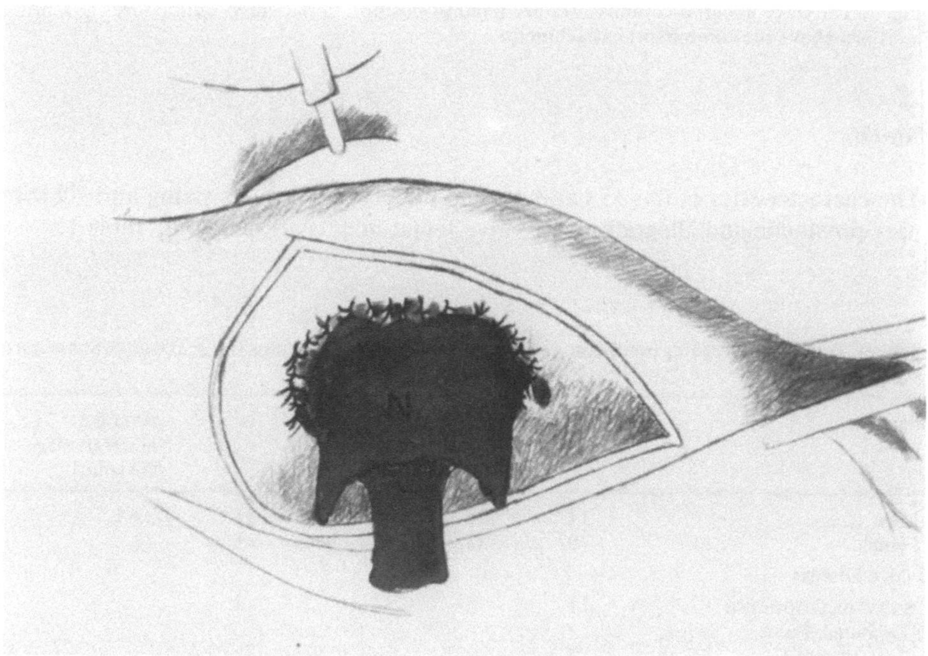

Fig. 6a + 6b. After all the sutures have been placed, the allograft is lowered into the subcoronary position and tied down.

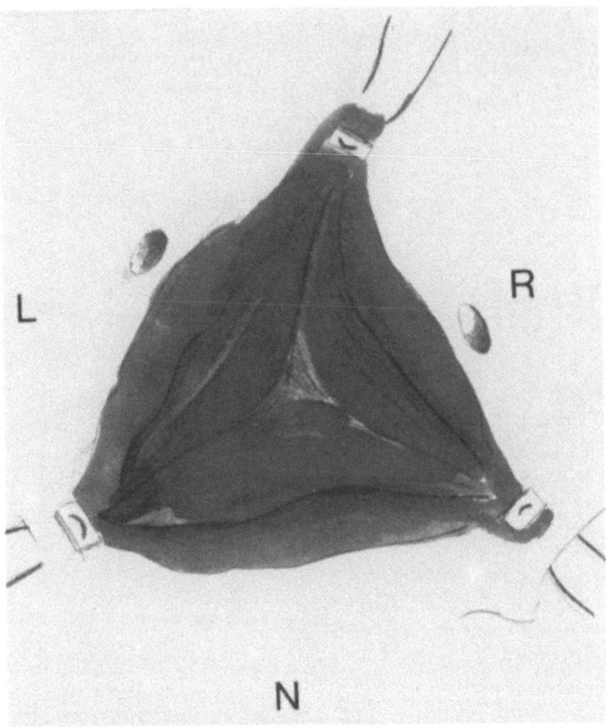

Fig. 7. The three allograft commissures are fixed in position to patient's commissures at a proper level just above the commissural attachments.

Results

The characteristics of the 35 patients who underwent annulus sizing and subcoronary prosthetic and allograft aortic valve replacements are shown in Table 1.

Table 1. Patients undergoing preoperative measurement of aortic annulus size and subcoronary aortic valve replacements.

Sex	N	Average prosthesis size OD (mm)	N	Average allograft size ID (mm)
Male	14	26,5	11	23.4
Female	9	23,2	1	22
Valve Disease				
Aortic incompetence	11		4	
Combined lesion	7		5	
Aortic stenosis	5		3	

OD = Outer diameter, ID = internal diameter, N = number of patients.

118

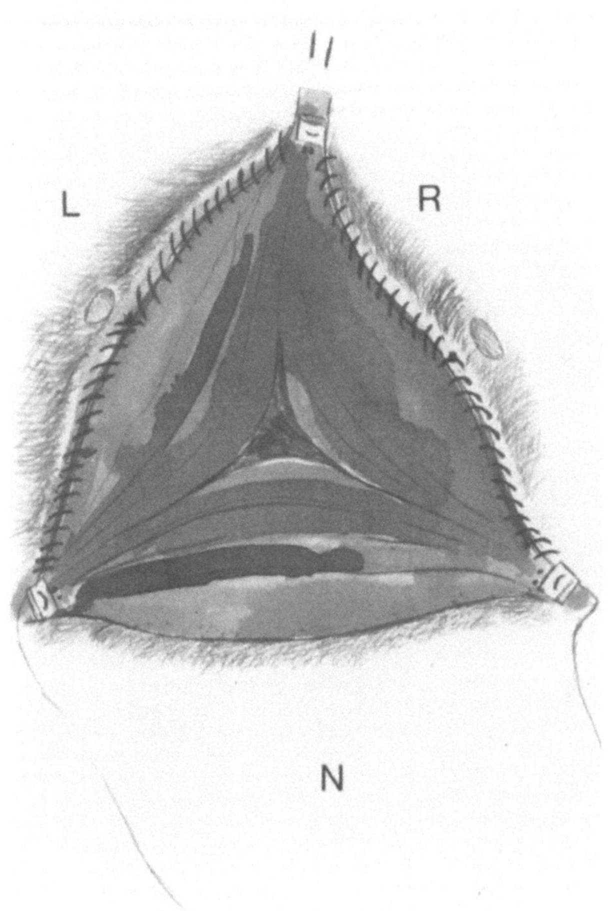

The type of valve was decided on the basis of annulus size, patient age and lifestyle, possible contra-indications to anticoagulants and surgeon preference. Valves were significantly smaller in women than in men. Patients with pure aortic incompetence or combined lesions had larger valves but the difference was not significant.

The comparison of preoperatively measured valve annulus size to angiographically measured size is shown in Fig. 10.

In 21 of 35 (60%) patients, the measured preoperative and intraoperative annulus size correlated exactly. In 14 of 35 (40%) they were within ± 1.0—2.0 mm of each other. All the allografts selected on the basis of the angiographic measurement fitted well in the subcoronary position after trimming redundant fatty and myocardial tissues. Initial studies on this work made in Kiel University have shown similar results (5).

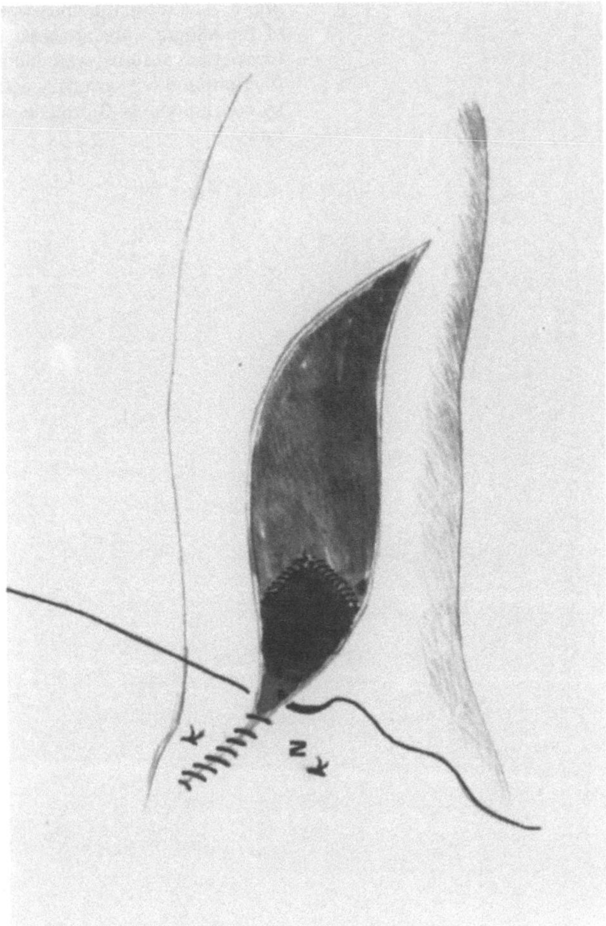

Fig. 9a. Closure of the aortomy is accomplished by incorporating the non-coronary sinus of the allograft to reinforce the suture line and obliterate the space between the allograft and patient's sinus wall with single interrupted sutures.

Discussion

Currently, the cardiac surgeon has a valid choice of armamentarium of valves for a given patient. The experience at our own institution indicates that 22% of the aortic valve recipients had a valve prosthesis of 23 mm in diameter. This is the range in which significant gradients can occur at normal flow rates across the valve (Table 2, Fig. 2). The relation between valve orifice area and body habitus have not been clearly defined for patients with heart disease (4). Without a reliable guide to the optimal prosthetic orifice area for a given patient there is a tendency that a relative prosthesis-patient mismatch (2) may result in suboptimal haemodynamics on exercise after an otherwise satisfactory valve replacement.

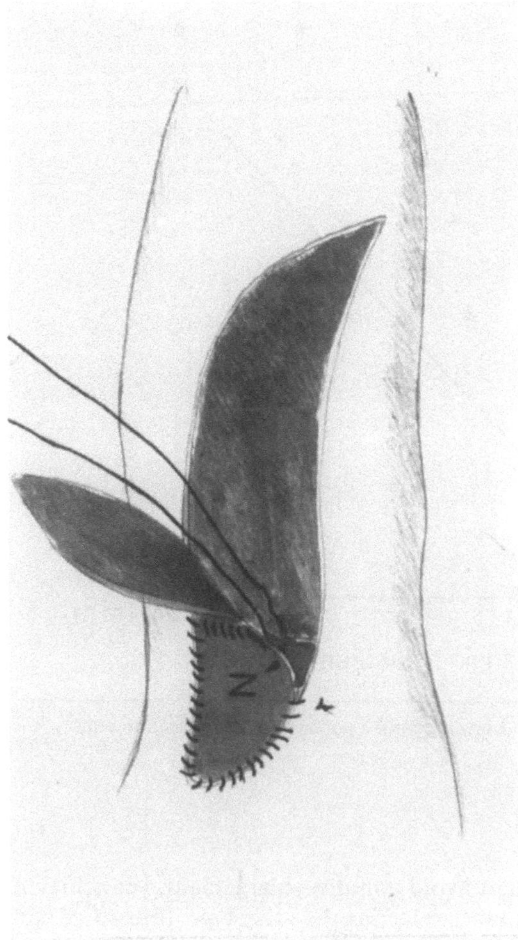

Fig. 9b. If the aortic root is small and the direct closure of the aortotomy with the non-coronary sinus might retract the valve cusp, enlargement of the patient's non-coronary sinus by autologous pericardium is made to allow proper and secured fixation and sometimes repositioning of the right commissural attachment is necessary.

Table 2. Relation between mean native valve area and prosthetic valve area for annulus of equivalent diameter.

	Mean native valve diameter (mm)	Area (cm²)	Manufacturer's calculated area (cm²) of 23 mm prosthesis		
			CE	IS	SJM
Aortic	23	4.8	3.5	2.96	2.55

CE = Carpentier-Edwarts, IS = Ionescu-Shiley, SJM = St. Jude Medical prostheses.

The ability to predict prosthesis size would allow the surgeon to plan for subcoronary allograft valve replacement, aortic root replacement or an annulus-enlarging procecure (3) and discuss the surgical techniques with the patient preoperatively. In

121

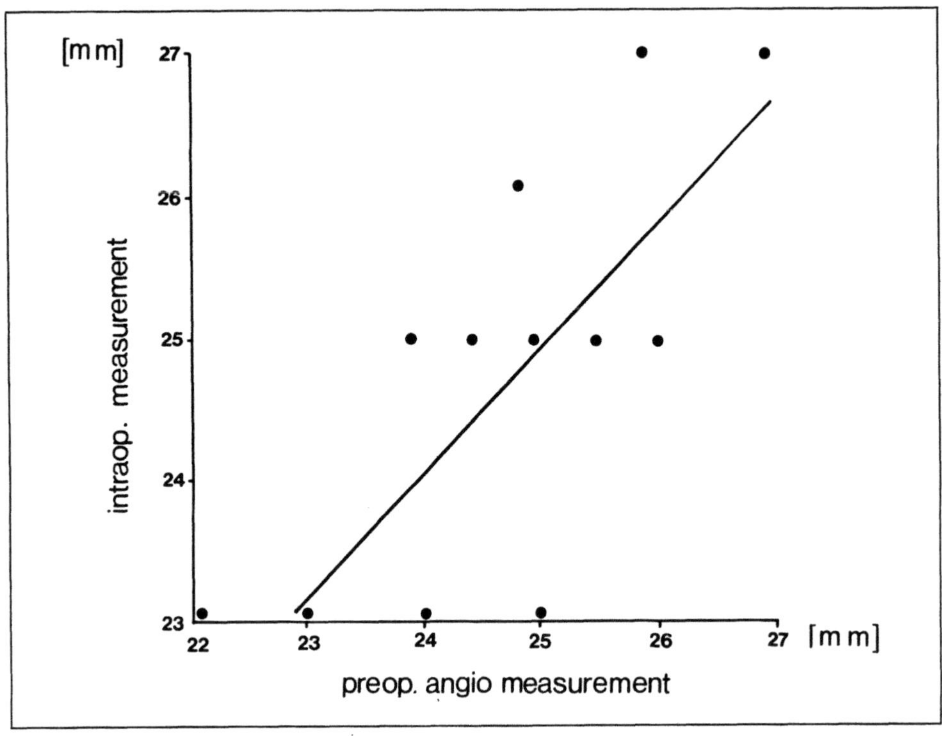

Fig. 10. Correlation between preoperative and intraoperative aortic annulus measurement.

most cases, the use of an allograft might avoid annulus-enlargement, yet achieving maximum acceptable unobstructive flow. In selecting the valve type, the orifice area, as well as the durability and necessity for long-term anticoagulation, should be considered.

There were two drawbacks in the technique which caused imperfection in the measurement, namely the presence of heavy calcified valve and the variation of the intrathoracic aortic root position from patient to patient (1). However, the inherent errors did not exceed 1—2 mm and were acceptable for allografts. This technique has been shown to be useful in selecting appropriate cryopreserved allograft valve size, and in planning surgery for patients with small aortic root, despite methodological limitations. The technique might not simplify the surgical technique, but could help in achieving satisfactory surgical results.

Acknowledgement

We are grateful to Mrs. Lee for her technical assistance in the preparation of the manuscript.

122

References

1. Babb JD, Parr GVS, O'Neill J (1981) Predicting aortic valve prosthesis size. J Thorac Cardiovasc Surg 81: 450—454
2. Rahimtoola SH (1978) The problem of valve prosthesis-patient mismatch. Circulation 58: 20—24
3. Sud A, Parker F, Magilligan DJ, Jr (1984) Anatomy of the aortic root. Ann Thorac Surg 38: 76—79
4. Westaby S, Karp Rb, Blackstone EH, et al (1984) Adult human valve dimensions and their surgical significance. Am J Cardiol 53: 552—556
5. Yankah AC, Wottge HU, Müller-Hermelink HK, et al (1987) Transplantation of aortic and pulmonary allografts, enhanced viability of endothelial cells by cryopreservation, importance of histocompatibility. J Cardiac Surg I, No 3, Suppl: 209—220

Authors' address:
A. C. Yankah, M.D.
German Heart Center
Augustenburger Platz 1
1000 Berlin (West) 65
Germany

"Fresh" free-hand, non-viable allografts for aortic valve replacement: Operative techniques and 15-year results

C. E. Moreno-Cabral, D. C. Miller, and N. E. Shumway

Department of Cardiovascular Surgery, Stanford University School of Medicine, U.S.A.

Introduction

The first unstented allograft valve inserted orthotopically for replacement of the aortic valve (AVR) was performed by Duran and Gunning working with Mr. Donald Ross in London; these pioneering attempts were reported by Ross in 1962 (11) and by Barratt-Boyes in 1964 (1). These investigators, and others, have continued using this method for AVR in selected patients for nearly three decades, and have recently updated their long-term results (2, 7, 8, 9, 10, 12). At Stanford, our initial experience with free-hand allograft AVR was accumulated between 1964 and 1971. A hiatus of 11 years followed; renewed interest in the use of allografts for AVR in children and adolescents started in 1982 at Stanford, due to dissatisfaction with the $5\frac{1}{n}$ 10-year durability of porcine xenograft valves in young patients, reports of reasonable long-term durability using both antibiotic stored (non-viable) and cryopreserved ("viable") valves (7, 8), and the demonstration of cell viability in cryopreserved allograft valves (4) (although this latter hypothesis continues at the present time, in our opinion, to be unproved in terms of clinical significance). We have subsequently expanded the use of "fresh" (4 °C antibiotic storage for $\leq 24\frac{1}{n}$ 48 h) allograft valves obtained locally from organ donors whose hearts cannot be used for transplantation and commercially marketed cryopreserved allografts (CryoLife, Inc.) for AVR in carefully selected patients in a cautious manner.

A report from Stanford in 1975 (13) stating that the durability of allograft valves was not satisfactory had included all patients receiving allograft valves, and had not discriminated between the various subgroups of allografts (mitral vs. aortic position, stented vs. unstented, "fresh" vs. preserved in many different ways); consequently, our negative conclusions at that time based on 5—10 years of observation may have been somewhat misleading. From that original experience, a subgroup of 83 patients who received free-hand (unstented), "fresh" (antibiotically stored at 4 °C between 1 and 24 days) allograft valves implanted in the aortic position has been studied to 15—18 years postoperatively. These valves were mostly non-viable due to the duration of storage. The subsequent widespread availability of satisfactory mechanical and xenograft bioprosthetic valves, in addition to the logistic difficulties inherent in procurement of "fresh" allograft valves and the unclear advantages of the allograft valve, considering its more demanding implantation technique, resulted in a decline in enthusiasm for its use for AVR in the 1970s at Stanford and elsewhere.

A large number of different operative techniques are in use today for freehand allograft AVR (5, 6, 7, 12), and there is probably no substantial difference in outcome according to the particular operative techniques employed. Nevertheless, we believe allograft AVR is a procedure associated with little or no margin for technical error and is more technically demanding than conventional AVR methods using mechanical prostheses or bioprostheses. In this assay, our surgical technique will be detailed, and the long-term results of allograft AVR at Stanford will be described and compared.

Clinical materials

Between 1964 and 1971, 83 patients received "fresh", free-hand allograft valves at Stanford University Medical Center. The term "fresh" is placed in quotation marks since our present definition is far more stringent than it was at that time; currently, an allograft valve is described as *fresh* only if it is implanted within 24 h or procurement. Our older experience included antibiotic-treated allografts that were stored at 4 °C for up to 24 days; today, we feel that those grafts were mostly nonviable. No cryopreserved valves were inserted during that period. Follow-up was performed in August 1986 and was 96% complete; the total cumulative follow-up interval was 773 patient-years. The median and the average follow-up times were approximately 9 years. Importantly, 37 patients were still alive with their original allograft valve after 10 years, and 12 patients after 17 years.

Surgical technique
Allograft valve procurement and preparation

An assiduous effort is made to match the recipient with the allograft donor ABO blood group in all cases. The patient's aortic annular size is measured directly from the left ventriculogram (with due regard to magnification factors) or the sino-tubular ridge diameter and annulus from a two-dimensional echocardiogram. Locally-obtained allograft valves are not rigorously sized, but donor and recipient body weights should be similar. For cryopreserved valves, an allograft that is 3—5 mm smaller than the recipient's aortic annulus or sino-tubular ridge diameter is selected, since the commercially-prepared valves are sized according to internal diameter. To date, we have used only allograft aortic valves for AVR, but allograft pulmonary valves can be used based on theoretical considerations (3) (less calcification and primary tissue failure) and the limited supply of aortic allograft valves, which are used widely as conduits in children with congenital heart disease. When the allograft is procured by our team for use as a fresh graft, the donor valve is excised in the operating room using sterile technique in a manner identical to that used for procurement of a donor heart for transplantation. The antibiotic concentrations recommended by Kirklin and Barratt-Boyes (3, 5) are used. The allograft valve is stored at 4 °C in tissue culture solution and implanted within 24 h. Otherwise, suitable allograft aortic and pulmonary valves (including those obtained from cardiac transplant recipients) are forwarded to a commercial laboratory for cryopreservation. When a commercially-prepared cryopreserved allograft is used, the graft is ABO matched and thawed according to the processor's instructions.

126

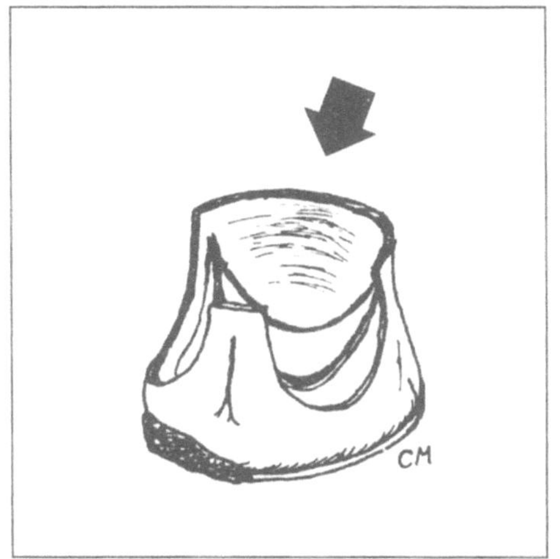

Fig. 1. Allograft aortic valve prepared and ready for implantation. The non-coronary sinus of Valsalva is not trimmed (arrow), which simplifies the procedure and can facilitate closure of the ascending aorta.

The allograft aortic valve is trimmed by sharply excising excess left ventricular free wall and septal muscle and the anterior mitral valve leaflet, carefully preserving the valve annulus. The muscle has little tensile strength and autolyzes after implantation, but it is not removed totally to avoid damaging the aortic leaflets and annulus. Superiorly, the right and left sinuses of Valsalva are excised in a scalloped manner following the curve of leaflet insertion leaving a 2—4 mm rim of aorta. Additional aortic wall can be excised from the bases of the sinuses later, if necessary, to avoid compromise of the recipient's coronary ostia. Following Ross's lead (12), the non-coronary sinus of Valsalva is usually not excised, such that the aorta is transected transversely 5 mm superior to the sino-tubular ridge, as shown in Fig. 1; this simplifies the procedure, expedites the subsequent cephalad anchoring of these two commissures, and can facilitate closure of the aortotomy (e.g. functioning as an aortic gusset) to avoid distortion of the valve in certain cases (6, 12).

Valve implantation technique

A longitudinal aortotomy is made and extended inferiorly to within 1 cm of the right coronary artery ostium. The aortic incision must be planned carefully such that it avoids the areas where the allograft valve commissures will be sutured. After the diseased valve is removed, the annulus is debrided and then ringed with 15—18 horizontal mattress sutures of 4—0 braided polyester (Ethibond or Tevdek) on a small needle (RB-2 or AT-1, respectively) (Fig. 2). The width of these mattress sutures is only 3—4 mm to avoid gathering or bunching of the proximal edge of the allograft. These sutures are placed from the ventricle upwards to the aortic aspect of the annulus *in a single spatial plane*, which is frequently actually located immediately *below* the native annulus. It is helpful to visualize this plane as being parallel with the plane of the sino-tubular ridge and of identical diameter, both of which will minimize the chances of distorting the valve. Importantly, this proximal suture

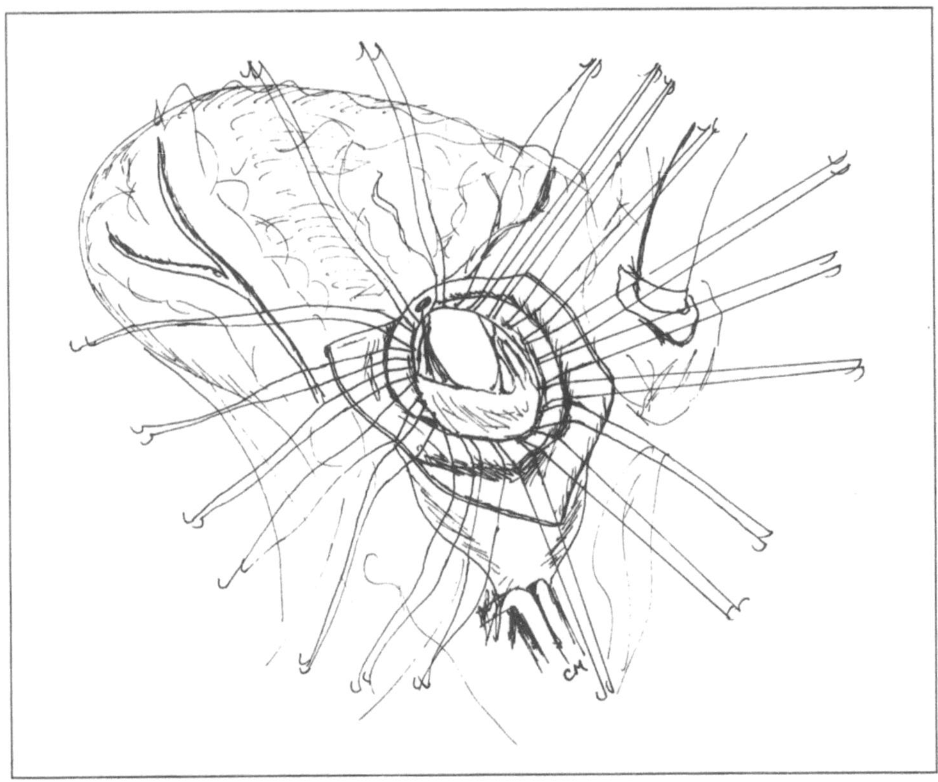

Fig. 2. The proximal suture line (aortic annulus) starts with the placement of 15—18 interrupted horizontal mattress sutures passed from the ventricular to the aortic aspect. These sutures are individually tagged to enhance exposure of both the patient's annulus and the allograft annulus during the next step.

line should not curve upwards to any great degree in order to conform to a highly scalloped annulus; it also should be placed far enough below the coronary ostia (particularly if they are located close to the annulus) to ensure that coronary compromise does not occur when the allograft valve is lowered into place. This interrupted suture method makes exact placement of the proximal suture line easier and enhances subsequent exposure, as illustrated in Fig. 2. We have found it preferable to a continuous proximal suture line technique.

The allograft valve is inverted on itself by pushing the commissural "posts" toward the central opening; the leaflets are now on the outside, and should be carefully protected. With this manoeuvre, the junction between the allograft leaflets and thin annulus can be seen clearly (Fig. 3). The inverted valve is stabilize by inserting the first assistant's index finger or a Hegar dilator through the allograft valve, which aids precise suture placement. The valve is then oriented properly; the sinuses of Valsalva (and respective leaflets) are usually kept in their normal anatomical relationship, i.e. allograft left coronary sinus corresponds to the patient's left coronary sinus, in contrast to other techniques which rotate the allograft 120 ° clockwise (5).

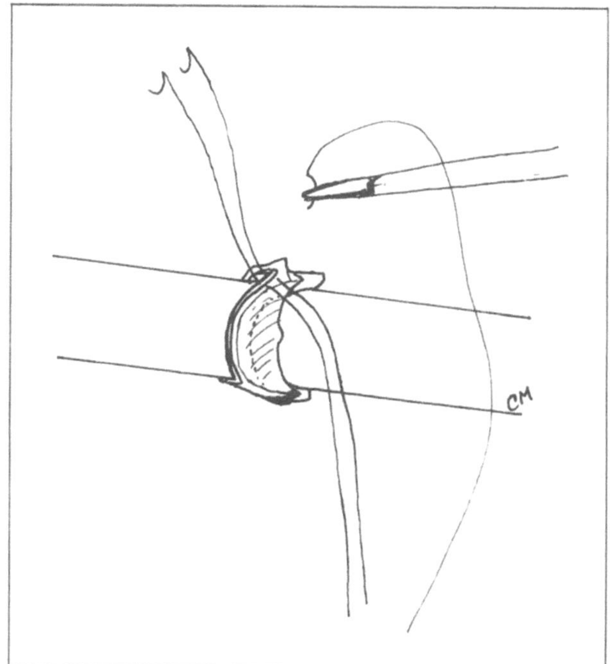

Fig. 3. Second part of the proximal suture line. The inverted allograft valve is supported on a Hegar dilator, which exposes the thin annulus. One of the leaflets can be seen on the "outside". The proximal horizontal mattress sutures are passed through the allograft annulus form "outside"-to-"inside".

The proximal valve sutures are then passed through the allograft from "outside-to-inside" (but the sutures have actually passed from the inside to the outside of the allograft, such that the knots can be tied and buried on the distal aspect). The needle entry point is just "above" the line of leaflet insertion (as the allograft annulus can be very thin); deep, but relatively small, bites are important (Fig. 3). Attention is necessary during this step to be certain that the needle incorporates the allograft annulus and/or external aspect of the allograft aorta, and not just excessive allograft muscle tissue. After all the sutures have been passed through the allograft annulus, the still-inverted valve is lowered into the left ventricle (Fig. 4), and the sutures are carefully tied and cut (Fig. 5).

The valve is then everted by pulling up on the "posts" subtending the allograft commissures. The proximal suture line is then completely hidden between the allograft annulus and the patient's aorta (Figs. 6 and 7). The commissural "posts" of the allograft are then suspended at the appropriate level and location by starting three pledgeted, double armed 4—0 polypropylene RB-1 (Prolene) horizontal mattress sutures. These three sutures are passed through the tops of the allograft commissural "posts" and a small oval pledget (Fig. 6). Positioning of the top of the commissures and valve competence is then assessed using saline irrigation; visual inspection of the allograft valve (with the edges of the aortotomy temporarily apposed) is also helpful to guarantee that the valve is not distorted and that the level and location of the commissural support sutures are correct. This is a critically important detail; insufficient tension supporting the commissures will result in valvular regurgitation due to leaflet prolapse. Occasionally, it may be necessary to re-

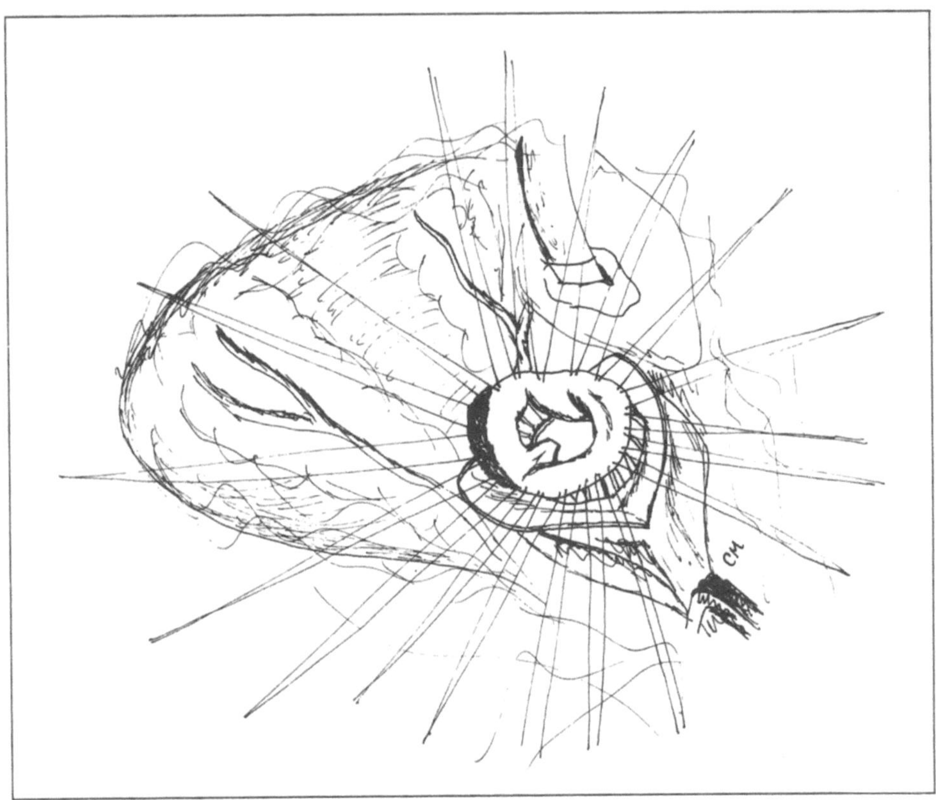

Fig. 4. The valve (still inverted) is lowered into the left ventricle.

position one or more of the commissural "post" stitches or to widden the aortic root with a gusset (separate patch of allograft aorta or incorporating the intact non-coronary sinus of Valsalva of the allograft) in order to achieve normal valvular architecture. Once adequate commissural placement is confirmed, the "post" sutures are tied and then used in a continuous fashion to approximate the distal edge of the allograft to the aortic wall, as shown in Fig. 7. Small 2—3 mm bites (carefully avoiding the valve leaflets) are taken in the allograft. This completes the distal suture line (Fig. 7). Valvular competence is tested again, and the aortotomy is closed with a running 4—0 polypropylene suture. Neither warfarin anticoagulation nor antiplatelet agents are routinely prescribed postoperatively.

Results

Among the 83 patients included in this study, two-thirds had aortic stenosis; regurgitation was present in 31 patients. Hospital mortality rate was 6%. To allow a broader perspective, we will review the late results of "fresh" unstented allograft aortic valve replacement from five different reports (2, 6, 8, 10, 12). These series

130

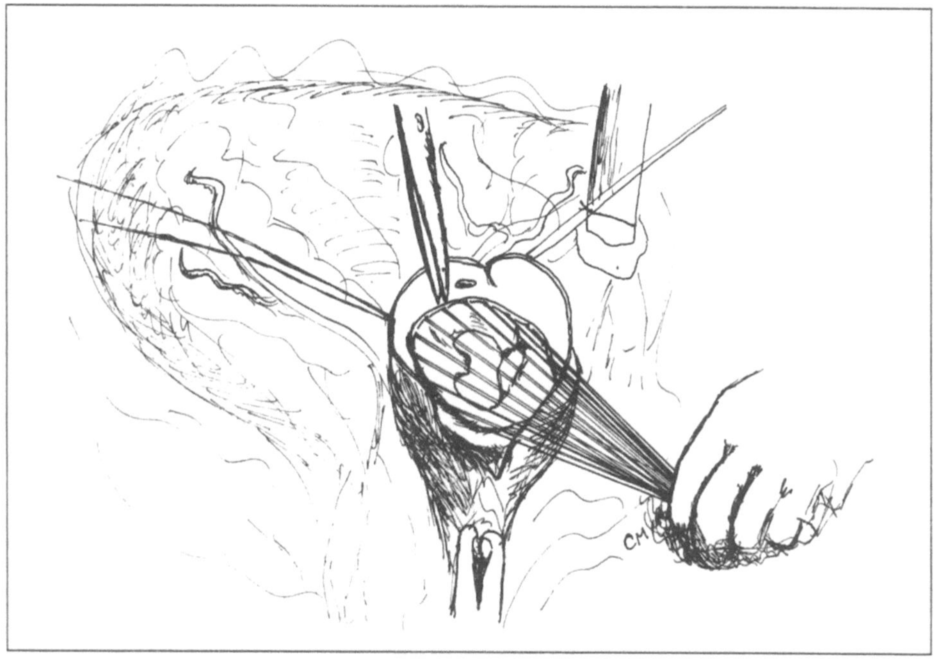

Fig. 5. The interrupted horizontal mattress sutures are tied and cut while the allograft valve is still inverted and inside the left ventricle, which completes the proximal suture line.

should not be considered strictly comparable, mainly due to lack of standardisation in the methods of valve preservation and differences in patient characteristics. (The technical aspects of valve implantation probably do not substantially alter the late results, and differences in techniques will not be discussed further.) Table 1 summarizes the long-term results from these different institutions. Not all authors report the same morbid events, but all such events are included when available. It is unfortunate that more information is not available in our series from Stanford to identify more clearly the factors and might portend valve failure, for instance ABO typing or length of time of valve storage before use. Multivariate analysis of Yacoub's results (9, 10) identified advancing age and development of left bundle branch block to affect adversely long-term survival; older age, female gender, haemodynamic valvular lesion (stenosis), and time interval between death and graft procurement were predictors of valve failure. Barratt-Boyes et al. (2) noted donor valve age (> 55 years), recipient age (< 15 years), and large aortic diameter (> 30 mm) as independent factors which significantly increased the probability of valve failure using multivariate statistical methods.

Morbidity

Eight thromboembolic events occurred in our series (1.0%/patient-year [%/pt-yr]). Although it is unlikely that these emboli originated from the aortic allograft valve,

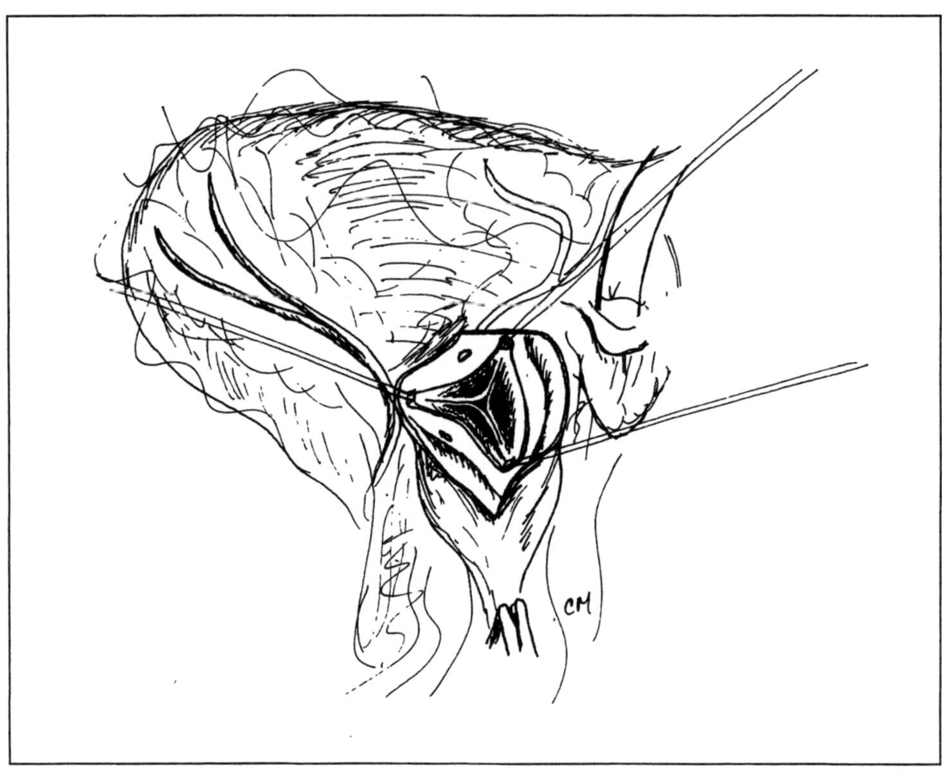

Fig. 6. The allograft valve is then everted, which causes the proximal suture line (and knots) to be totally hidden between the allograft and the patient's annulus. The three commissural posts are suspended and anchored to the ascending aorta with pledgeted sutures.

the source of emboli is not known with certainty. Barratt-Boyes (2) and Yacoub (9) have reported no episodes of thromboembolism. O'Brien (7) noted that 90 ± 3% of patients were free of thromboembolism at 10 years. There was one bleeding episode in our experience (0.18%/pt-yr); however, it is unclear why this patient was on anticoagulation. None of the other studies reported an analysis of bleeding complications, probably because almost all patients were not given anticoagulants.

The linearized rate of prosthetic valve endocarditis in our patients was 0.5%/pt-yr; actuarial rates of freedom from this event were 96% and 92% at 5 and 14 years, respectively, in Barratt-Boyes' experience; 94% at 10 years in O'Brien series, and 93% and 88% after 5 and 10 years, respectively, in Yacoub's experience. Thus, the incidence of prosthetic valve endocarditis is low (and remarkably similar) in all of these reports. Four of our patients, however, died of endocarditis. This was somewhat disconcerting, because we were hopeful that the use of allograft valves would reduce or maybe even eliminate late infectious valve complications. Although no controlled studies are available, there is a some evidence that endocarditis occurring in a patient with a free-hand allograft valve may be controlled by antibiotic treatment alone (2).

132

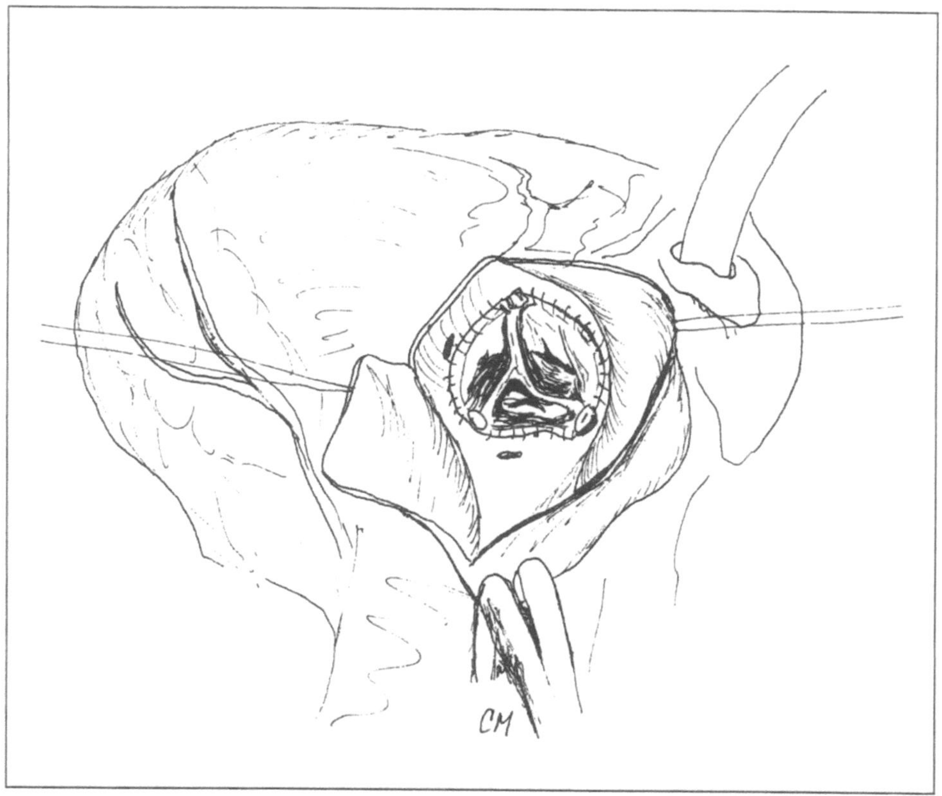

Fig. 7. The second continuous suture line is finished. Closing the aortotomy then completes implantation of the allograft valve.

Other valve-related complications were defined using our standard, conservative criteria. When these criteria were originally devised, the substrate being analyzed included patients with allograft valves. Even though we consider a new regurgitant murmur to be valve failure (unless proven to be a periprosthetic leak), we exclude patients who have a Grade 1 aortic regurgitation murmur if it is heard early post-operatively and is non-progressive over time. We do not believe this entity represents valve failure per se; it's more likely a technical failure, but probably does not portend less than average long-term functional durability.

In our experience, 73% of all allograft valve failures were due to fibrocalcific degeneration, similar to the fraction observed in all long-term allograft valve series. Degenerative valve failure occurred with increasing frequency over time. After 10 years, 70 ± 6% of patients were free of this complication; the actuarial estimate was 51 ± 7% at 15 years (Fig. 8). As seen in Table 1, freedom from valve failure ranged from between 55—78% at 10 years and 23—61% at 15 years in the different reports. Under the "best of circumstances", i.e. excluding patients found to be at high risk of valve failure by Barratt-Boyes (2) (donor age > 55 years, recipient age < 15 years, and/or aortic root diameter > 30 mm), the freedom from valve failure was 98% at 5 years, 94% at 9 years, and 56% at 13 years.

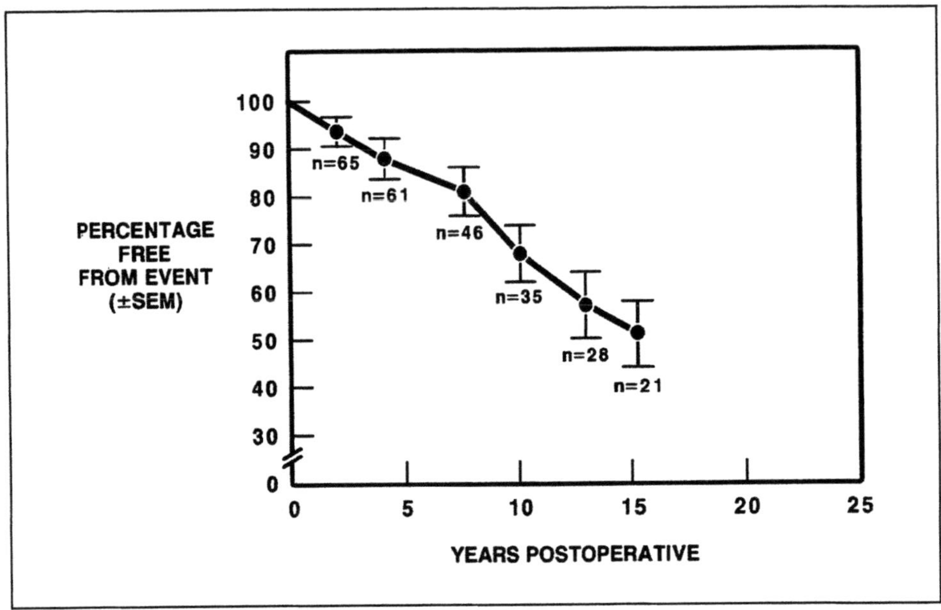

Fig. 8. Actuarial curve demonstrating freedom from degenerative valve failure. Error bars indicate ± 1 standard error of the mean probability estimate; n = number of patients remaining at risk at that time. With permission from ref. (6).

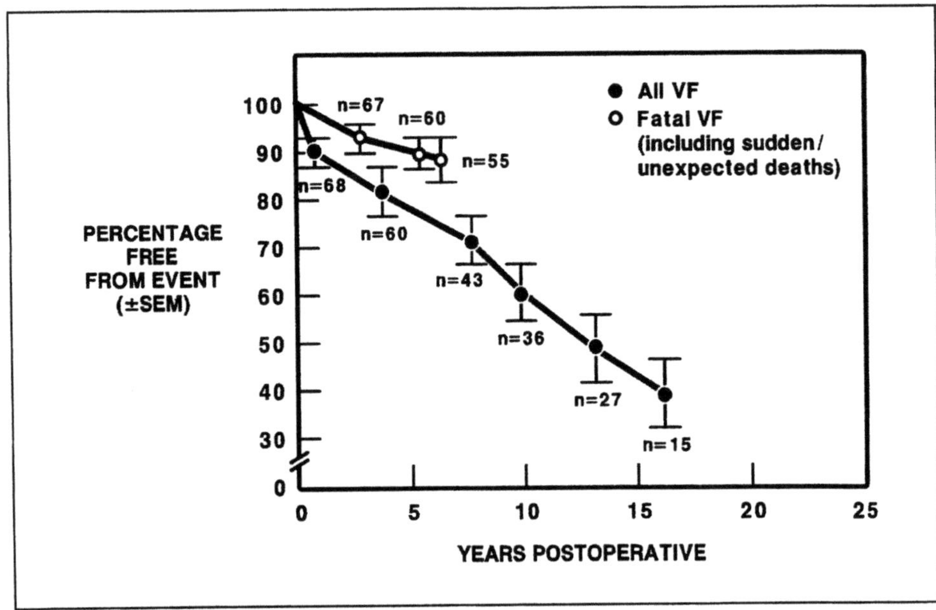

Fig. 9. Incidence of all modes of valve failure (●) and fatal valve failure (○) calculated by the actuarial method. Error bars and n as in Fig. 8. With permission from ref. (6).

134

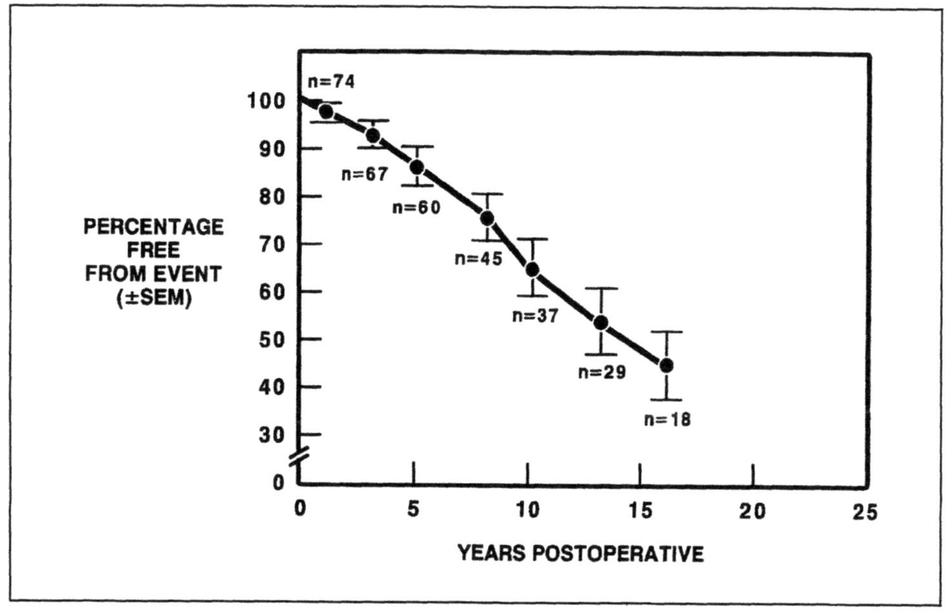

Fig. 10. Actuarial curve showing probability of freedom from reoperation. Error bars and n as in Fig. 8. With permission from ref. (6).

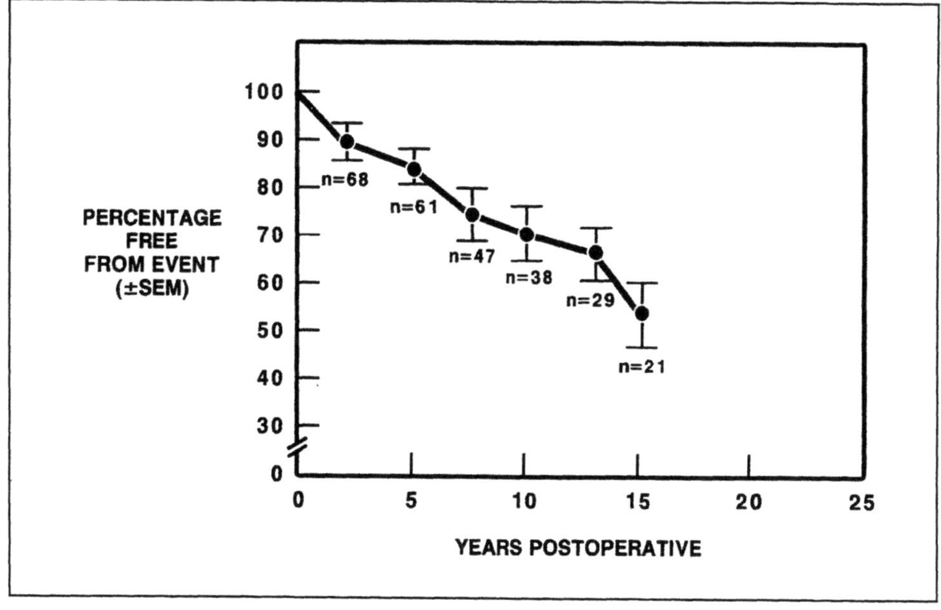

Fig. 11. Actuarial estimates of probability of late survival in discharged patients. Error bars and n as in Fig. 8. With permission from ref. (6).

Focusing on valve failure due to all causes (Fig. 9) — including endocarditis and sudden, unexplained deaths —, 62 ± 6% of our patients were estimated to be free of this event at 10 years, and 43 ± 7% at 15 years. Fatal valve failure (again, including all sudden, unexplained late deaths) occurred at a low, but finite, rate of 11 ± 4% at 6 years. This comprehensive inclusion of all causes of valve failure in our analysis was not used in the other series for comparison. It is difficult to draw conclusions based on fatal valve failure over the long-term because the last valve-related death occurred 6 years postoperatively; while we do not know what this curve is going to look like at 15 years, the absence of valve-related deaths occurring beyond 6 years is certainly promising.

Reoperation occurred at a progressively increasing rate (Fig. 10). At 10 years, 67 ± 6% of our patients were free of reoperation; at 15 years, this figure was 48 ± 7%. Barratt-Boyes (2) reports estimates of freedom from reoperation of 93%, 79% and 54% at 5, 10, and 15 years, respectively. O'Brien's estimates (8) for anti-biotic stored, non-viable allografts are 85 ± 4% of patients free from reoperation at 10 years and 53% at 15 years. While still unproved due to lack of controlled, pro-spective studies and limited follow-up (11—12 years), many investigators believe that the use of viable (cryopreserved) allograft valves will be associated with sub-stantially lower reoperation rates between 10 and 20 years (7).

Late survival

Figure 11 illustrates actuarial late survival rates in these 83 patients from Stanford; 70% of patients were alive at 10 years and 55% at 15 years. Table 1 summarizes late survival rates in other series, which are similar to our results with the exception of Barratt-Boyes's statistics (2), where only 38% of patients were alive 15 years post-operatively. Any real difference in late survival is a moot point, however, since late deaths are essentially independent of the type of valve used; late survival is much more a function of the patient population undergoing operation. Late survival av-erages 57—70% after 10 years and 38—55% after 15 years. In Yacoub's series (9), multivariate analysis revealed that advanced age and the appearance of postopera-tive left bundle branch block were independent variables which adversely affected late survival.

Discussion

Most features regarding the use of allografts for AVR have been well known for many years, but the 15-year long-term durability and clinical performance charac-teristics have not been well defined until recently (2, 3, 6, 7, 9, 12). It is still difficult to compare long-term results according to the method of allograft procurement and preservation because there was little uniformity in the early years of allograft valve use. Cryopreservation techniques appear to maintain the allografts as a viable graft, but to what extent this viability is of clinical importance in terms of potentially prolonged durability currently remains unknown. The very low incidence of thromboembolism and bleeding is a well-known advantage associated with the use of allograft valves (Table 1), and represents a clear advantage over the use of mechanical valves. The use of other types of tissue valves, e.g., porcine bioprostheses, in the aortic position is also associated with very low rates of these complications. Allograft valves are not free of infectious complications, as 4—7% of patients will develop endocarditis by the end of 5 years, and up to 12% by 10 years (Table 1). This is somewhat disappointing, since no synthetic material is implanted; nonetheless, the incidence of endocarditis is quite low, and such cases can be treated successfully, frequently without the need for reoperation (2, 7).

Long-term durability remains the most important unanswered issue surrounding the use of allograft valve substitutes. In the 5 and 10-year time "windows", nonviable (antibiotically stored) allografts appear to have no distinct advantage over porcine bioprostheses. Current 5-year estimated freedom from failure is > 90%; at 10 years, results vary between 55% and 78%; the 15-year results have only recently appeared, and range from a low of 23% of patients free of valve failure in Ross's experience (12) to a high of 61% in Yacoub's patients (10). In our experience, 51% of patients were free from degenerative allograft valve failure 15 years postoperatively; this figure is reasonable, considering the rudimentary methods of preservation and the lack of more rigorous control of storage time and other donor and recipient variables in this remote era. To compare these results with the 15-year results with porcine substitutes may be of historic interest only, since it is believed - albeit unproved - that the long-term results after free-hand allograft AVR currently (improved, more controlled procurement and preservation techniques, better donor and patient matching, and the recognition and elimination of adverse patient and valve risk

Table 1. Morbid events, operative mortality rates, and late death in five series of patients undergoing "fresh" free-hand allograft replacement of the aortic valve. The actuarial rates of freedom from an event are shown; the linearized rates indicate the incidence of an event.

	Thrombo-embolism	Endocarditis		Degenerative valve failure		Reoperation		Hospital mortality %	Late survival	
		% free	at n years	% free	at n years	% free	at n years		%	at n years
Barratt-Boyes (2)	0	96	5	95	5	93	5	6	77	5
		92	14	78	10	79	10		57	10
				42	15	54	14		38	15
O'Brien (7, 8)	90±3%	94	10	NA		85±4	10	9	67±5	10
						53	15		<50	15
Ross (12)	0	NA		55	10	NA		<3	NA	
				23	15					
Yacoub (9, 10)	0	93	5	90	5	NA		<3	83	5
		88	10	72	10				67	10
				61	15				52	15
Stanford University	1.0%/pt-yr	0.5%/pt-yr		70±6	10	67±6	10	6	70	10
				51±7	15	48±7	15		55	15

factors) will be superior in terms of valve failure. We postulate that the 15-year performance characteristics with non-viable, free-hand allografts for AVR reported herein from our institution may actually be very similar to those using (first generation) porcine bioprosthesis after 15 years; this sobering possibility underscores the importance today - in our opinion - of confining the use of allograft valves only to those patients with a disproportionately high risk of xenograft valve fibrocalcification (e.g., children, young adults, patients with renal failure) and selected other patients with special considerations, viz., very small annulus, prosthetic valve endocarditis, etc.

To date, the best results with "fresh" (now considered in retrospect to be non-viable), free-hand allograft valves for AVR are those reported by Barratt-Boyes and colleagues (2), especially when their "high risk patients" were excluded. Multivariate analysis revealed several risk factors which portended premature degenerative valve failure and/or reoperation, including donor age > 50 years, recipient age < 15 years (but the very small numbers in this subgroup preclude conclusive interpretation of this finding), and aortic root diameter > 30 mm. After 5, 9 and 13 years, the estimated proportions of "low risk" patients free from valve failure were 98%, 94%, and 56%, respectively. The 5 and 10-year figures appear to be superior to clinical results obtained with porcine xenograft valves, but after 15 years (a time where concrete information with large numbers of bioprostheses is not yet available), a situation in which approximately 50% of patients are free from valve degeneration would make the performance of the glutaraldehyde-preserved xenograft valves comparable to that of these non-viable allografts. In another study by Penta et al. (9), four independent variables were found to predict valve failure: older recipient age, female sex, type of valve lesion (stenosis > regurgitation), and longer time between death and removal of the allograft valve. Of these factors, only the latter one can be modified to any extent preoperatively.

It is apparent, therefore, that "fresh" allograft valves inserted free-hand for AVR have performed satisfactorily over the past 15—20 years, but these results are clearly not optimal. When compared with porcine bioprostheses, we speculate that the long term results of these older, non-viable allograft valves may not be associated with any distinct advantage in terms of valve degeneration or reoperation. This is one of the reasons why improved tissue (allograft, autograft, or xenograft) valves are needed. A theoretical advantage would be to implant allograft pulmonary valves in the aortic position (3), as the use of pulmonary autograft valves for AVR has been shown by Ross and colleagues to be quite successful for at least 15 years (3). The second, and currently most widely debated issue, pertains to allograft cell viability, where many unanswered questions remain. Do the "truly fresh" valves (stored for $\leq$ 24 h) remain viable? If so, for how long? Does such "viability" pertain to cells other than fibroblasts, e.g. endothelial cells, smooth muscle cells? If the valves remain viable, is this beneficial or detrimental in terms of long-term durability? Will the viable valves elicit immunological reactions that might alter long-term results or, at the least, mandate more rigorous donor-recipient tissue matching? Obviously, at the present time we can only speculate concerning these questions. Theoretically, viable valves should grow and function as part of the body, and have a very low failure rate, but at this time no convincing proof of this hypothesis exists.

Tissue matching may have an important effect, not only in terms of ABO red blood cell type but perhaps also for Class I and Class II HLA alloantigens. The answers to all of these questions await further investigation.

Recent reports of excellent long-term results with cryopreserved allograft valves have aroused renewed scientific interest in this technique of preserving mammalian tissues, and the viability of donor fibroblasts has been demonstrated (4, 7). In O'Brien's series, freedom from reoperation at 10 years for patients receiving cryopreserved allograft valves was 92 ± 3%, and the 10-year survival rate was 70 ± 5%. These results, however, are closely comparable to those attained in Barratt-Boyes's "low risk" patient population (94% freedom from valve failure at 9 years) who received non-viable, antibiotically stored allografts (2).

While the rates of valve degeneration and reoperation are necessarily related, they are not identical, due to the fact that some patients tolerate the gradual onset of mild to moderate aortic regurgitation well and not uncommonly postpone elective reoperation until symptoms appear or become worse or left ventricular dimensions increase. Two-thirds of our patients were free of reoperation at 10 years, and 48% at 15 years. Somewhat better statistics were reported by Barratt-Boyes (2) and by O'Brien (8) (see Table 1). The operative mortality rate for a second allograft AVR operation has been reported to vary between 9% (2) and 13% (9).

In summary, current analysis of this older information from Stanford has lead us to conclude that the long-term results using free-hand, "fresh" aortic valve allografts for AVR are relatively satisfactory, although far from optimal. The incidence of valve-related complications was acceptable, but still amenable to improvement. Although promising results up to 11—12 years after AVR with cryopreserved allograft valves have been reported recently, it remains unproved, in our opinion, whether or not the durability of cryopreserved allograft valves will be superior to that of non-viable allografts. We hope that better, more refined procurement and preservation methods will yield better long-term results. We should recognize, however, that it will take several years to learn if an "improvement" really is better — the second decade after implantation of free-hand allograft valves, treated and procured a specific way, will tell us if newer methods have really made any difference. Patient selection criteria also have an important role in improving long-term outcome, e.g. excluding patients with a large aortic annulus, ABO and HLA matching, etc., and should be addressed in the future.

References

1. Barratt-Boyes BG (1964) Homograft aortic valve replacement in aortic incompetence and stenosis. Thorax 19: 131—150
2. Barratt-Boyes BG, Roche AGH, Subramanyan R et al (1987) Long-term follow up of patients with the antibiotic-sterilized aortic homograft value inserted freehand in the aortic position. Circulation 75: 768—777
3. Bodnar E (1987) Pulmonary autografts, viable and non-viable aortic homografts in the subcoronary position: A comparative study. In: This volume, pp 261—264
4. Brockbank KGM, Bank HL (1987) Measurement of post cryopreservation viability. J Cardiac Surg 2 (Suppl): 145—151
5. Kirklin JW, Barratt-Boyes BG (1986) Cardiac Surgery. John Wiley and Sons Inc, New York, pp 379—388 and 421—422

6. Miller DC, Shumway NE (1987) "Fresh" aortic allografts: long-term results with free-hand aortic valve replacement. J Cardiac Surg 2 (Suppl): 185—191
7. O'Brien MF, Stafford G, Gardner M et al (1987) The viable cryopreserved allograft aortic valve. J Cardiac Surg 2 (Suppl): 153—167
8. O'Brien MF et al. (1988) Cryopreserved viable allograft aortic valves. In: This volume, pp 311—322
9. Penta A, Qureshi S, Radley-Smith R, Yacoub MH (1984) Patient status 10 or more years after "fresh" homograft replacement of the aortic valve. Circulation 70 (Suppl I): I-182—186
10. Radley-Smith R, Yacoub MH (1988) Long-term function of antibiotic treated allografts in the subcoronary position. In: This volume, pp 265—272
11. Ross DN (1962) Homograft replacement of the aortic valve. Lancet 2: 487
12. Ross DN (1987) Application of homografts in clinical surgery. J Cardiac Surg 2 (Suppl): 175—182
13. Stinson EB, Griepp RB, Shumway NE (1977) Long-term results of isolated aortic and mitral valve replacement with fresh aortic allografts. In: Davila JC (ed) Second Henry Ford Hospital International Symposium on Cardiac Surgery. Appleton-Century Crofts, New York, pp 502—510

Authors' address:

D. C. Miller M.D.
Department of Cardiovascular Surgery
Cardiovascular Research Center
Stanford University Medical Center
Stanford, California 94305
U.S.A.

Modified techniques for subcoronary insertion of allografts

A. J. Dziatkowiak, R. Pfitzner, J. Andres, P. Podolec, Z. Marek, M. Zarska

Institute of Cardiology, N. Copernicus University, School of Medicine, Cracow, Poland

Introduction

The choice of optimal substitute, mechanical or biological, for aortic valve replacement is still discussed (4, 7, 8, 14, 15). The use of fresh, unstented, antibiotic-sterilised allografts (homografts) for replacement of aortic valve, aortic root or for correction of some complex congenital malformations, is emphasized by many authors (4—6, 9, 13—15, 17). The method was introduced into clinical practice in the early 1960s, particularly by Ross and Barratt-Boyes (2, 12). The well documented follow-up studies demonstrate that the results of allograft implantation are comparable or better than those of mechanical valves (5, 8, 11).
Allografts are well tolerated and behave like the native valves. The further advantages are no need for anticoagulation, no thromboembolic complications, higher security in cases with severe tissue damage because of active endocarditis, and significantly less bleeding during the aortic root replacement for aneurysms. However, degenerative changes and calcifications occur. Fortunately, in the majority of cases, they are not of clinical importance for many years (5, 6, 9, 11, 16, 17).
Allografts have been used in Poland since 1974 when M. H. Yacoub implanted in Łódź an antibiotic-sterilised, free-hand aortic valve allograft in a male (4). At the present time, after 13 years, the function of this allograft is still good and the patient is functioning normally.

Materials and Methods

From 1980 to July 1987, we inserted 240 antibiotic-sterilised, unstented aortic valve allografts in subcoronary position for aortic valve replacement including ascending aortic aneurysms replacement (because of annulo-aortic ectasia and acquired or congenital malformations) on 46 occasions. The patients comprised 190 men and 50 women, aged 15 to 64 years.

Grafts collection

All grafts were received from the Dept. of Forensic Medicine, University School of Medicine in Cracow. They were removed during the elective post-mortem examinations of previously healthy, accidentally deceased persons under 40 years of age, not later than 48 h after death.

Preparation and storage

Grafts were transferred to our department and prepared at the Bank of Allografts. The overbounded tissue was excised and the specimens consisting of the ascending aorta and arch with aortic valve, stumps of coronary arteries and a border of tissue (muscle and mitral leaflet), preserved in sterilising medium at + 4 °C with some fragments of aortic tissue, used for microbiological examinations. The sterilising medium contained such antibiotics as Fungisone, Neomycin, Ceporin, Polymyxin, and Pyopen diluted in Hanks' solution. Subsequently, if the microbiological examinations were reproducibly negative, after 2—3 days the specimens were transferred into the nutrient medium, containing Nystatin, Streptomycin, Penicillin, natrium bicarbonate and calf serum diluted the Hanks' solution, and stored at + 4 °C for 3 weeks. The microbiological examinations were repeated. In practice, the grafts were implanted within 10—14 days after acquisition. The definitive preparation and trimming was performed by the surgeon after the aorta was opened and the graft was perhaps selected by size and quality. The blood group compatibility of the donor and recipient was not obligatory.

Techniques

All grafts were implanted subcoronary after the removal of the affected native aortic valve but in the cases of annulo-aortic ectasia the aortic leaflets of the patients were usually left intact.
1. Initially, the grafts were trimmed and implanted after the Ross (12) and rarely Barratt-Boyes (2) techniques (Fig. 1a, b). The proximal suture line (annular) was performed using single straight or mattress Mersilene 4/0 sutures. The commissures were fixed by three single mattress Mersilene 3/0 sutures, and the distal margin of the donor's aorta was sutured into the sinuses of Valsalva using 4/0 running suture.
2. The last 150 grafts were implanted using our modified technique. It consists of implantation of total aortic bulb with valve and the side-to-side anastomosis of the coronary ostia. The annular part of the graft is trimmed similarly as in the Ross and Barratt-Boyes technique and sutured (proximal or annulo-annular anastomosis) with single stitches. Then, the cylinder of aortic bulb about 3 cm in length is cut off. The coronary orifices of the graft are adapted to the native ostia and sutured side-to-side using running Prolene 5/0 suture. The cylinder is fixed with 3—4 mattress sutures knotted outside the patient's aorta, and the distal margin of the graft is sew to the inner side of the patient's aortic wall with a running 4/0 suture. The aorta is closed with a Blalock or a single running Prolene 4/0 suture (Fig. 1c).
3. 46 of 61 patients with ascending aortic aneurysms received allografts. The technique of implantation is similar to our cylinder-graft technique but the allograft is longer and comprises total ascending aorta. The coronary ostia of the graft and the

142

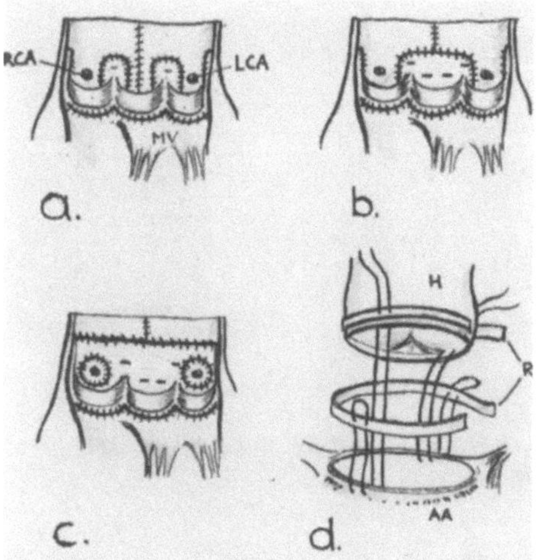

Fig. 1. Schematic presentation of aortic valve replacement with an allograft, after: (a) Barratt-Boyes, (b) Ross, (c) our own technique of total aortic bulb implantation, (d) our own method of ascending aorta and valve replacement with aortic annulus reinforcement. (RCA) Right coronary ostium; (LCA) left coronary ostium; (MV) mitral valve leaflet; (AA) aortic annulus; (R) fabric felt ring; (H) allograft.

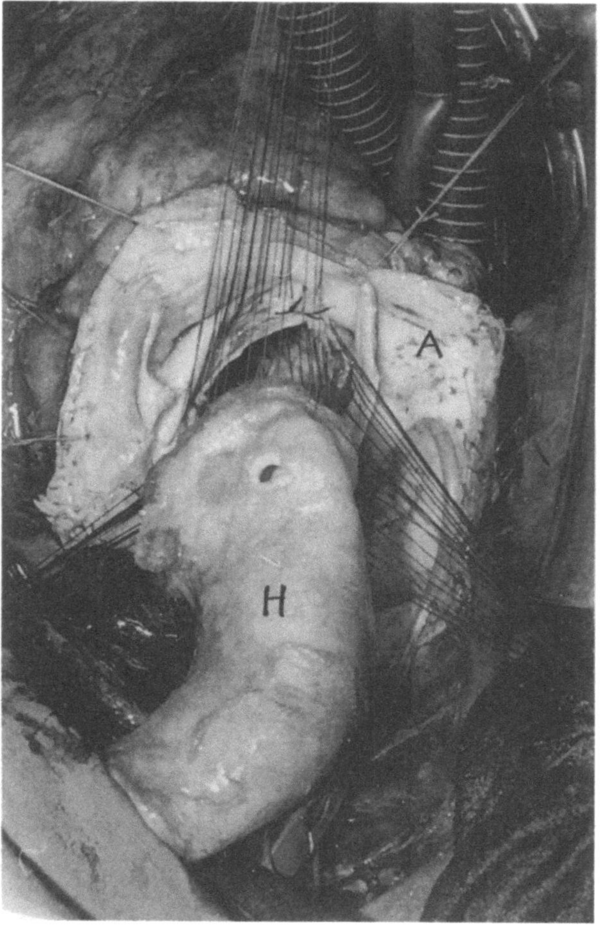

Fig. 2. Technique of aortic root replacement with an allograft — proximal (annulo-annular) anastomosis: (A) aortic wall; (H) allograft.

143

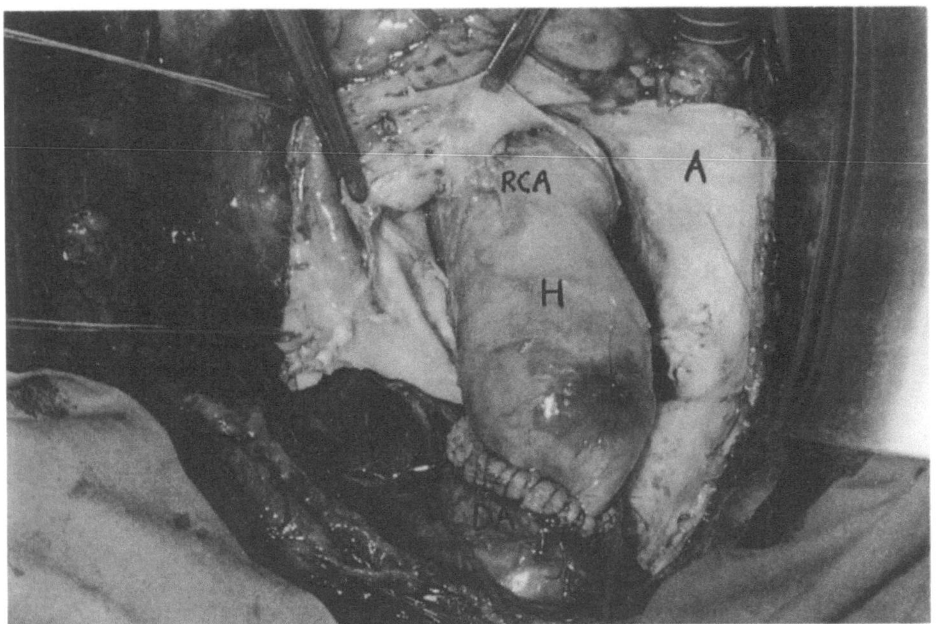

Fig. 3. Technique of aortic root replacement with an allograft: (A) aortic wall; (H) allograft; (RCA) right coronary ostium anastomosed side-to-side with the graft; (DA) distal anastomosis with the patient's aorta.

recipient are carefully adapted. In the large aneurysms the native ostia are considerably displaced, consequently the coronary ostia of the graft must be sutured and the new orifices cut out distally. Additional 3 or 4 single Prolene 5/0 reinforcing sutures are placed around the anastomoses to release the tension of the coronary junction. The distal anastomosis is a routine end-to-end anastomosis or the allograft is placed and anastomosed inside the lumen of the patient's aorta like a telescope with a continuous Prolene 4/0 suture. In cases with weak aortic wall, to reinforce the suture line against bleeding or tear, the sutures passed through the externally-located fabric felt tape. In the events of aortic wall dissection it is sutured with running Prolene 4/0 prior the distal anastomosis is made.

In annulo-aortic ectasia the aortic annulus should be constricted by single or double fabric ring, inserted around the patient's and the graft's annuli with Mersilene 4/0 single straight or mattress sutures. The fabric annuli may be circle in shape or as a tape with 3 indicated distances of the graft commissures, and finally, after the sutures are placed, they are formed in a closed circle (5) (Fig. 1d, 2, 3).

The allografts are usually wrapped around by the remaining aneurysmal wall and to avoid hypertension of blood commulated in the "dead-space", usually a small hole is left for venting. When residual bleeding is evident, the anastomosis between the "dead-space" and the right appendage was made in two instances to release the tension on the coronary anastomoses.

The patients were cannulated for the cardiopulmonary bypass through the external iliac artery to avoid cannula insertion into the false lumen at ascending aorta level.

144

Results

From among 240 patients with aortic valve allografts the hospital mortality rate was 4.2% (ten patients). Only one patient (2.2 %) died after the ascending aortic aneurysm replacement. There were no early deaths over the last 2 years. During mean follow-up of 4 years (1 month to over 7 years) the cumulative late mortality was 8.9%.

In 26% of patients there are in echocardiography some thickenings of the aortic leaflets, with symptomatic regurgitation in two cases. The calcification of implanted aorta of different intensity in echo occurred in about 30 % of instances. There were no signs of aortic valve incompetency immediately after the "cylinder" graft implantation but in about 15% of patients after "classic" operation a murmur was present.

None of the nine patients with annulo-aortic ectasia with annular reinforcement after our method demonstrate further annular dilatation and/or aortic valve regurgitation. One patient after dissected aneurysm replacement showed, in aortography, a discrete rest communication between the graft and false lumen of the aorta.

Five patients were reoperated on: three for early valve endocarditis and two for chronic regurgitation due to massive calcifications. All survivors demonstrate clinical improvement.

Discussion

Our experience — 13 years in Poland and 8 years in our Institution — favours fresh, free-hand antibiotic-sterilised allografts as a good substitute for aortic valve and root replacement.

Our results are similar to those of others authors, and the early and late mortality is acceptable and comparable or lower than that after mechanical or bioprosthetic valve implantation (3—6, 10, 14, 16, 17). The rate and intensification of degenerative changes of the graft and complications are lower than after insertion of bioprostheses (6, 11, 14). Probably, among the factors influencing this phenomenon, the preservation in nutrient antibiotic solution instead of glutaraldehyde may be important. The cryopreservation of allografts has not been widely propagated as yet (1, 6, 11, 18, 19).

However, implantation of allografts is more difficult than that of stented mechanical or biological valves and needs perfect technique. The most important technical factors influencing the results and further fate of the grafts and patients are:

Perfect size and geometry of the implant;

Adequate coronary ostia anastomoses;

Prevention of annular dilatation.

A small distortion of graft's annulus and leaflets, possible using both Barratt-Boyes' and Ross's techniques, may produce discrete or larger regurgitation. In about 15% of our patients, a murmur was stated postoperatively. Our method, consisting of application of a cylindrical graft comprising the total aortic bulb which is less susceptible to rotation or distortion, may efficaciously prevent graft incompetency.

The problem of adequate coronary ostia anastomoses occurs particularly in patients with large ascending aortic aneurysms. The native coronary ostia are often distantly displaced but may appear to be near the annulus. Therefore, the places for holes in the graft for coronary ostia anastomoses should be precisely measured and adapted. All techniques leading to release the tension of coronary junction, as additional sutures around the anastomosis, prevent the dissection and bleeding, which may be difficult to efficaciously manage, particularly in patients with weak aortic wall. Our technique of reinforcing the aortic annulus against further dilatation in annulo-aortic ectasia has been previously described (5). The observation of nine patients confirm the expediency of this manoeuvre.

References

1. Al-Janabi N, Ross DN (1973) Enhanced viability of fresh aortic homografts stored in nutrient medium. Cardiovasc Res 7: 813
2. Barratt-Boyes BG (1964) Homograft aortic valve replacement in aortic incompetence and stenosis. Thorax 19: 131
3. Bodnar E, Wain WH, Martelli V, Ross DN (1979) Long-term performance of 580 homografts and autograft valves used for aortic valve replacement. J Thorac Cardiovasc Surg 27: 51
4. Dziatkowiak A, Moll J, Musiał W, Tracz W, Zienkiewicz J, Zasłonka J, Leśniak K, Oszczygieł S, Tyburska I, Kęsiak J (1977) Fresh homogenous aortic valves in treatment of aortic valve diseases (in Polish). Kard Pol 20: 189—199
5. Dziatkowiak A, Pfitzner R, Sadowski J, Tracz WD, Koziorowska B, Marek Z, Zacny E (1986) Aortic root replacement using antibiotic sterilized "fresh" unstented homografts: modification of annulus reinforcement. In: Bodnar E, Yacoub M (eds) Biologic and bioprosthetic valves. Yorke Medical Books, pp 14—21
6. Fontan F, Choussat A, Deville C, Doutremøpuich C, Coupillaud J, Vosa C (1984) Aortic valve homografts in the surgical treatment of complex cardiac malformations. J Thorac Cardiovasc Surg 87: 649—657
7. Hammond GL, Geha AS, Kopf GS, Hashim SW (1987) Biological versus mechanical valves. Analysis of 1116 valves inserted in 1012 adult patients with a 4,818 patient-year and a 5,327 valve year follow-up. J Thorac Cardiovasc Surg 93: 182—198
8. Horstkotte D, Rovelli F (1986) Choosing between mechanical and tissue valves for the treatment of valvular heart disease. In: Horstkotte D, Loogen F (eds) Update in heart valve replacement. Steinkopff-Darmstadt, Springer-New York, pp 15—22
9. Lau JKH, Robles A, Cheridan A, Ross DN (1984) Surgical treatment of prosthetic endocarditis. Aortic root replacement using a homograft. J Thorac Cardiovasc Surg 87: 712—716
10. Lillehei CW (1986) The St. Jude Medical prosthetic heart valve. Results from a five year multicenter experience. In: Horstkotte D, Loogen F (eds) Update in heart valve replacement. Steinkopff-Darmstadt, Springer-New York, pp 3—13
11. Moore CH, Martelli V, Al-Janabi N, Ross DN (1975) Analysis of homograft valve failure in 311 patients followed-up to 10 years. Ann Thorac Surg 3: 274—281
12. Ross DN (1962) Homograft replacement of the aortic valve. Lancet 2: 487
13. Saravalli OA, Somerville J, Jefferson KE (1980) Calcification of aortic homografts used for reconstruction of the right ventricular outflow tract. J Thorac Cardiovasc Surg 80: 909—920
14. Somerville J, Ross DN (1982) Homograft replacement of aortic root woth reimplantation of coronary arteries. Results of one to five years. Br Heart J 47: 473—482
15. Struck E, Meisner H, Hagl S, Paek S, Sebening F (1986) Preferred use of allografts in the treatment of valvular heart disease. In: Horstkotte D, Loogen F (eds) Update in Heart Valve Replacement. Steinkopff-Darmstadt, Springer-New York, pp 25—29
16. Thompson R, Yacoub M, Ahmed M, Somerville W, Towers M (1980) The use of "fresh" unstented homograft valves for replacement of the aortic valve. Analysis of 8 years' experience. J Thorac Cardiovasc Surg 79: 896—903

146

17. Tracz M, Seabra-Gomes R, Thompson R, Yacoub R, Yacoub M (1979) Left-ventricular function investigations before and after implantation of homologous aortic valve (in Polish). Kard Pol 22: 205—213
18. Van der Kamp AWM, Visser WJ, van Dongen LM, Nauta J, Galjaard H (1981) Preservation of aortic heart valves with maintenance of cell viability. J Surg Res 30: 47—56
19. Yacoub M, Kittle CF (1979) Sterilization of valve homografts by antibiotic solution. Circulation 41, suppl 2: 29

Authors' address:
A. J. Dziatkowiak
Institute of Cardiology
N. Copernicus University School of Medicine in Cracow
Pradnicka Str. 80
31-202 Cracow
Poland

Allograft aortic root replacement

M. H. Yacoub

Harefield Hospital, Harefield, National Heart and Brompton Hospital, London, U.K.

Since 1975 we have developed and used a technique of excising the aortic root and replacing it with a cylindrical segment of aortic homograft, including the aortic valve and root (1). After excision of the diseased aortic valve, the lower end of the homograft root is anastomosed to the aortic annulus by multiple interrupted sutures. The mobilised coronary ostia with 2 mm of surrounding aortic wall are then anastomosed to the site of the coronary ostia of the homograft using continuous monofilament sutures. The top end of the homograft is then anastomosed to the ascending aorta. No prosthetic material is used to support any of the anastomoses. This technique preserves the functional integrity and spatial relationship of the different components of the homograft valve and allows reconstruction of the aortic root and left ventricular outflow in a variety of conditions. The principle indications in our series included (Fig. 1):

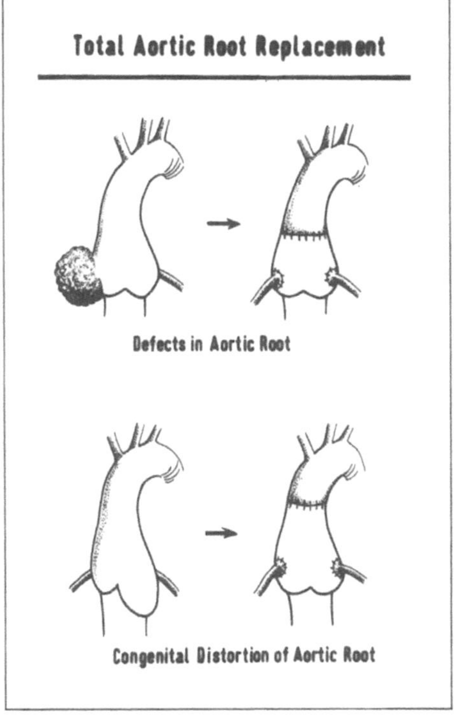

Fig. 1a.

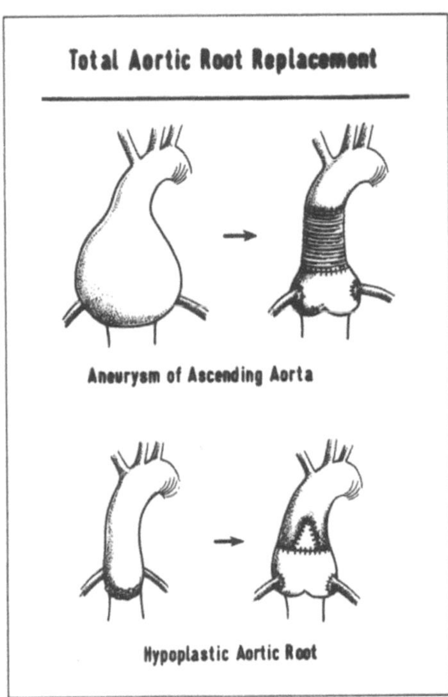

Fig. 1b.

Fig. 1a, b. Diagramatic representation of technique and principal indications for aortic root replacement.

1. Mismatch between the size and shape of the homograft and the aortic root.
2. Hypoplastic aortic root, particularly in children.
3. Aneurysms of the ascending aorta.
4. Aneurysmal dilatation of one or more aortic sinuses.
5. Destruction of the root secondary to infective endocarditis with abscess formation.

Patients and Methods

Between 1975 and 1986, 131 patients underwent aortic root replacement at Harefield Hospital. Their age and sex distribution are shown in Fig. 2. The principal indications and aetiology of valve and root disease are summarised in Table I. Additional procedures were performed in 49 patients (37%) and included excision of aortic aneurysm or dissection in 20 patients, mitral valve repair in 15, mitral valve replacement in two, coronary artery bypass grafting in eight, correction of anomalous origin of coronary arteries in two and closure of ventricular septal defect in two.

150

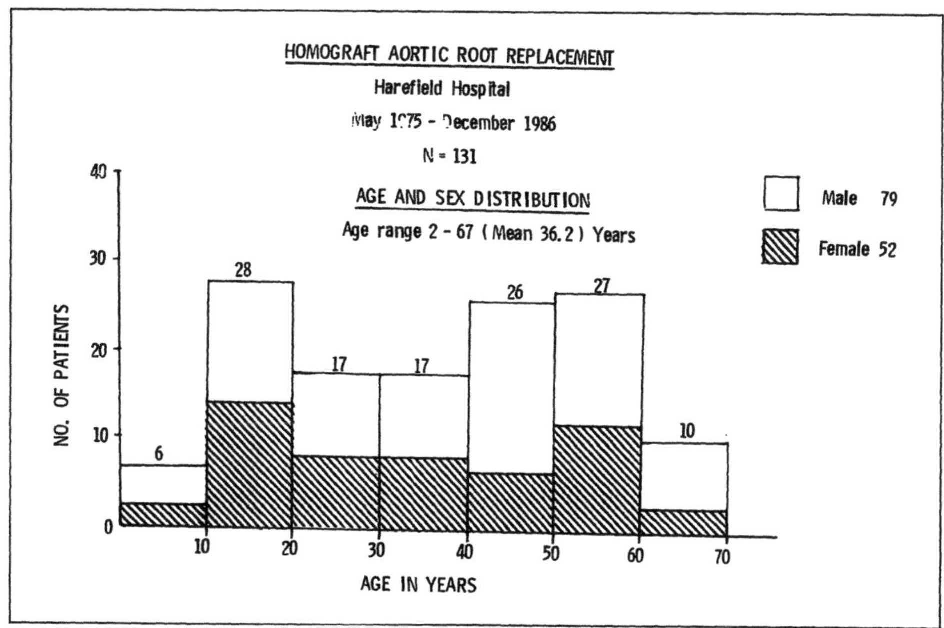

Fig. 2. Age and sex distribution of patients undergoing aortic root replacement.

Preparation of the homografts

The valves were obtained, under sterile conditions, from cardiac transplant recipients in 32 patients. These valves were kept at 4 °C in Hartmann's solution or tissue culture medium (TC 199) and used within 48 h. The remaining valves were obtained from routine postmortem material within 48 h of death, sterilised in antibiotic solution and stored in tissue culture medium (2). The age distribution of valve donors is shown in Fig. 3.

Early and late mortality

In all, there were 11 early deaths (8.4%): six of these occurred in the 14 patients undergoing emergency operations. The early mortality for elective, isolated aortic root replacement was 2.6%. During a period of follow-up ranging from 3—127 (mean 76) months, there were 12 (9%) late deaths. The causes of late deaths are shown in Table 2. The actuarial survival was 87% at 5 years and 80% at 12 years (Fig. 4). This compares favourably with patients undergoing homograft valve replacement by the conventional intra-aortic two-suture technique (3). Multivariant analysis of the possible influence of several patient, disease, graft or procedure related factors on survival showed that older age of the patient and additional procedures adversely affected survival.

Table 1. Indications and aetiology of aortic valve and root disease.

		No.
I	Small or distorted aortic root	
	a. bicuspid aortic valves	76
	b. rheumatic valves	12
	c. malfunctioning prosthetic valves	
	Bjork Shiley	1
	Hancock porcine xenografts	2
	Aortic valve homografts	9
		100 (77%)
II	Dilated aortic root (aneurysm)	
	a. Marfan syndrome	14
	b. atherosclerosis	6
		20 (15%)
III	Active infection of aortic root and valve	
	a. on native valve	8
	b. aortic homograft	2
	c. prosthetic valve (Starr-Edwards)	1
		11 (8%)

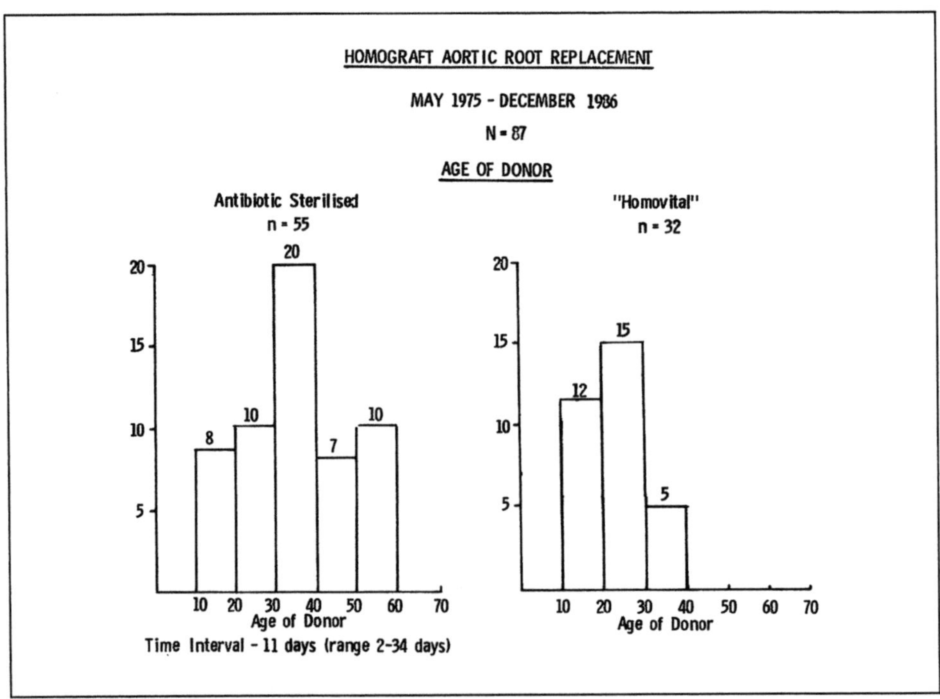

Fig. 3. Age distributions of donors of antibiotic (a) and homovital aortic homografts.

Table 2. Causes of late deaths after allograft aortic root replacement.

	No.	Age	Interval (months)	
Coronary heart disease	4	64	65	
Endocarditis	1	60	2	} 3 valve
Valve degeneration	2	46	66	} related
Suicide	1	22	107	
Rupture Type III dissection	1	29	60	
Cerebrovascular disease	1	70	57	
Chest infection	1	69	88	
Sudden death	1	7	80	
Total	12	(9%)		

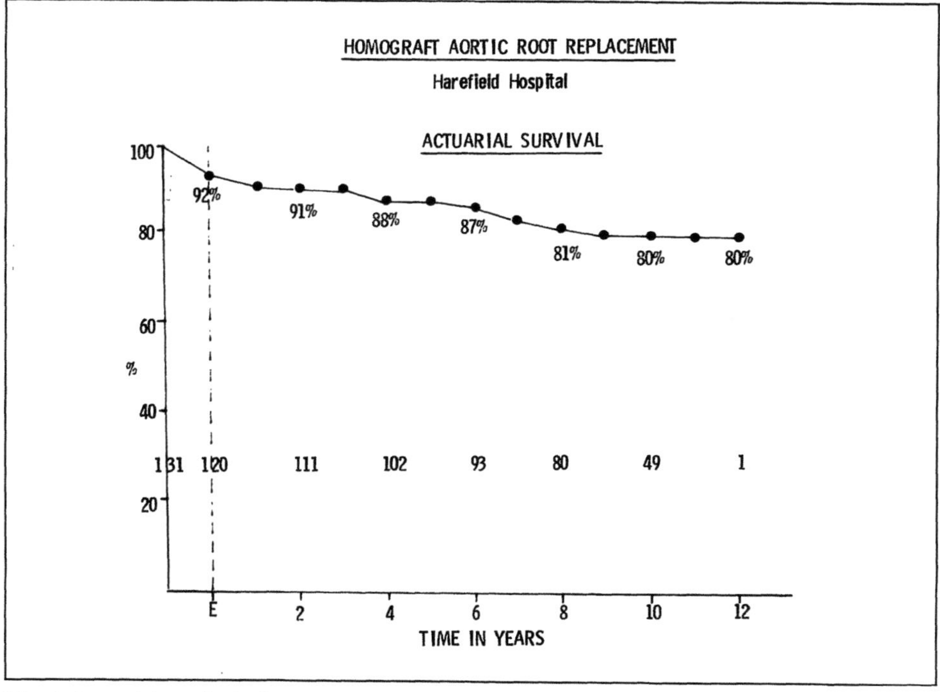

Fig. 4. Actuarial survival after allograft aortic root replacement.

Endocarditis

There were two instances of endocarditis during the period of follow-up defined above, one at 2 and the other at 73 months. The cumulative probability of freedom from endocarditis at 10 years was 98%.

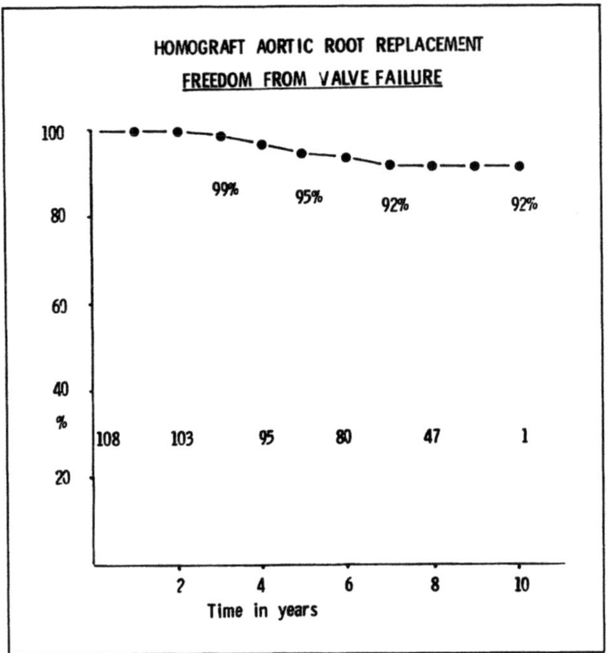

Fig. 5. Actuarial curve showing the cumulative probability of freedom from valve failure after allograft aortic root replacement.

Valve failure

During the period of follow-up (ranging from 3—127 months with a mean of 76 months), nine patients developed valve failure — this was secondary to endocarditis in two and valve degeneration in 7. Valve degeneration was observed at intervals varying from 43—120 months. The cumulative probability of freedom from valve failure was 95% at 5 years and 92% at 10 years (Fig. 5).

Reoperation

Seven patients underwent re-operation for valve failure at intervals varying from 48—120 months. In all patients there was good healing of the homograft wall to the patient's tissues with widely patent coronary ostia and no evidence of dilatation of the aortic wall of the homograft. Cusp tissue was replaced without a need for re-replacement of the aortic root. There was one death related to re-operation.

Discussion

This experience has shown that homograft aortic root replacement is an effective means of treating patients with complex forms of aortic root disease. This has encouraged us to cautiously widen the indications for this operation.

154

References

1. Gula G, Ahmed MS, Thompson RH, Yacoub MH (1976) Combined homograft replacement of the valve and aortic root with reimplantation of the coronary arteries. (Abs) Circulation 54 (Suppl II): 150
2. Yacoub MH, Kittle CF. Sterilisation of valve homografts using antibiotic solutions. Circulation 61 (Suppl II), 29, 170
3. Penta A, Qureshi SA, Radley-Smith R, Yacoub M (1984) Patient status 10 or more years after "fresh" homograft replacement of the aortic valve. Circulation 70 (Suppl I), 182

Author's address:
Magdi H. Yacoub, M.D.
Professor, Consultant Cardiac Surgeon
Harefield Hospital
Harefield
Uxbridge, Middlesex
U.K.

Extended aortic root replacement in 12 patients with complex left ventricular outflow tract obstruction

D. R. Clarke

Cardiovascular and Thoracic Surgery, The Childrens Hospital, Denver, Colorado, U.S.A.

Introduction

Complex left ventricular outflow tract obstruction (LVOTO) with its involved pathology represents a particularly difficult problem for paediatric cardiac surgeons. Aortic valve replacement in such cases can be complicated by associated aortic insufficiency, hypoplastic annulus, or multiple levels of obstruction. Aortic subvalvular stenosis accounts for as much as 20% of all LVOTO and can present in a variety of forms from discrete membranous to diffuse tunnel stenosis (1, 4, 10). Furthermore, in 25% of cases, subvalvular stenosis recurs and the usual mode of recurrence is fibromuscular tunnel obstruction, often with valvular regurgitation which proves an even more complicated surgical challenge.

In the mid 1970s, Rastan and Konno (3, 7, 8) each reported their use of aortoventriculoplasty for the treatment of complex LVOTO (Fig. 1). Beginning in 1978, we used the procedure in the surgical treatment of 18 children ranging in age from 5 months to 17 years. Operative mortality was 17% and 13 of 15 survivors are currently asymptomatic. There were two late deaths; both were complications of the valvular prosthesis. One patient acquired prosthetic valve fungal endocarditis and the second developed calcification of a bovine pericardial valve.

The use of cryopreserved allografts provides a feasible alternative to bioprosthetic or mechanical valve implantation with their late complications and/or attendant need for anticoagulation.

Aortoventriculoplasty was thus combined with the concept of aortic root replacement proposed by Somerville and Ross (9). The resultant operation is known as extended aortic root replacement and is described below.

Patients

12 patients underwent extended aortic root replacement between September, 1985 and August, 1987. The group comprised six males and six females who ranged in age from 3 months to 22 years (mean: 8 years). Cardiac catheterization confirmed the presence of LVOTO in every case and seven of 12 patients (58%) exhibited concomitant aortic insufficiency. Indication for operation was subvalvular aortic stenosis associated with valvular insufficiency in four cases (33%). There were also four incidences (33%) of combined valvular and subvalvular aortic stenosis, three patients (25%) presented with valvular stenosis and insufficiency, and one (8%) had

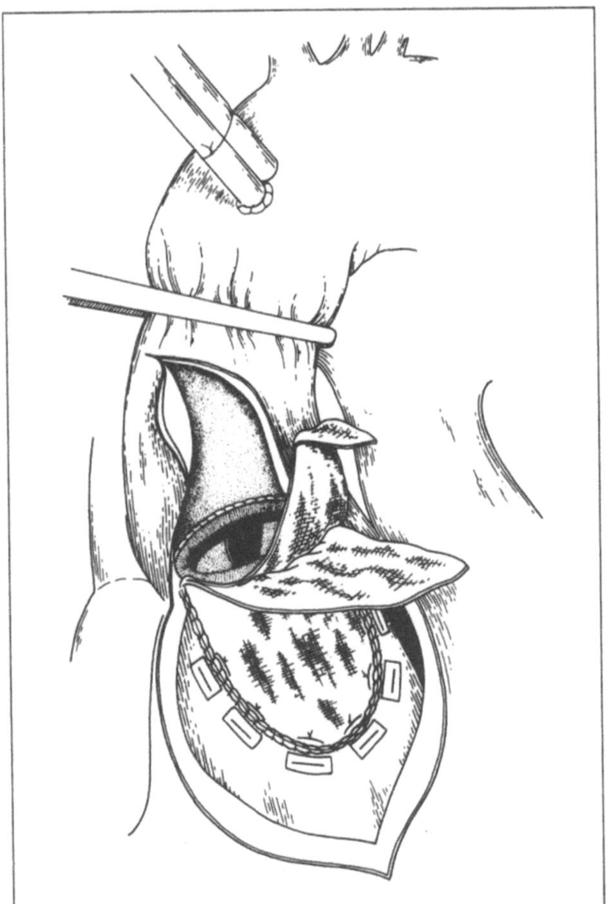

Fig. 1. Technique for aortoventriculoplasty. (From (1a) with permission from J Cardiac Surg.)

aortic stenosis and valvular dysplasia. Preoperative aortic gradients by cardiac catheterization ranged from 22 to 100 mmHg (mean: 65 mmHg).

All 12 patients had undergone prior procedures. Of the 12 patients, ten (84%) had previously undergone one or more procedures to relieve aortic stenosis. Five patients had seven subvalvular membrane resections which were performed at ages 7 months to 11 years (mean: 5 years) before undergoing EARR. Four children had a prior surgical aortic valvulotomy and one a balloon valvuloplasty. All previous surgeries are listed in Table 1.

Operative technique

An aortic valved allograft of appropriate size was selected prior to surgery. Valve sizes in our patient group ranged from 12 to 25 mm in internal diameter (mean: 19 mm). Conduit size was determined by patient weight, as illustrated in Fig. 2.

158

Table 1. Prior procedures in 12 patients undergoing extended aortic root replacement.

Resect subvalvular membrane/myectomy	7
Aortic valvotomy	4
Balloon valvuloplasty	1
Repair aortic coarctation	2
Repair interrupted aortic arch	1
ASD & VSD repair with PDA ligation	1
Portacaval shunt	1
(for type II hyperlipidemia)	
Total number of procedures:	17

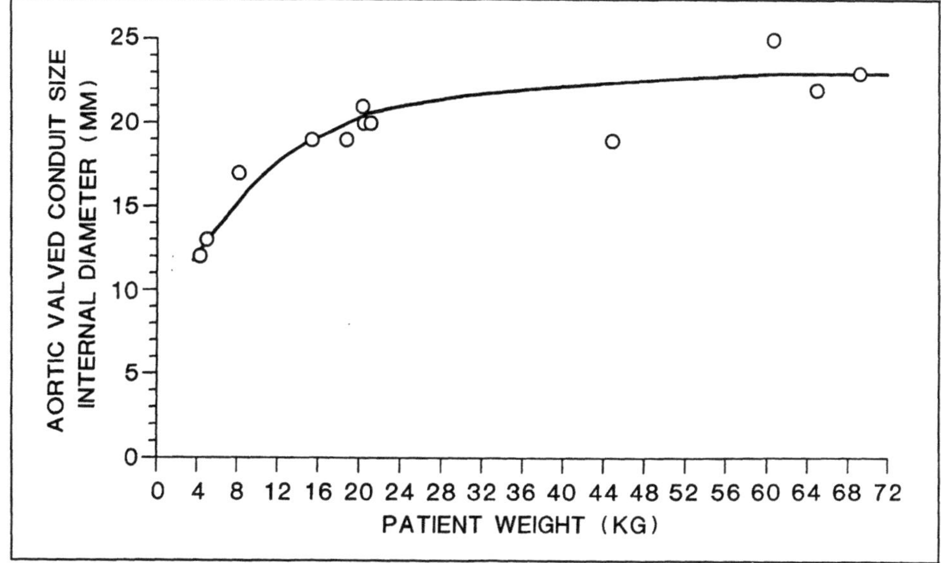

Fig. 2. Conduit size related to patient weight.

Upon entering the sternum, standard preparations are made for cardiopulmonary bypass. The aorta is cannulated near the origin of the innominate artery. The superior vena cava and inferior vena cava are cannulated with right angle cannulae and total bypass is established. The patient is subsequently cooled to 20 °C and blood cardioplegia is infused to preserve the myocardium.

During the initial phase of the operation, the allograft, still in its foil pouch, is removed from liquid nitrogen storage and placed in a 37 °C water bath to thaw for approximately 20 min. It is then removed from the pouch, passed onto the sterile field and is rinsed sequentially in three basins of fetal calf serum which contain decreasing amounts of dimethylsulphoxide. Allograft preparation is completed with a final rinse in saline (Fig. 3).

An oblique incision across the right ventricular outflow tract and a vertical incision along the ascending aorta, similar to those used in aortoventriculoplasty, meet at

159

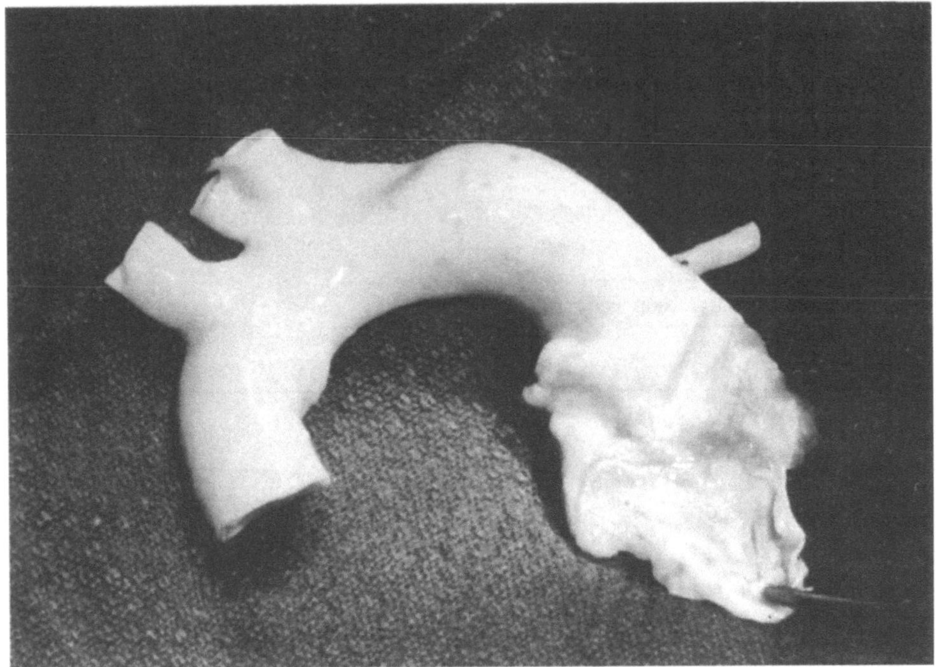

Fig. 3. Prepared aortic allograft ready for implantation. (From (1a) with permission.)

the aortic annulus between the left and right coronary ostia. At this point, the incision is carried across the annulus and into the infundibular interventricular septum. The ascending aorta is transected and the coronary ostia, with buttons of aortic wall, are then excised in preparation for their reimplantation into the conduit (Fig. 4). The aortic valve leaflets are removed and the annulus is thus prepared for allograft insertion.

The allograft is trimmed of excess muscle to within a few millimeters of the annulus and this area is thinned to prevent a bulky proximal suture line. With running monofilament suture, the proximal anastomosis is carried out posteriorly approximating the allograft annulus to the recipient's annulus and proximal aortic wall. Suture lines are continued to the right and left until the interventricular septum is encountered (Fig. 5a). The anterior leaflet of the donor mitral valve is then trimmed to fill the septal incision exactly and is used to enlarge the area as the proximal suture line is brought around the right ventricular edge of the incised septum. Horizontal mattress sutures buttressed with Teflon felt pledgets are used to reinforce this portion of the suture line (Fig. 5b).

The allograft is then transected to the precise length necessary to complete the connection to the ascending aorta. The donor aortic valve leaflets are thus clearly visualized and can be protected during the creation of holes produced by a 5- or 6-mm-diameter hole punch into which the coronary ostia buttons are sutured (Fig. 5b). The distal aortic anastomosis is sutured posteriorly with running suture from inside the lumen and the suture line is completed anteriorly and laterally from the outside. At this point in the procedure, the aortic cross-clamp can be released.

160

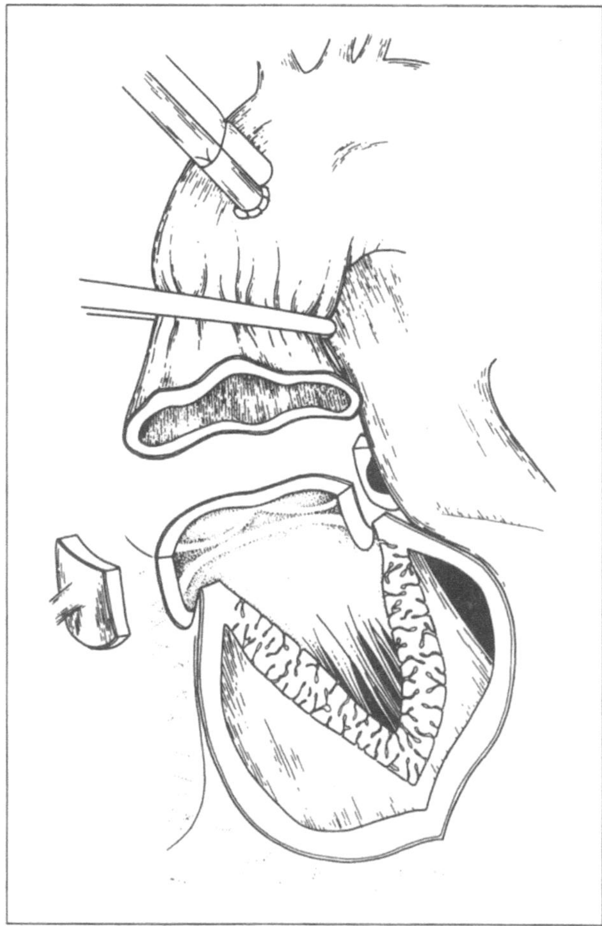

Fig. 4. The incision is carried into the interventricular septum, the aorta is transected and coronary buttons are excised, the valve leaflets are removed. (From (1a) with permission.)

The right ventricular outflow tract is mended with a triangular-shaped patch constructed from a piece of distal allograft aorta. The base of the triangle is sutured, again with running suture, to the donor aortic root at the annular level. The corners between right ventricular myocardium and allograft should be sutured with care to avoid bleeding (Fig. 6). The right ventricular suture line can then be completed with the heart beating. Pacemaker wires are attached to the right atrium and anterior surface of the right ventricle for postoperative management. The surgery is completed in standard fashion after the patient has been weaned from cardiopulmonary bypass and decannulated.

Results

Of 12 patients, two (17%) experienced a completely benign postoperative course. The most serious complication was a case of Serratia marcescens mediastinitis and

161

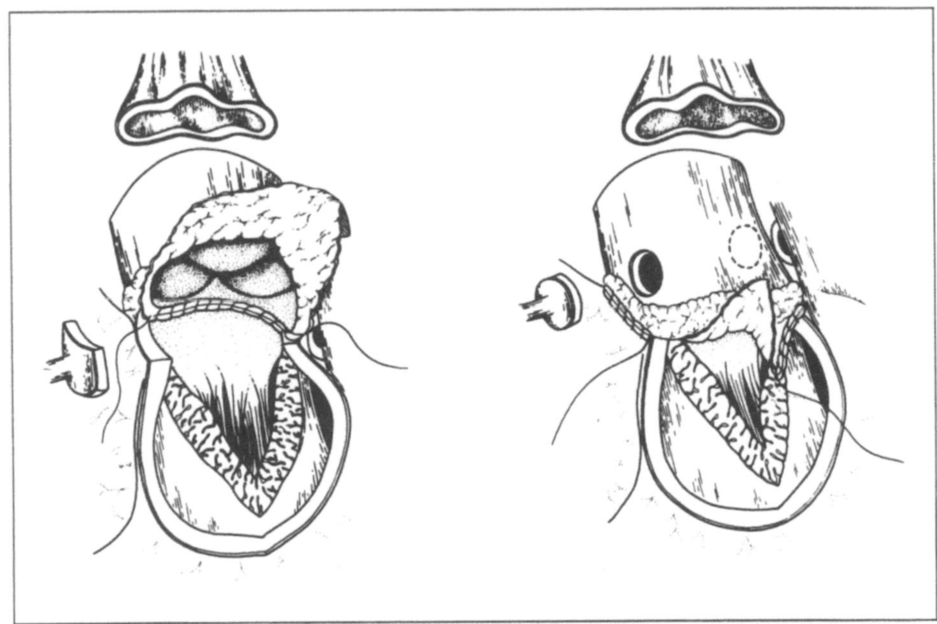

Fig. 5a. The proximal allograft anastomosis is begun posteriorly. (From (1a) with permission.)

Fig. 5b. The anterior mitral leaflet is sewn into the interventricular septal incision to enlarge the area. (From (1a) with permission).

bacteremia which required debridement, drainage and long-term antibiotics but ultimately did not affect the allograft function. Other postoperative complications included three incidents of transient complete heart block, all of which resolved completely. Two patients were reoperated for postoperative bleeding and two experienced postpericardiotomy syndrome. There were singular incidences of superficial wound infection, incisional hernia, and right phrenic nerve palsy (Table 2). All patients were discharged from the hospital doing well.

One patient required further surgery 6 months after EARR when he presented with angina pectoris. Cardiac catheterization demonstrated an 80% obstruction of the left main coronary artery as well as narrowing of the distal allograft-aorta anastomotic site. The coronary artery lesion was attributed to progression of the patient's familial hyperlipidemia since the stenosis was 2 cm from the ostia. During surgery, the allograft valve appeared normal but lipid deposits were noted on the aortic allograft intima. Late follow-up on the remaining 11 patients has thus far been without incident.

Discussion

Konno (3) and Rastan (8), pioneers in aortoventriculoplasty, reported their use of the technique in 1975 and 1976, respectively. Rastan subsequently published his experience with 21 patients treated with aortoventriculoplasty. All were anticoagulated and nine (43%) developed varying degrees of heart block.

162

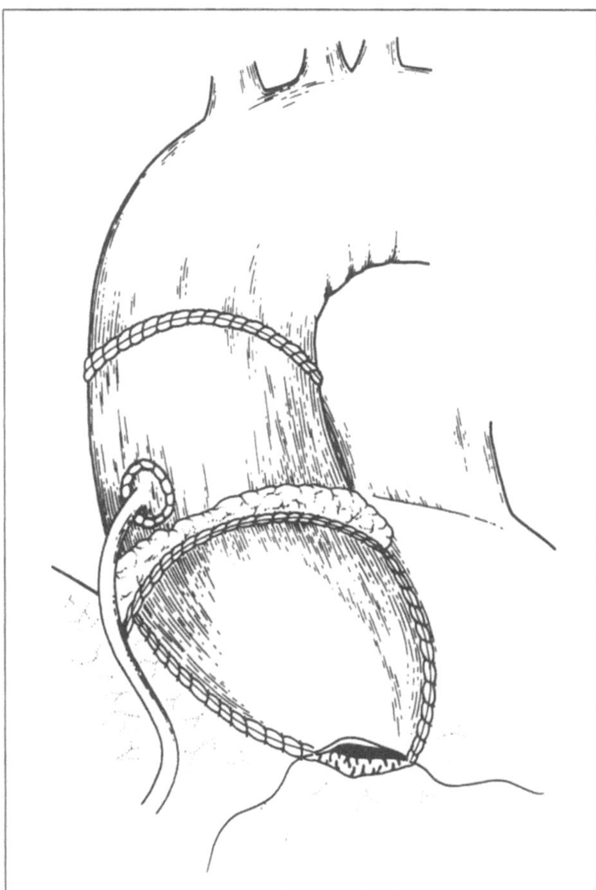

Table 2. Complications following extended aortic root replacement.

Transient heart block	3
Postpericardiotomy syndrome	2
Reoperation for bleeding	2
Reoperation for hyperlipidemia complications	1
Serratia marcescens mediastinitis	1
Superficial wound infection	1
Incisional ventral hernia	1
Right phrenic palsey	1
No complications	2

Ross (9) used allograft aortic root replacement and coronary reimplantation to treat complex LVOTO in a series of 26 patients operated on between 1976 and 1980. The technique involves extensive excision of subvalvular tissue, thus placing in jeopardy the anterior leaflet of the mitral valve and atrioventricular conduction tissue. Fifteen

163

percent of patients who underwent this form of treatment experienced permanent postsurgical heart block.

EARR allows placement of an adult size aortic valve in most children and offers an alternative to aortic valve replacement in infants too small to accept the smallest prosthesis, even with aortoventriculoplasty. EARR also avoids the problems inherent in aortoventriculoplasty since a mechanical valve and therefore anticoagulation are avoided. In addition, infectious complications may be less devastating, as indicated by the single patient in this series. Obviation of the need for extensive subvalvular resection greatly lessens the risk of damage to structures surrounding the left ventricular outflow tract. All of the patients in this series have remained in normal sinus rhythm since hospital discharge.

Long-term follow-up of "fresh" aortic allografts appears promising. Thompson (11) reported 4-year follow-up of 411 patients, of which 24 (5.9%) experienced valve failure and another 24 had additional valve-related complications. The fact that allograft failure occurred only in valves procured from donors older than 65 is noteworthy. Postoperative aortic diastolic murmurs were commonly noted, but did not increase over time. Another series of 140 "fresh" isolated allograft aortic valve replacements was analysed by Penta (6) who revealed a 5-year failure rate of 10%. More recently, O'Brien (5) has indicated the superiority of cryopreserved aortic allografts. In a series of 308 allograft aortic valve replacement patients (124 fresh "nonviable" and 184 cryopreserved "viable"), comparative follow-up at 10 years after implantation was analysed actuarially. Patients who received fresh allografts showed 73 % freedom from all valve-related complications, while those with cryopreserved valves were 92% free of problems.

Conclusion

Extended aortic root replacement appears to be a valuable surgical technique for the treatment of complex LVOTO. Advantages over other procedures include: (1) EARR is effective in dealing with cases of LVOTO complicated by subvalvular aortic stenosis or a hypoplastic annulus in which aortic valve replacement is required. (2) A larger, often adult size, aortic valve may be implanted in children by enlarging the annulus. (3) The technique avoids complications and disadvantages inherent in aortoventriculoplasty by avoiding the use of mechanical prostheses and anticoagulation in children. (4) EARR obviates the need for extensive damaging subvalvular resection. (5) Cryopreserved allografts which are antibiotically sterilized appear to be superior to allografts preserved by other methods.

In our limited but promising experience, we have seen excellent clinical results following EARR. We therefore recommend the procedure for patients with complex LVOTO.

References

1. Cain T, Campbell D, Paton B, Clarke D (1984) Operation for discrete subvalvular aortic stenosis. J Thorac Cardiovasc Surg 87: 366

1a. Clarke DR (1987) J Cardiac Surg 1, Suppl 3: 121–128
2. Donaldson RM, Ross DM (1984) Homograft aortic root replacement for complicated prosthetic valve endocarditis. Circulation 70: I–178
3. Kono S, Imai Y, Iida Y, et al (1975) A new method for prosthetic valve replacement in congential aortic stenosis associated with hypoplasia of the aortic valve ring. J Thorac Cardiovasc Surg 70: 909
4. Moses RD, Barnhart GR, Jones M (1984) The late prognosis after localized resection for fixed (discrete and tunnel) left ventricular outflow tract obstruction. J Thorac Cardiovasc Surg 87: 410
5. O'Brien MF, Stafford EG, Gardner MAH, et al. (1987) A comparison of aortic valve replacement with viable cryopreserved and fresh allograft valves with a note on chromosomal studies. J Thorac Cardiovasc Surg (in press)
6. Penta A, Qureshi S, Radley-Smith R, Yacoub MH (1984) Patient status 10 or more years after "fresh" homograft replacement of the aortic valve. Circulation 70: I-182
7. Rastan H, Abu-Aishah N, Rastan D, et al (1978) Results of aortoventriculoplasty in 21 consecutive patients with left ventricular outflow tract obstruction. J Thorac Cardiovasc Surg 75: 659
8. Rastan H, Koncz J (1976) A new technique for the treatment of left ventricular outflow tract obstruction. J Thorac Cardiovasc Surg 71: 920
9. Somerville J, Ross D (1982) Homograft replacement of aortic root with reimplantation of coronary arteries. Br Heart J 47: 473
10. Somerville J, Stone S, Ross D (1980) Fate of patients with fixed subaortic stenosis after surgical removal. Br Heart J 43: 629
11. Thompson R, Yacoub M, Ahmed M, et al (1980) The use of "fresh" unstented homograft valves for replacement of the aortic valve. J Thorac Cardiovasc Surg 79: 896

Author's address:
David R. Clarke, M.D.
Chief, Cardiovascular and Thoracic Surgery
The Childrens Hospital
1056 East 19th Avenue
Denver, Colorado 80218
U.S.A.

Aortic root replacement with a cardiac allograft: The infected aortic root

D. N. Ross

The National Heart Hospital, London, U.K.

The aortic valve continues to be the most commonly affected in both native endo-carditis and the post-prosthetic variety. The chief surgically treatable complication of native endocarditis is valve regurgitation and the onset of ventricular failure during treatment is the usual indication for surgical intervention.

Post-prosthetic endocarditis is more insidious in onset and with an organism of low virulence, like Staphylococcus epidermidis, the course of the disease is likely to be complicated by burrowing root abscesses particularly around the aortic ring (Fig. 1).

The resulting abscesses of the aortic root pose severe anatomical and therapeutic problems, not the least of which is the fact that there have usually been preceding operations.

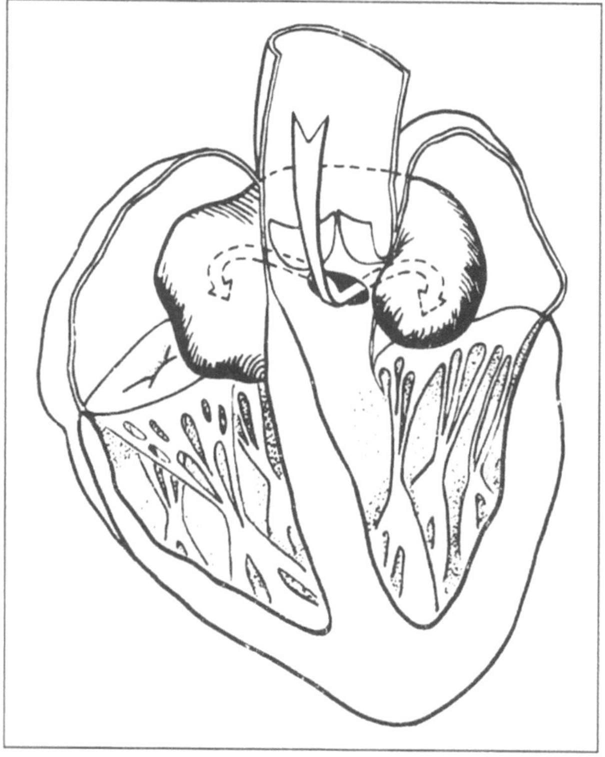

Fig. 1. The commonly found aortic root abscess starting in the anterior mitral valve cusp.

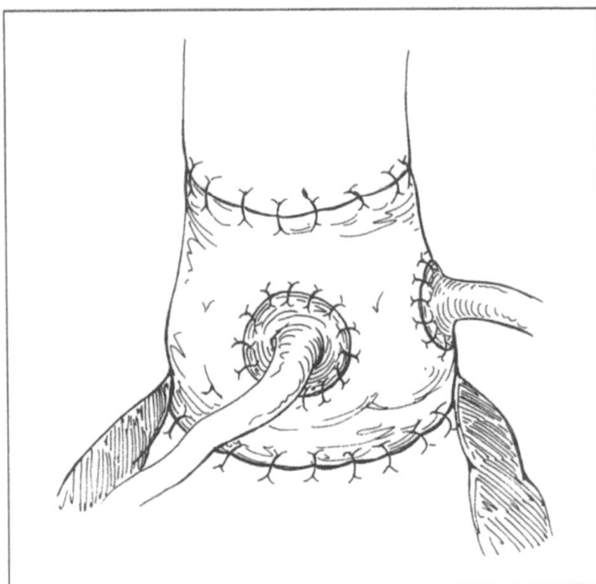

Fig. 2. Root replacement with an antibiotic-sterilised homograft. The coronary arteries have been re-implanted.

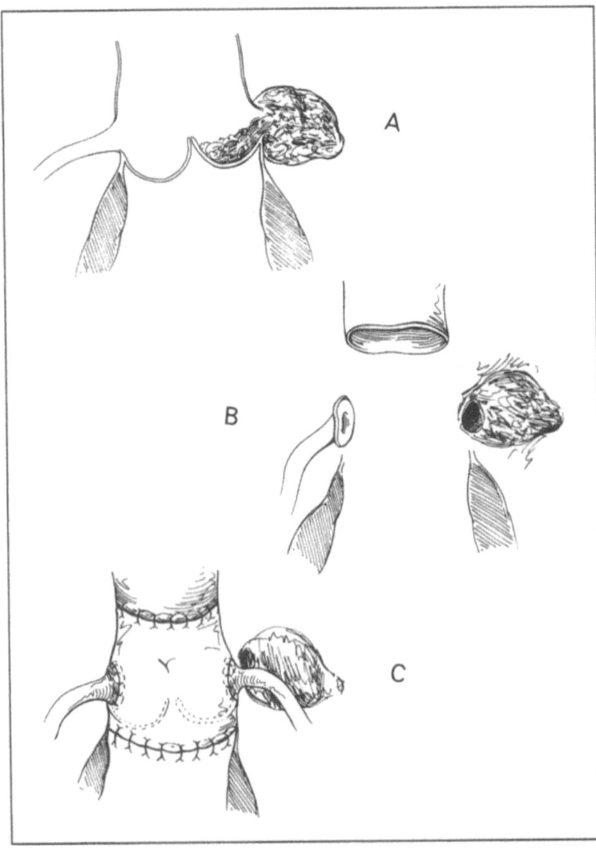

Fig. 3. The infected root is excised down to healthy tissue allowing the abscess cavities to drain into the mediastinum.

On more than one occasion there has been complete separation of the aorta and left ventricle within an abscess cavity over a distance of about 6 cm.

Operations designed simply to replace the infected valve or prosthesis plus local debridement are likely to fail due to the persistence of residual infected material retained within the circulation. To exclude such material from the blood stream and to debride the annulus effectively usually involves excision of the whole aortic root and its replacement with a homograft root (Fig. 2).

The primary aim of homograft root replacement is therefore to exclude all infected material from the circulation and to allow free drainage of abscess cavities and infected material into the mediastinum. The secondary aim is to replace the valve with antibiotic-impregnated tissue, resistant to infection and one which exudes antibiotics into the surrounding tissues during the immediate post-operative period.

The operation has followed the general principles of homograft aortic root replacement which we have practised since 1972 when a totally destroyed root embedded in pus was replaced with a homograft. The operation was subsequently developed primarily for enlargement of the small tunnel type aortic root (3) and we have now returned to its application in root abscess (1, 2).

In infected cases, the general plan is to excise the whole root including the valve and its immediate supra- and subvalvar structures leaving the well-mobilised coronaries attached to buttons of aortic wall. Abscess cavities are opened fully and infected tissue is excised so as to expose a healthy viable sewing margin (Fig. 3).

An adult-sized antibiotic-sterilised homograft is then fixed in place in the aortic root attaching it in a corresponding exact anatomical position with multiple interrupted 4/0 sutures. The anterior mitral cusp of the homograft can be used to make good the commonly found destruction of the recipient mitral leaflet.

The left coronary is attached first, then the upper suture line is completed before the right coronary is attached to an appropriate position anteriorly on the homograft.

A total of 120 aortic homograft roots have been inserted over the past 15 years. There has been an average of 2.2 previous surgical operations per case or previous surgery in 78% of patients (Table 1).

The overall hospital mortality has been 19.1%, but significantly among the patients not having previous surgery the mortality is zero.

Overall survival for root replacement at 10 years is 72% with 88% freedom from infective endocarditis. As with most homografts, tissue failure first becomes apparent around 7 years (Fig. 4).

Table 1. Aortic root replacement (homograft).

	Cases	Deaths
Hypoplastic tunnel obstr.	42	6
Small aortic annulus	17	3
Endocarditis and root abscess	33	10
Calcified root	28	4
	120	23

Previous ops: 78%; overall mortality: 19.1% (no prev. op.-zero).

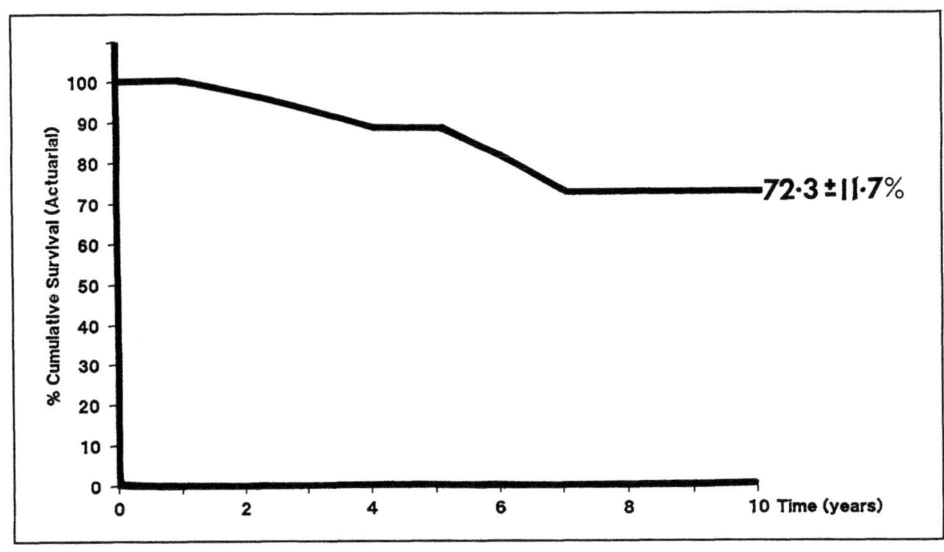

Fig. 4. Homograft aortic root replacement: overall survival.

47 patients have had antibiotic-preserved homografts for infective endocarditis of the aortic valve and 33 of these had total root replacement. There were 12 deaths and ten of these were in the root replacement group (30%). All the root replacements had extensive abscesses, considerable toxicity and at least two, and up to four previous operations. Two late deaths occurred at $6\frac{1}{2}$ and 10 years.

Table 2. Infected aortic root.

Homograft	14
Homograft root	33
	47

10 Deaths
  2 Late deaths ($6\frac{1}{2}$ and 10 years)   } root replacement
  1 Recurrent endocarditis (richettsia)

There has been only one case of recurrence of the endocarditis and that was due to undiagnosed rickettsial disease. The patient was subsequently successfully re-operated upon with a further root replacement.

Although the mortality is high, the disease is a chronic and intractible one. We are encouraged to continue to use root replacement in post-prosthetic endocarditis by the overall good results of homografts roots in general, the absence of recurrent infection, apart from the one rickettsial case, and the prospect of a low or zero mortality where there has been no previous surgery. These considerations underline the need for early surgery in post-prosthetic endocarditis.

170

References

1. Donaldson RM, Ross DN (1982) Homograft aortic root replacement for complicated prosthetic valve endocarditis. Circulation 70 (Suppl 1): 178—182
2. Lau JKH, Robles A, Cherian A, Ross DN (1984) Surgical treatment of prosthetic endocarditis. Aortic root replacement using a homograft. J Thorac Cardiovasc Surg 87: 712—716
3. Somerville J, Ross DN (1988) Homograft replacement of aortic root with re-implantation of coronary arteries. Br Heart J 47: 473—482

Author's address:
Donald N. Ross
The National Heart Hospital
Westmoreland Street
London W1
U.K.

Indications and surgical technique of aortic valve replacement with the autologous pulmonary valve

L. Gonzalez-Lavin, D. Graf, D. N. Ross

Introduction

The pulmonary valve has been utilized to replace the diseased aortic valve since 1967 by Donald Ross and associates at the National Heart Hospital in London. This approach stemmed from the experimental work Lower and associates, indicating the possibility of using the autologous pulmonary valve for aortic or mitral valve replacement. Ross reported the first clinical trial in 1967 and since that time over 250 patients have undergone this operation. Based on this experience, as well as a limited experience from Gonzalez-Lavin, the indications and surgical technique for this procedure are described.

Indications

The indications for aortic valve replacement with the autologous pulmonary valve have been expanding throughout the last two decades. Originally, it was recommended for young patients with isolated aortic valve replacement; however, as experience with the technique increased, patients in the sixth decade of life with isolated aortic valve disease were accepted and more recently young patients in the hope that the valve will grow with the patient. Initially the presence of multi-valve

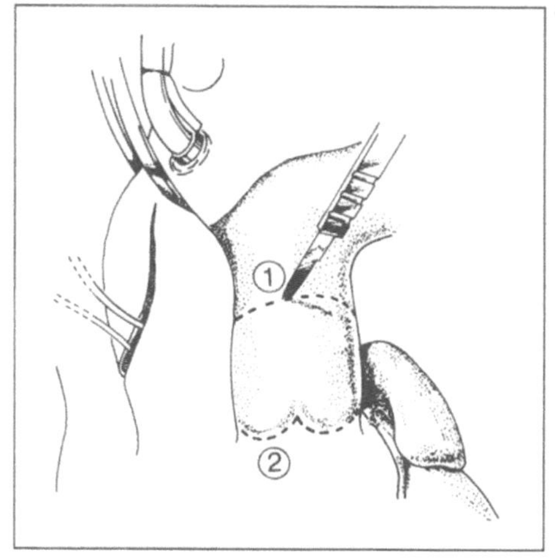

Fig. 1. Step 1 and 2

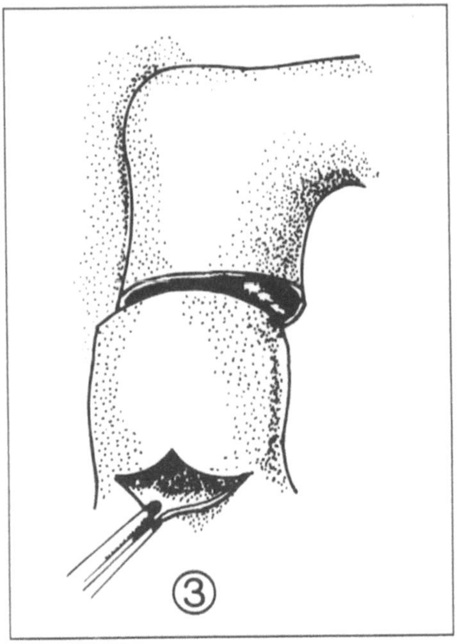

Fig. 2. Step 3

involvement was a contra-indication. More recently, however, following conservative mitral valve repair rather than replacement, the indication for this operation has been extended to suitable patients having aortic and mitral valve disease. Contra-indications for this operation are elderly patients with multi-valvular disease as well as associated coronary artery disease, due to the fact that the length of the surgical procedure would probably increase operative morbidity and mortality.

The pre-operative evaluation of patients selected to have this procedure should consist of routine pre-operative measures; with 2-D echo to measure the annulus of the pulmonary artery and compare the size with that of the aortic annulus. Use of this study has not been well documented; however, from experience there is rarely a severe disparity between the size of the pulmonary and aortic annulus. It is important to have coronary arteriography in patients over 40 years of age to exclude coronary artery disease. A left ventriculogram and an aortogram are indispensable invasive studies in the preparation and pre-operative evaluation of these patients.

Surgical technique (Steps 1—13)

The chest is opened through a midline sternotomy and routine cannulation of the heart is performed. A single RA cannulation is adequate in most cases. After heparinisation (2 mg/kg) bypass is started and the ascending aorta is opened vertically and both coronary orifices are cannulated.

174

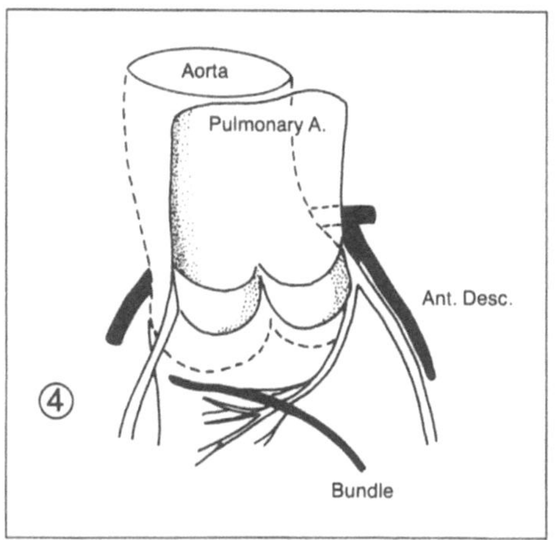

Fig. 3. Step 4

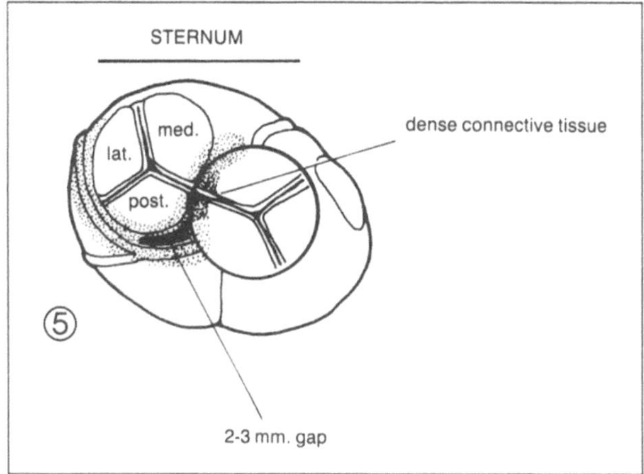

Fig. 4. Step 5

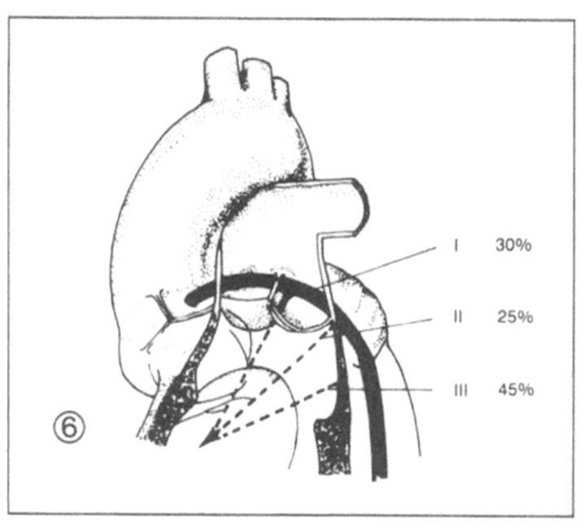

Fig. 5. Step 6

175

With the coronaries perfusing it is easy to avoid damaging a major coronary branch. Dissection of the pulmonary artery from the aorta is performed by sharp scissors dissection and all bleeding points are controlled using a low-current cautery.

The pulmonary artery is first transected and dissected from above down till RV muscle is visible along the posterior margin of the dissection. After freeing the posterior wall, a short incision is now made in the anterior right ventricle wall just below the valve sinuses as seen from within the PA. This incision is continued transversely across the RV outflow just below the sinuses. The pulmonary valve is now enucleated carefully from the muscle taking care to avoid the first septal branch of the left anterior descending coronary artery. The excised autograft is then allowed to rest in the pericardial cavity immersed in blood.

The aortic valve is now excised and coronary perfusion can be continued, but it is more convenient at this stage to have a bloodless field and a cardioplegic solution, preferably blood cardioplegia, is used. The first dose contains 20 millequivalents of potassium and subsequent doses only 5 mEq potassium per litre. A thermistor probe is placed at the apex near the septum and the myocardial temperature is measured in that area, which is usually between 10° and 12°C. The use of topical cold saline or even slush is added. Any residual calcium in the aortic ring should now be removed.

Attention is now directed to the RV outflow tract which is reconstituted either with an aortic or pulmonary homograft. Nowadays a pulmonary homograft is used electively.

The muscle bed of the excised right ventricular area is inspected for bleeding and any residual bleeding points are again treated with diathermy.

Any excess muscle on the pulmonary homograft is trimmed leaving about 2—3 mm attached to the base of the leaflets to use for the lower suture line. The homograft

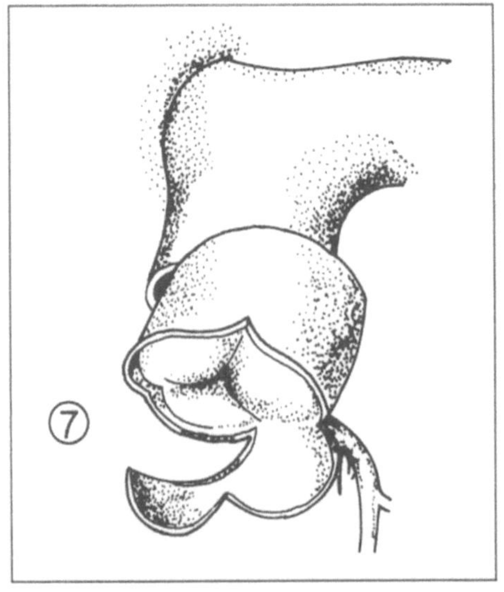

Fig. 6. Step 7

176

is oriented in such a way that the posterior cusp and sinus will match exactly with that of the excised posterior cusp of the pulmonary valve. After orienting the homograft in this manner, the distal suture line is placed with a continuous over and over stitch of 4-0 polypropylene attaching the upper part of the aortic homograft to the native pulmonary artery including the adventitia of this vessel (Step 8).

The suture line starts posteriorly in the midline and is continued to right and left, until they meet anteriorly. It is advisable to interrupt this suture line with a locking stitch at least twice to prevent a pursestring effect.

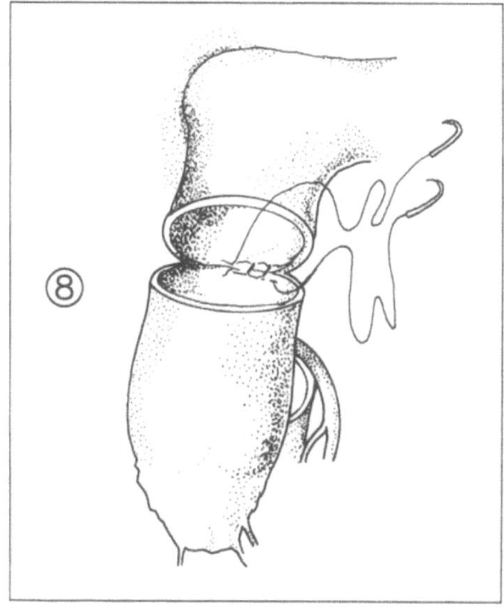

Fig. 7. Step 8

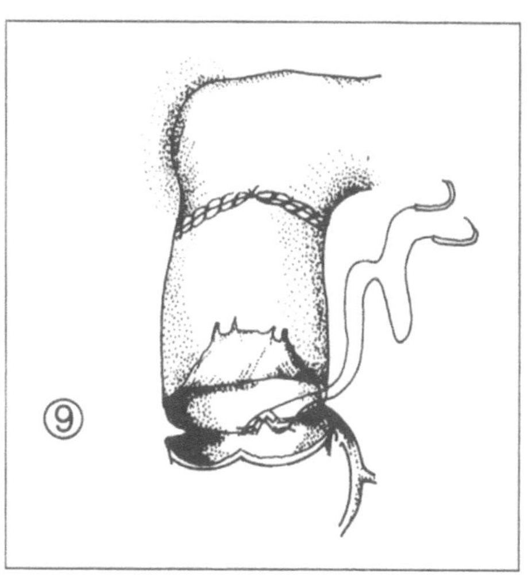

Fig. 8. Step 9

The proximal suture line which joins the right ventricular outflow tract is begun by reorienting the valve and the aortic sinuses of the homograft to the bed of the pulmonary valve as it lay in the right ventricular outflow tract. This suture line starts in the posterior rim and is run proximally towards the surgeon in the first instance and locked in order to take all tension off of the more vulnerable distally-placed segment of suture line. This further lessens the danger to the septal coronary artery.

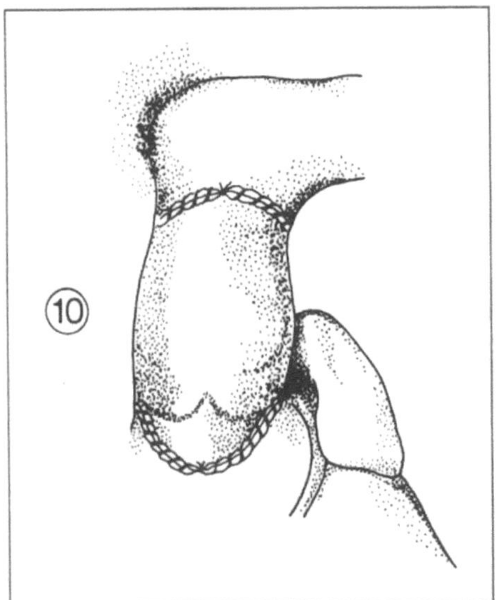

Fig. 9. Step 10

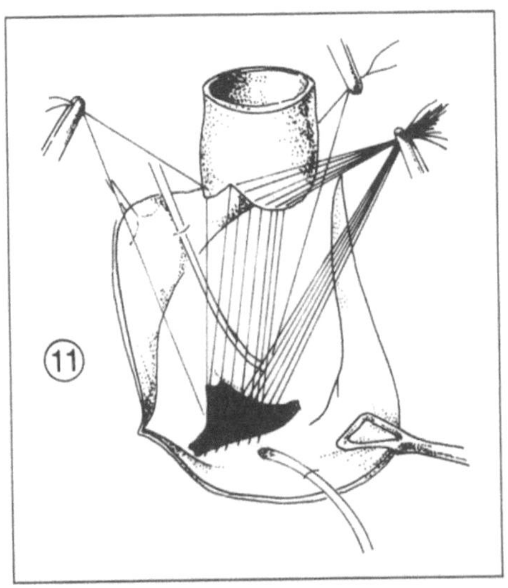

Fig. 10. Step 11

The pulmonary valve autograft is then inserted into the aortic root with two suture lines. Interrupted 4/0 sutures are used for the lower suture line and a continuous running suture is used above after suspending the commissures with three 3/0 mattress sutures (Steps 12 and 13).

The lower interrupted suture line is placed horizontally between the lower margins of the excised aortic valve and not following the scalloped line of the excised valve (as indicated in Step 11). The suspending sutures of 3/0 Prolene are placed slightly above the point of attachment of the commissures and are under moderate tension. This is an important point in achieving a competent valve. The wall of the pulmonary artery is then tailored and scalloped to avoid the right and left coronary orifices (Step 12).

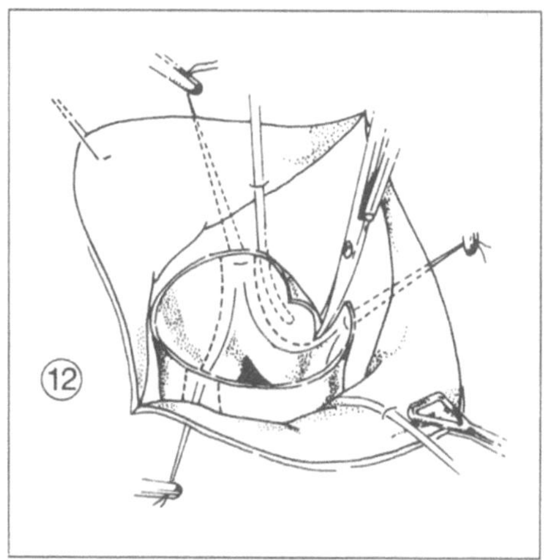

Fig. 11. Step 12

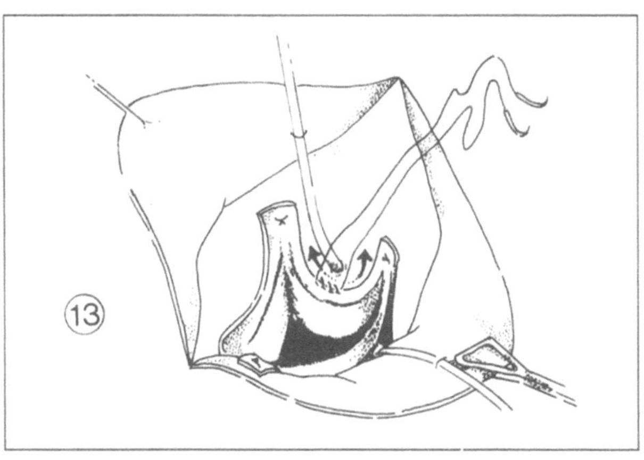

Fig. 12. Step 13

The non-coronary sinus is not scalloped but is incorporated in the closure of the aortotomy helping to ensure that there will be no leak and maintaining the spatial relationships of the adjacent commissures.

On coming off cardiopulmonary bypass, the diastolic pressure is measured and the closing shock of the valve can be felt within the surgeon's index finger. Additional evidence of valve competence is assessed by noting whether there is a drop of perfusion pressure on opening the aortic closing and by noting whether there is a leak of blood from the apical needle used to aspirate air.

It is also wise when coming off bypass cardiopulmonary bypass, to make sure that there is no bleeding from the right ventricular suture lines which are otherwise difficult to secure once bypass has been discontinued.

Authors' address:
Lorenzo Gonzalez-Lavin, M.D.
Chairman, Department of Surgery
Deborah Heart and Lung Center
Brown Mills
New Jersey 08015
U.S.A.

The morphology of tricuspid atresia, pulmonary atresia and truncus arteriosus

S. P. Allwork

Department of Surgery, Royal Postgraduate Medical School, Hammersmith Hospital, London, U.K.

Tricuspid atresia

Tricuspid atresia is an abnormal mode of atrioventricular connection characterised by absence of both the valve and the valve ring. It is generally considered to represent part of the spectrum of univentricular heart.

The right atrium is dilated and there is always an interatrial communication. Both systemic and pulmonary venous connection are usually normal but a left SVC entering the coronary sinus may aggravate dilatation of the right atrium. The chamber beneath the right atrium is in variable size but the morphology is readily identifiable as that of the trabecular and smooth outflow portions of the right ventricle, but the inlet portion, carrying the tricuspid valve, is not represented. This chamber communicates with the morphologically normal left ventricle through a foramen of variable size. This opening is often called a defect of the ventricular septum (VSD), but it is usually the remnant of the embryonic interventricular foramen. This foramen is placed either low in the chamber, at the junction of the trabecular and infundibular musculature, or it may be situated close to the arterial outlet. In either case the foramen may reduce in size or close altogether.

Both obstruction of the outlet and anomalies of ventriculoarterial connection occur with some frequency. In a series of 31 examples studied by the author (1), only 9 had normal ventriculoarterial connection; pulmonary stenosis or atresia occured in 18 and arterial transposition in nine, while malposition was associated in a further three hearts. (In the remainder there was either no "outlet chamber" or truncus arteriosus was associated.)

Coarctation of the aorta and/or valvar aortic stenosis occurred in six of the hearts with transposition, while patency of the ductus arteriosus was present in most of the hearts.

A rare type of tricuspid atresia is exemplified when the valve is present but imperforate. In such hearts all the elements of the right ventricle (inlet, trabecular and outlet zones), are present and indeed the right ventricle may be of normal size, although it is usually small and dysplastic. Pulmonary outflow tract obstruction and anomalies of arterial connection and position are rare.

Pulmonary atresia

Pulmonary atresia is expressed in a spectrum of anomalies ranging from an imperforate valve in an otherwise normal heart to that state in which the only mode of supply to the lungs is by way of a collateral circulation originating from elaborated intersegmental arteries arising from the descending aorta.

The conditions occurs in both intact ventricular septum and in the presence of VSD but there are striking morphological differences between the two groups.

Pulmonary atresia with intact ventricular septum

This anomaly is usually divided into two groups, those with a poorly-developed right ventricle (Type 1) and those with a well-developed right ventricle (Type 2). Type 1 is more common although the malformation is a continuum from Type 2 to Type 1, so that the severity of the disease is variable (2).

Type 1: Large intramyocardial sinusoids can usually be demonstrated in hearts with hypoplastic right ventricles, irrespective of the severity of the lesion (which is variable), suggesting that the maldevelopment occurred early in organogenesis (2, 3).

Type 2: Those with Type 2 (well-developed right ventricle), have a well-developed, sometimes quite large pulmonary valve which is imperforate, indicating that the anomaly occurred late in organogenesis. Persistent patency of the ductus arteriosus occurs in both types, but anastomotic collateral channels, for example by way of enlarged bronchial arteries or vessels from the descending aorta, are not found in pulmonary atresia with intact ventricular septum.

Pulmonary atresia with VSD

VSD: In pulmonary atresia with VSD the defect is usually of the "perimembranous/ malalignment" type when the infundibulum, albeit atretic, is recognised in its normal anterior position and a thread-like pulmonary artery is confluent with recognisable left and right pulmonary arteries.

In the much rarer hearts (usually with atrioventricular discordance), in which the atretic outflow tract and pulmonary artery are posteriorly placed, the VSD is of the infundibular muscular kind and lies subjacent to the anteriorly placed aorta.

The ductus arteriosus: Where the atretic main pulmonary artery is confluent with left and right pulmonary arteries these are supplied by a ductus arteriosus. If the left and right branches are hypoplastic the duct may be absent, in which case pulmonary blood supply is by way of tortuous systemic arteries originating from the descending aorta. Uncommonly, one lung may be supplied by systemic collaterals while the other takes its supply from an ipsilateral duct. The two modes do not coexist in the same lung (5).

The collateral blood supply: The major aorticopulmonary collateral arteries, two or three in number, originate from the descending aorta close to the inferior margin of the left main bronchus when the aortic arch is left-sided, and immediately below and to the right of the carina when the aorta arches to the right (6).

(These vessels are sometimes referred to as "bronchial" arteries (7), which is both inaccurate and confusing. The bronchial arteries are constant in position (close together and immediately proximal to the first pair of intercostal arteries), and are always to be found in normal individuals. The collateral supply is derived from the

182

primitive intersegmental branches of the paired dorsal aortae of the embryo which supplied the lung buds [8, 9].)

Other sites of origin of collateral arteries are the underside of the aortic arch and the proximal parts of the brachiocephalic arteries as well as the aorta below the diaphragm (7).

Truncus arteriosus

There is some confusion between Collet & Edwards type IV truncus arteriosus and pulmonary atresia with VSD (10, 11), but the two are distinguishable.

As Thiene et al. have stated (5), it is mandatory to discriminate between atresia and agenesis of an artery. Where the embryonic sixth arch arteries (the ductuus arteriosi), do not develop (agenesis), there is no anatomical arterial connection between the heart and the lungs. When a fibrous cord connects the two there is anatomical evidence that there had been a distal sixth arch in the past (atresia).

Pulmonary atresia with VSD represents exaggerated malseptation of the cardiac outflow tract at the expense of the pulmonary artery, whereas in truncus arteriosus the outflow is unseptated. It has been postulated that non-septation of the cardiac outflow tract may make redundant the establishment of a (second) connection between the ventral and dorsal aortae (i.e. the growth of the distal sixth arches, the ductuus arteriosi). This sequence of ontogenic events determines that the intersegmental arteries (the first connection) persist, thus becoming the sole arterial supply to the lungs (5).

The morphology of truncus arteriosus

Truncus arteriosus is that condition in which the coronary, pulmonary and systemic arteries arise from a common source. In the light of the foregoing paragraphs we may add that no derivatives of the sixth arch arteries (the ductuus arteriosi), are to be identified within the pericardial cavity.

There is always an interventricular communication and it is always pear-shaped, outlining the absent infundibular septum. The semilunar valve of the trunk overrides the VSD (or, more precisely, the absent septum), and is itself often abnormal. The truncal valve may be bi- or quadricuspid, stenotic, regurgitant or both. Anomalies of the coronary arteries, especially single coronary artery, occur with some frequency. The single artery may arise from either sinus in the case of a two-leaflet valve, but in three- or four-leaflet valves the "non-coronary" sinus tends to be the most anterior.

The origin of the pulmonary arteries is variable, but with the exception considered above, these always spring from the trunk, usually from the proximal, ascending portion.

References

1. Allwork SP (1979) The univentricular heart in man: A comparative and morphological study. PhD Thesis, University of London

2. Davignon AL, Greenwold WE, DuShane JW, Edwards JE (1961) Congenital pulmonary atresia with intact ventricular septum. Clinicopathologic correlation of two anatomic types. Am H J 62: 591—602

3. Lauer RM, Fink HP, Pery EL, Dunn MI, Diehl AM (1964) Angiographic demonstration of intramyocardial sinusoids in pulmonary atresia with intact ventricular septum and hypoplastic right ventricle. New Engl J Med 271: 68—72

4. Gersony WM, Bernhard WF, Nadas AS, Gross RE (1967) Diagnosis and surgical treatment of infants with critical pulmonary outflow obstruction. Circulation 35: 765—776

5. Theine G, Bortolotti U, Gallucci V, Valenta ML, Dalla Volta S (1977) Pulmonary atresia with ventricular septal defect. Further anatomical observations. Br Heart J 39: 1223—1233

6. Haworth SG, Macartney FJ (1980) Growth and development of pulmonary circulation in pulmonary atresia with ventricular defect and major aortopulmonary collateral arteries. Br Heart J 44: 14—24

7. McGoon DC, Baird DK, Davis GD (1975) Surgical management of large bronchial collateral arteries with pulmonary stenosis or atresia. Circulation 52: 109—118

8. Congdon ED (1922) Transformation of the aortic arch system during the development of the human embryo. Contrib Embryol (Carnegie Institute) 14: 47—110

9. Boyden EA (1970) The time lag in the development of the bronchial arteries. Anat Rec 166: 611—614

10. Taussig HB, Momberger N, Kink H (1973) Long-time observations on the Blalock-Taussig operation. VI, Truncus Arteriosus Type IV. Johns Hopkins Med J 133: 123—147

11. Stockey D, Bowdler JD, Reye RDK (1968) Absent sixth aortic arch; a form of pulmonary atresia. Br Heart J 30: 258—264

Author's address:
Sally P. Allwork
Department of Surgery
Royal Postgraduate Medical School
Hammersmith Hospital
Ducane Road
London W12 OHS
U.K.

Population-based requirements for allograft surgery in children

J. T. Davis, F. A. Baciewicz Jr., R. Ehrlich, J. Hennessy, M. Levine

Medical College of Ohio at Toledo, Toledo, Ohio, U.S.A.

This paper will attempt to set into perspective the magnitude of the problem of homograft procurement for the paediatric population. We thought it would be useful to have an estimate of how many homografts and of what size might be required for a given population. While we cannot speak of the use of homografts for aortic valve replacement in the adult population, we are able to speak of the potential use of this tissue in the paediatric age group.

This paper will present a retrospective review of 575 consecutive paediatric open-heart procedures over 8.5 years, for the purpose of estimating requirements for homografts in a defined population. At the Medical College of Ohio at Toledo, we have only recently begun using homografts in our congenital heart program. However, it was possible, in reviewing our series, to select out those cases in which xenografts or mechanical valves were used; and, with certain assumptions, decide whether a homograft would have been employed, given current indications.

Such a study in our type of service area could be useful because of its clear definition and known population of 1.2 million people. We serve a 20-county area of Northwest Ohio. To the north and west are state lines which, while not inviolate, do form relatively unchanging lines of demarcation. Well-defined and stable referral patterns separate us from the areas served by the programs ot our south and east. Because of these factors, only a few cases are transferred out of or into our area for surgical care. Therefore, our caseload is not terribly skewed by referral patterns, but rather represents a reasonable approximation of the incidence and prevalence of surgical disease in the area. Therefore, we believe that the homograft requirements for our population could be extrapolated to other regions to estimate the needs of a given geographical area based on its population. It would seem that such approximate requirements might be useful in estimating procurement needs as well as forming a rational base for regional distribution or local stockpiling.

Figure 1 shows our surgical caseload over the years of the study and is simply intended to show a reasonably steady state after the starting up period. The slight recent decline reflects the cardiologist's use of balloons where operations would have been done previously. This should not influence homograft requirements.

Table 1 lists the procedures which, in retrospect, would have been performed using homografts at present. This group represents 5.2 % of our total paediatric open heart procedures. We assumed that a homograft would be the conduit of choice for right ventricular outflow reconstruction and listed those cases where a porcine xenograft had been used.

Severe tetralogy of Fallot requiring a Rastelli procedure was the most common. Four cases of recurrent left ventricular outflow obstruction had been treated by a Konno procedure or an apical aortic shunt. We currently would employ an extended aortic

""

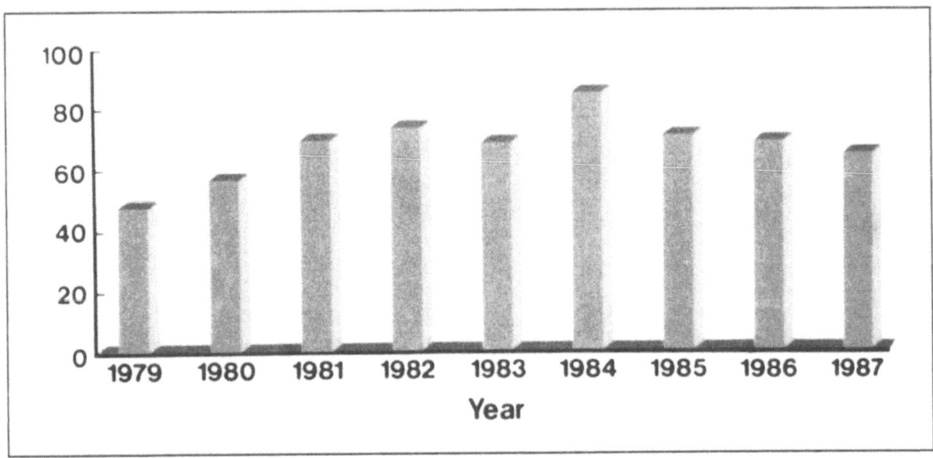

Fig. 1. Surgical caseload for paediatric open heart surgery.

Table 1. Procedures which would have required homografts (see text).

Tetralogy of Fallot	5
Recurrent LV Outflow Obstruction	4
Truncus Arteriosus	4
Truncus Arteriosus/Interrupted Arch	2
Double Outlet Right Ventricle	3
Pulmonary Atresia/VSD	2
Transposition Great Vessels/Subpulmonic Stenosis	2
L-Transposition Great Vessels/Subpulmonic Stenosis	2
Conduit Replacement	6
Total	30

root replacement with a homograft for this purpose. Truncus arteriosus, with or without interrupted aortic arch, was another common indication, mostly in infancy. Double outlet right ventricle, pulmonary atresia with VSD, and the transposition family of defects make up the rest of the primary procedures. Finally, conduit replacements were undertaken in cases of outgrown or obstructed conduits. We excluded a number of cases where conduits had been used as part of a Fontan procedure, since we currently do not employ conduits in this position but prefer direct anastomosis.

We catalogued the sizes of conduits used, thinking that this might give us an indication of what size homografts would be most useful. Figure 2 plots the sizes used against the year. It is not surprising that larger sizes were needed in later years as we moved into the stage of replacing conduits in children originally operated as infants. A baseline requirement for smaller conduits seems to continue through the years, as expected, mostly for infant truncus repairs.

Therefore, over 8.5 years, a total of 30 procedures were performed in which homografts would have been used given current indications. This equals 2.9 homografts per year per million person population base, and we feel represents the underlying needs of the paediatric population. This requirement would be increased in pro-

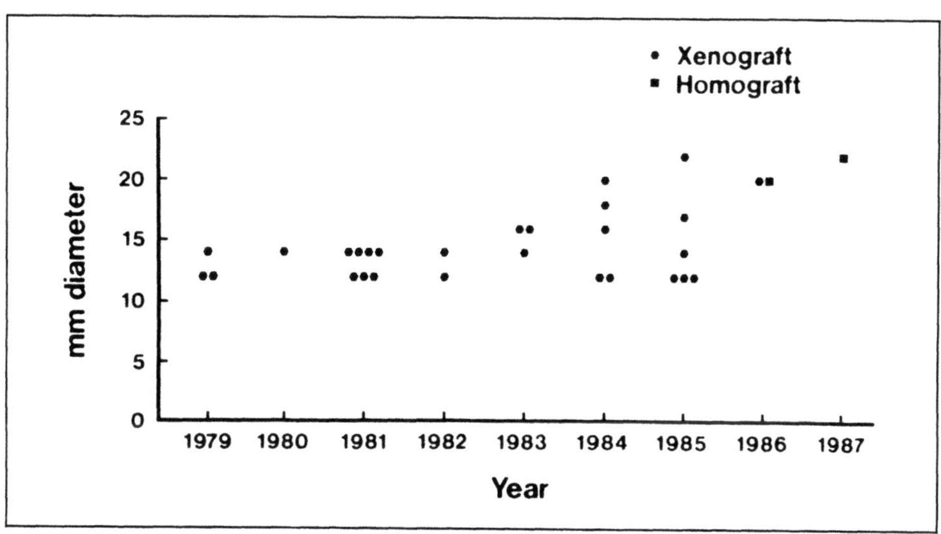

Fig. 2. Diameter of conduits used by year (outer diameter for xenografts; inner diameter for homografts).

grams where large numbers of patients are referred for care. In addition, this number does not take into account the utilization of homografts for aortic valve replacement in the adult population. It is also apparent that larger size homografts were more frequently required as our program matured. It is realized, of course, that indications will vary with time and among surgeons. This data, therefore, is presented only for interest and as a baseline to assess developing needs.

Authors' address:
J. T. Davis, M.D.
Medical College of Ohio at Toledo
Department of Surgery
C.S. 10008
Toledo, Ohio 43699
U.S.A.

The pulmonary allograft for right ventricular outflow tract reconstruction

P. H. Kay, U. Livi, R. Parker, D. N. Ross

The National Heart Hospital, London, U.K.

Introduction

In 1966, Ross and Somerville (14) pioneered the use of the aortic allograft for right ventricular outflow tract reconstruction. Excellent results have been reported by several authors (2, 4, 6, 7) who stress the advantages of antibiotic sterilised allografts over porcine valve conduits (10, 16). Indeed, in our own series only 13% patients required conduit replacement for obstruction at 10 years (7).

In addition, we have used the aortic allograft for right ventricular outflow tract reconstruction in adult patients with aortic valve disease who have undergone aortic valve replacement using a pulmonary autograft. Again results in this group have been excellent with 19% patients requiring further right ventricular outflow reconstruction for allograft dysfunction at 10 years (13).

However, despite these excellent results, the aortic allograft has several disadvantages. Approximately 20% aortic allografts are imperfect and have to be discarded. Furthermore, the thick arterial wall is prone to early calcification (15). These limitations led us to consider the pulmonary allograft as a possible and perhaps superior alternative.

We have performed experimental studies to compare the morphology and viability of aortic and pulmonary allografts (9). As a result of these studies, we now prefer to use a pulmonary allograft and present our initial clinical results.

Experimental studies

Aortic and pulmonary allografts were harvested from ten cadaveric hearts within 60 h of death. Morphometric measurements of diameter at both the level of the valve ring and the trunk were made, together with wall thickness.

Three samples of aortic and pulmonary walls were taken at the time of dissection and after 2 and 4 weeks of storage in nutrient antibiotic solution (1). An assessment of viability was made using the tritiated thymidine autoradiographic technique described by Al Janabi (1). Calcium content was measured by single beam atomic absorption spectrometry (9). The third samples were fixed in 10% neutral buffered formalin, processed in paraffin wax and sectioned at 5 μm. These were then stained with haematoxylin-eosin and Miller's elastic van Gieson method to highlight any differences in collagen and elastin content (8).

Patients and methods

The first pulmonary allograft was inserted in July 1983. Since that time, 51 pulmonary allografts have been used for right ventricular outflow reconstruction.

Congenital lesions

21 patients with cyanotic congenital heart disease underwent right ventricular out-flow reconstruction using a pulmonary allograft (11). 15 patients had pulmonary atresia, two Fallot's tetralogy, two transposition of the great arteries and two tricuspid atresia. In 11 cases (six pulmonary atresia, two Fallot, one transposition, two Fontan) the operation was to replace a previously calcified and obstructed aortic allograft. The mean age of the patients was 20 years (range 1—40 years); of the patients, eight were male.

Acquired lesions

30 patients with aortic valve disease received a pulmonary autograft, the pulmonary allograft being used to reconstruct the right ventricular outflow tract (5). The mean age of these patients was 27 years (range 3—55 years); of the patients, 26 were male.

Surgical technique

The operations of right ventricular outflow tract reconstruction for congenital heart disease (11) and the pulmonary autograft (5) have previously been described in detail for the aortic allograft. When using the pulmonary allograft we believe that five important surgical principles of conduit placement must be adhered to:
1. Use as short and wide conduit as possible.
2. Countersink in the line of ejection of the ventricle.
3. Keep the conduit valve close to the point of delivery.
4. Use biological tissue to extend the conduit.
5. Keep to one side of the midline to avoid conduit compression.

Follow-up

The 46 long-term survivors have been followed-up for a mean of 23 months (range 3—43 months). All patients have recently undergone radiographic, echocardiographic and Doppler assessment of the pulmonary allograft. Four patients have undergone elective cardiac catheterisation to assess the gradient across the homograft.

Results

Experimental studies

Morphometric analysis

The pulmonary allograft (PA) clearly has an improved orientation over the aortic allograft (AA). In all cases the pulmonary allograft was larger than its aortic counterpart at both the level of the valve annulus (PA : AA = 1.08) and at the trunk

(PA : AA = 1.15). The wall of the pulmonary allograft was thinner in all cases (PA : AA = 0.6).

Viability

Tritiated thymidine autoradiography showed similar viability for fibroblasts in both aortic and pulmonary allografts (Fig. 1). Viability was strongly correlated to the interval between the death of the donor and harvesting of the valve. Over 75% fibroblasts took up thymidine when the harvesting interval was reduced below 36 h. Viability was also reduced at similar rates with increasing preservation time.

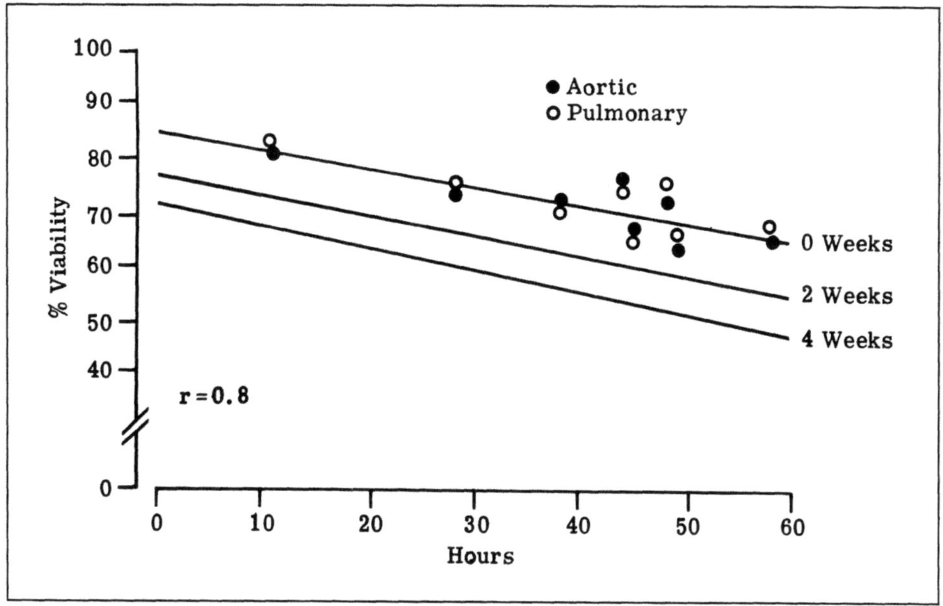

Fig. 1. Relationship between harvest time and homograft viability.

Calcium content

The calcium content ($\pm$ standard deviation) in the pulmonary allograft (105.9 $\pm$ 26.5 g/g tissue) was significantly lower than that in the aortic allograft (222.1 $\pm$ 88.9 g/g tissue) (p < 0.005 — paired t-test with Bessel's correction for small samples).

Histology

The elastic tissue in the media of the great vessels is arranged differently in the systemic and pulmonary circulations. In the aorta there is a regular arrangement of

191

long, uniform and parallel laminae. In the pulmonary trunk the arrangement is more sparse, irregular and fragmented. These arrangements did not change after 4 weeks' antibiotic preservation, nor was there evidence of collagen degeneration in either specimen.

Clinical studies

Operative mortality

There were two operative deaths. A 35-year-old man with pulmonary atresia and severe pulmonary hypertension died from low output cardiac failure. A second patient with similar pathology died of haemorrhage following complementary thoracotomy and ligation of collaterals.

Late mortality

There were three late deaths. Two patients died of infection following replacement of degenerate aortic allografts (one endocarditis, one mediastinitis). Both allografts were sterile at the time of implantation. The third patient had undergone two previous Fontan operations for tricuspid atresia. She died of low output cardiac failure following a third operation to isolate the outflow tract from the residual right ventricle. Thus, no deaths were directly related to the pulmonary allografts.

Follow-up

The 46 surviving patients have been followed-up for a mean of 23 months and are all in New York Heart Association Class I or II with regard to exercise tolerance. Current chest radiographs show no evidence of calcification. Doppler studies show that two patients have mild pulmonary regurgitation. Four patients have undergone repeat cardiac catheterisation which shows a mean transconduit gradient of less than 5 mmHg.

Discussion

The role of the pulmonary allograft in right ventricular outflow tract reconstruction was first suggested by Euguchi (3) during experimental work with dogs. Pierce (12) found smaller gradients across both proximal (ventricular-allograft) and distal (allograft-pulmonary artery) anastomoses for pulmonary compared with aortic allografts. The smaller gradients were due to the larger diameter and thinner wall of the pulmonary allograft, producing less fibrosis at the anastomotic site (3). In addition, there appeared to be less calcification in the wall at 1 year with the pulmonary allograft (17). This is predictable from the decreased elastin and intrinsic calcium content of the pulmonary allograft.

192

Our initial results with the pulmonary allograft have been excellent. Its principal advantage is the physiological orientation of the cusps which allows the conduit to lie better than its aortic counterpart. The thinner wall is not only less prone to calcification but also easier to suture. The pulmonary allograft is more freely available than its aortic counterpart, whilst its larger diameter leads to improved trans-conduit haemodynamics.

Though our experience with the aortic allograft has been good, we believe that the theoretical and practical advantages of the pulmonary allograft will lead to a significant improvement in the long-term. The pulmonary allograft is now our conduit of choice for right ventricular outflow tract reconstruction.

References

1. Al-Janabi N, Ross D (1973) Enhanced viability of fresh aortic homografts stored in nutrient medium. Cardiovasc Res 7: 817—823
2. Di Carlo D, De Leval M, Stark J (1984) "Fresh", antibiotic sterilised aortic homografts in extracardiac valved conduits: long-term results. Thorac Cardiovasc Surg 32: 10—14
3. Euguchi S, Asano K-I (1968) Homograft of pulmonary artery or ascending aorta with valve as right ventricular outflow. J Thorac Cardiovasc Surg 56: 413—420
4. Fontan F, Choussat A, Deville C, Doutremepuich C, Coupilland J, Vosa C (1984) Aortic valve homografts in the surgical treatment of complex cardiac malformations. J Thorac Cardiovasc Surg 87: 649—657
5. Gonzalez-Lavin L, Geens M, Ross D (1970) Aortic valve replacement with a pulmonary autograft. Indications and surgical technique. Surgery 68: 450—456
6. Jonas R, Freed M, Mayer J, Castaneda A (1985) Long-term follow-up of patients with synthetic right heart conduits. Circulation 72 (part 2): II 77—83
7. Kay P, Ross D (1985) Fifteen years experience with the aortic homograft: the conduit of choice for right ventricular outflow tract reconstruction. Ann Thorac Surg 40: 360—364
8. Kay P, Livi U, Robles A, Ross D (1986) In: Bodnar E, Yacoub M (eds) Biologic valve prostheses, procedings of the third international symposium. Yorke Medical Books, pp 58—63
9. Livi U, Abdulla A-K, Parker R, Olsen E, Ross D (1987) Viability and morphology of aortic and pulmonary homografts. J Thorac Cardiovasc Surg 93: 755—760
10. Miller D, Stinson E, Oyer P, et al (1982) The durability of porcine xenograft valves and conduits in children. Circulation 66 (part 2): II 72—85
11. Moore C, Martelli V, Ross D (1976) Reconstruction of right ventricular outflow tract with a valved conduit in 75 cases of congenital heart disease. J Thorac Cardiovasc Surg 71: 11—19
12. Pierce W, Thompson W, Kazami S, Waldhausen J (1971) Replacement of the pulmonary outflow tract and valve with a formalin treated porcine heterograft. J Thorac Cardiovasc Surg 61: 924—929
13. Robles A, Vaughan M, Lau J, Bodnar E, Ross D (1985) Long-term assessment of aortic valve replacement with autologous pulmonary valve. Ann Thorac Surg 39: 238—242
14. Ross D, Somerville J (1966) Correction of pulmonary atresia with a homograft aortic valve. Lancet 2: 1446—1447
15. Saravalli O, Somerville J, Jefferson K (1980) Calcification of aortic homografts used for reconstruction of the right ventricular outflow tract. J Thorac Cardiovasc Surg 80: 909—920
16. Schaff H, Di Donato R, Danielson G, et al (1984) Reoperation for obstructed pulmonary ventricle-pulmonary artery conduits. J Thorac Cardiovasc Surg 88: 334—343
17. Seki S, Rastelli G, McGoon D, Titus J (1970) Replacement of the pulmonary artery with a pulmonary arterial homograft. J Thorac Cardiovasc Surg 60: 853—859

Authors' address:
P. H. Kay
The National Heart Hospital
Westmoreland Street
London W1M 8BA
U.K.

Pulmonary valve allograft reconstruction of the right ventricular outflow tract

D. R. Clarke

Cardiovascular and Thoracic Surgery, The Childrens Hospital, Denver, Colorado, U.S.A.

Introduction

The development of procedures to reconstruct the right ventricular outflow tract has been a major advancement in the treatment of congenital heart disease. However, extensive reconstruction of the right ventricular outflow tract (RVOT) with porcine valved Dacron conduits is not ideal. Difficulties with insertion may arise since the often friable pulmonary artery is easily torn when sutured to non-pliable Dacron material. Secondly, conduit compression or compression of structures beneath the conduit on sternal closure is a frequent occurrence with serious consequences (2). Intimal peel formation and porcine valve degeneration or calcification have produced late problems resulting in the subsequent development of transconduit gradients (1, 5).

As an alternative, aortic allografts have been used with success for reconstruction of the RVOT (3, 8). However, availability of "fresh" allografts is limited since they must be used within a few weeks of procurement. With the introduction of cryopreservation, allograft valve banks have been established which allow prolonged storage of conduits and thus increase availability. Cryopreservation also provides viable tissue which may prove to be functionally durable for long periods (6) which is an extremely attractive feature with regard to the paediatric population. Pulmonary valve allografts further increase tissue availability and may be a more suitable replacement for the right ventricular outflow tract (4). During the past 28 months, 43 pulmonary valve allograft RVOT reconstructions have been performed and provide the basis for this study.

Patients

42 patients underwent 43 procedures for construction or repair of their right ventricular outflow tract. A pulmonary valve allograft was used in every case from April 1985 up to and including August 1987. The patient group comprised 22 males and 20 females who ranged in age from 9 weeks to 20 years (mean : 5 years). Three patients (7 %) had undergone no previous surgery, while the remaining 39 (93 %) had experienced 46 prior palliative or corrective procedures (Table 1).

18 patients carried an original diagnosis of tetralogy of Fallot; eight had undergone prior total repair. Nine had pulmonary atresia associated with VSD, five were diagnosed with complex transposition of the great arteries, three with double outlet right ventricle and two patients had truncus arteriosus. Six patients required surgery

Table 1. Prior procedures in 42 patients requiring right ventricular outflow tract reconstruction.

Unilateral systemic — PA shunt	20
Bilateral systemic — PA shunt	7
ToF repair	8
Ventricle — PA conduit	6
Other	5
No previous surgery	3

Table 2. Diagnoses in patients requiring right ventricular outflow tract reconstruction.

Complex ToF	18
Pulmonary atresia/VSD	9
Conduit replacement	6
Complex TGA	5
DORV	3
Truncus arteriosus	2

to replace previously inserted right ventricle to pulmonary artery conduits. Their original diagnoses included three tetralogies, two double outlet ventricles and one truncus arteriosus. One of the patients initially presented with tetralogy of Fallot but subsequently developed severe pulmonary allograft valve regurgitation requiring conduit replacement and is included in the latter group (Table 2).

Operative technique

In preparation for right ventricular outflow tract reconstruction, a pulmonary allograft of appropriate size is selected. Valve size can be approximated using the child's weight. Figure 1 illustrates the relationship between the two variables. Following a median sternotomy and while preparations are being made for cardiopulmonary bypass, the cryopreserved allograft is prepared for implantation. It is first thawed in its foil pouch in a 37 °C saline bath for 20 min. The allograft is then removed from the outer package and passed onto the sterile field where it is put through three rinse solutions containing fetal calf serum and decreasing concentrations of dimethylsulphoxide. Lastly, the valved conduit is rinsed in saline.

After cardiopulmonary bypass is established, the aorta is cross-clamped and blood cardioplegia is infused into the aortic root to provide myocardial protection. A vertical right ventriculotomy is made and extended into the main pulmonary artery if present. The distal main as well as right and left pulmonary arteries are inspected for areas of stenosis or dysplasia. Depending on the anatomy observed, one of three variations on the surgical procedure may be pursued. A standard circular anastomosis to the main pulmonary artery can be accomplished if the distal arteries are unobstructed (Fig. 2). If one of the distal pulmonary arteries is obstructed, an allograft flap can be extended onto that side to enlarge the area (Fig. 3). When central

196

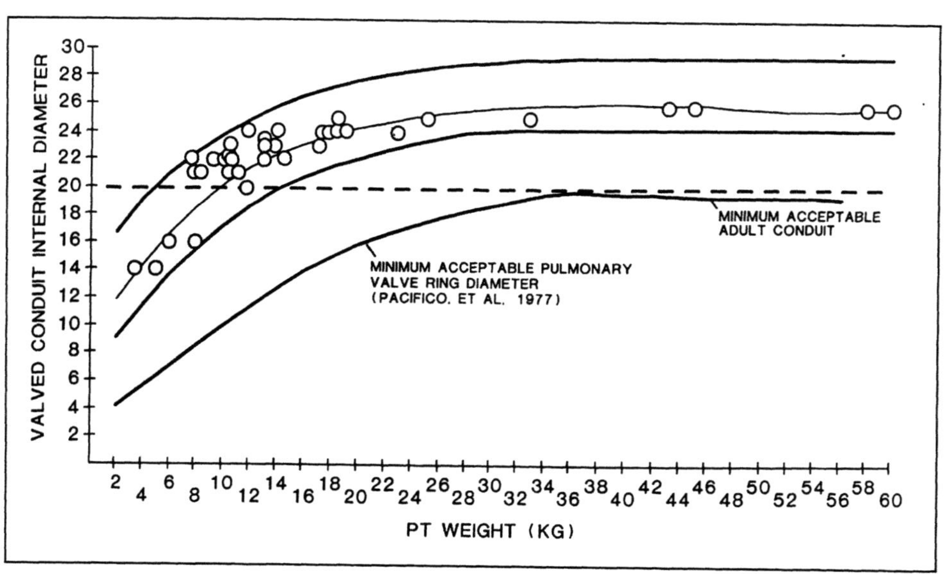

Fig. 1. Conduit size related to patient (pt) weight.

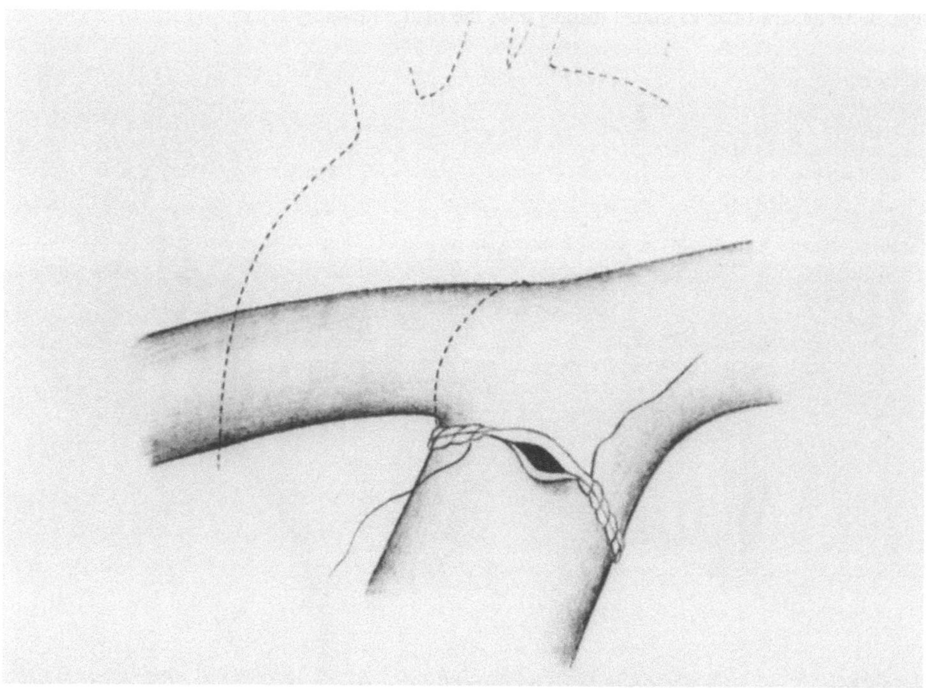

Fig. 2. A standard circular anastomosis of the distal pulmonary allograft to the main pulmonary artery.

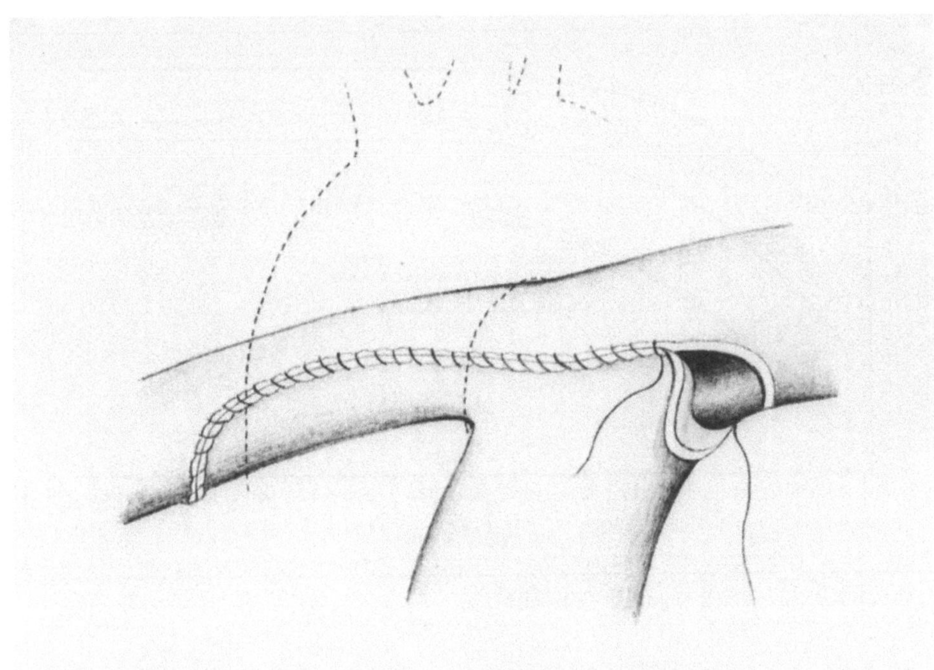

Fig. 3. An allograft flap extended distally onto the right pulmonary artery.

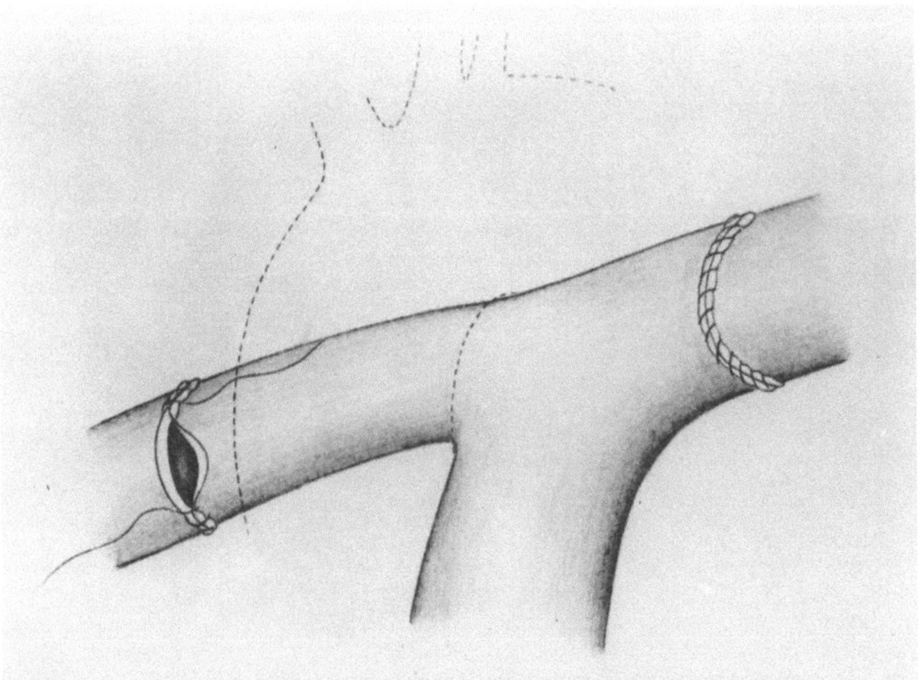

Fig. 4. Anastomosis of a bifurcated allograft to the right and left pulmonary arteries.

198

pulmonary artery distortion is severe, a bifurcated allograft is anastomosed to both right and left pulmonary arteries (Fig. 4).

Final preparation of the pulmonary allograft involves trimming excess muscle from below the valve and remaining muscle is thinned to provide less bulk around the suture line. Length is then determined by positioning the allograft and transecting excess tissue from the distal end. Care is taken to avoid excess length which might kink when the graft distends. The distal anastomosis is begun posteriorly by suturing from within the lumen. Laterally, the suture is brought outside to complete the anterior anastomosis. The proximal connection is subsequently made by suturing the posterior portion of the allograft either directly to the pulmonary valve annulus if present or to the superior margin of the right ventriculotomy (Fig. 5).

The remaining procedure can be readily accomplished on partial bypass. The aortic crossclamp is therefore removed and the myocardium revascularized. A triangular "shield"-shaped synthetic or biological patch is then fashioned and used to form a hood from anterior and lateral allograft to ventriculotomy (Fig. 6). The base of the patch is sutured distally to the proximal pulmonary allograft and the sides of the triangle sutured to the edges of the right ventriculotomy. Corners at which allograft, right ventricle and patch come together must be sutured carefully to avoid bleeding (Fig. 7). If allograft artery is used for the hood, it will stretch and balloon out if cut too large. At this point, the patient is warmed, gradually weaned from cardiopulmonary bypass and decannulated in routine fashion.

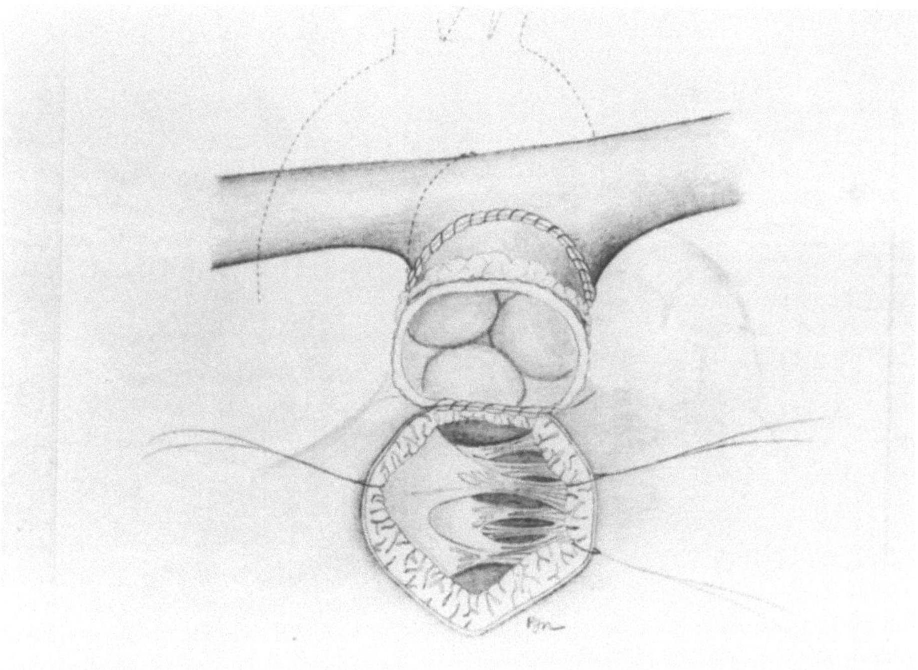

Fig. 5. The distal anastomosis has been completed. The proximal anastomosis is begun to the margin of the right ventriculotomy.

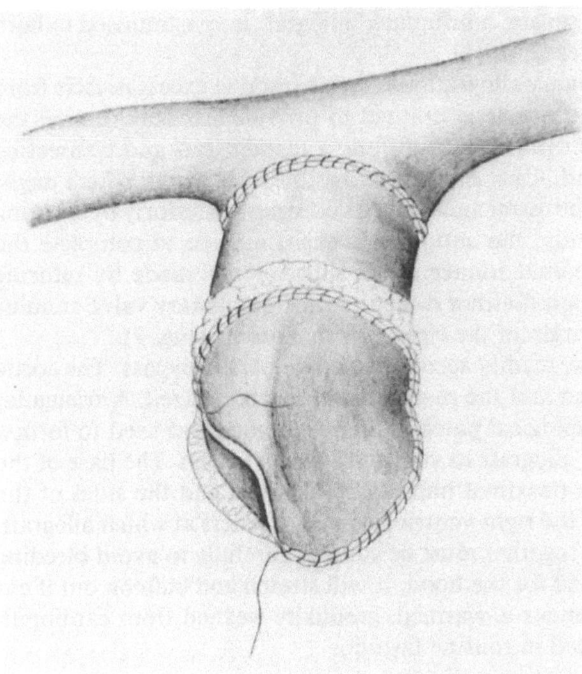

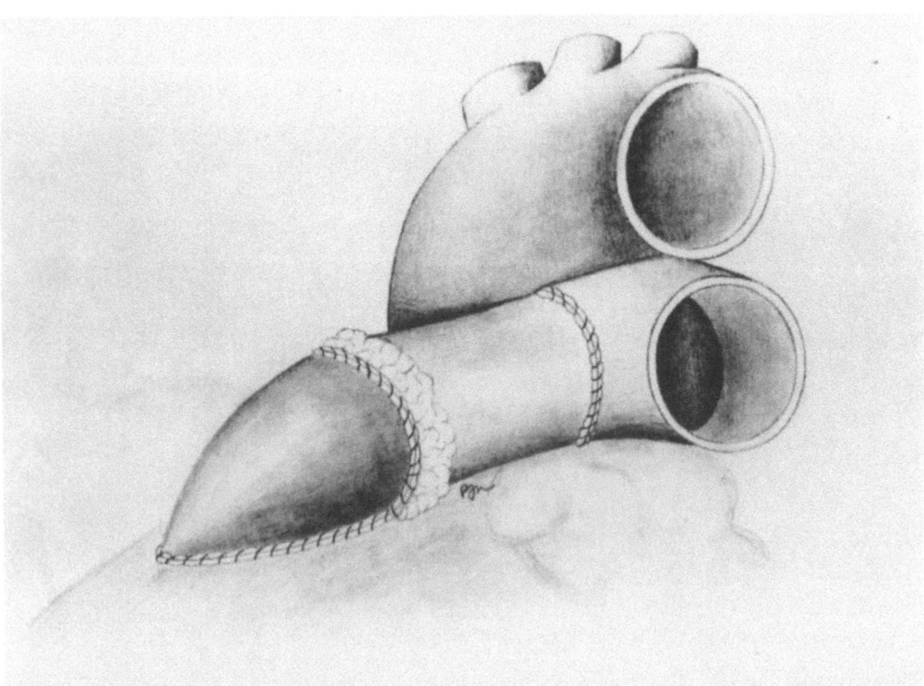

Fig. 7. Corners of the hood are sutured tightly to avoid bleeding and the pulmonary valve allograft repair of the right ventricular outflow tract is complete.

200

Results

Pulmonary valve allografts with 12 to 26 mm (mean: 22 mm) internal diameters were implanted. 35 patients (81 %) have received conduits 20 mm or larger which can be considered adult size (Fig. 1) (7). In 27 of 43 (63%) pulmonary allograft placement procedures, the allograft was extended to the distal pulmonary arteries. In the 16 remaining operations (37%), an allograft to main pulmonary artery anastomosis was sufficient. The hood was polytetrafluoroethane (PTFE) in 28 cases, allograft pulmonary artery in nine procedures, pericardium in five cases and there was one dacron hood (Fig. 8).

A variety of postoperative complications were encountered and they are listed, with their frequency of occurrence, in Table 3. The postoperative convalescence of 24 (56%) patients was completely benign. Four incidences of bleeding required surgical re-exploration. The three postoperative arrhythmias resolved spontaneously. Several patients experienced multiple complications. Two children who underwent reoperation for bleeding subsequently developed subglottic stenosis. A third patient with bleeding complications acquired postoperative Candida sepsis that resolved after a 6-week course of antibiotics. One 3½-year-old suffered brain damage (presumably anoxic), and subsequent arrhythmias. Neurological residuals were significantly improved by discharge and continued resolution was expected.

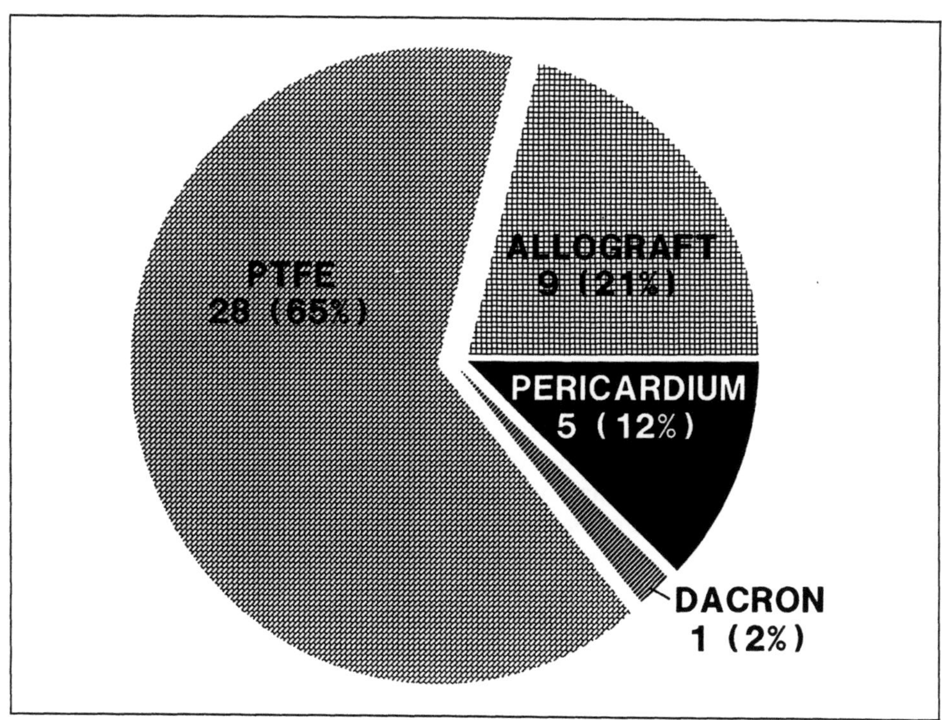

Fig. 8. Materials used in hood reconstruction.

Table 3. Complications following pulmonary valve allograft reconstruction of the right ventricular outflow tract.

Bleeding	4
Arrhythmia/heart block	3
Residual VSD	2
Neurological	2
Subglottic stenosis	2
Diaphragm paralysis	2
Candida sepsis	1
Allograft valve failure	1
Sternal osteomyelitis	1
Postpericardiotomy syndrome	1
Oesophageal perforation	1
Death (11.9%)	5

There were five postoperative deaths in our series; two had presented with pulmonary atresia, one with tetralogy of Fallot and one with double outlet right ventricle. All the children were under 2 years of age and had undergone previous operations for repair of their defects. Four (9%) deaths occurred early and were a result of cardiac failure. One death occurred 31 days postoperatively in a patient who experienced seizures and increasingly prolonged apnoeic episodes resulting from severe neurological dysfunction.

37 survivors have been followed for 3 to 31 months (mean: 16 months). There has been one allograft failure (2.7%). It occurred in a patient with an original diagnosis of tetralogy of Fallot. The initial procedure was a Blalock-Taussig performed at one month. At 3 years, the first pulmonary allograft was placed. 15 months later, reoperation was required for right ventricular failure secondary to stenosis of both pulmonary arteries at the distal anastomosis and allograft valvular insufficiency. At operation, one leaflet was found to be severely deformed by the previous proximal suture line. The conduit was replaced with another pulmonary valve allograft and the early result is favourable. Trivial pulmonary valve regurgitation is a common clinical finding in these patients but the severity has not increased with time. Overall functional results have been excellent.

Conclusion

For patients with complex congenital heart disease, the ability to reconstruct the right ventricular outflow tract is one of the most notable surgical advances in recent years. Experience with pulmonary valve allograft reconstruction is limited, but several advantages over the use of Dacron xenografts or aortic homografts are apparent: (1) Pulmonary allografts are not technically difficult to implant; (2) Cryopreservation has made pulmonary allografts readily available; (3) They provide an anatomically ideal replacement for the right ventricular outflow tract and central pulmonary arteries; (4) Since larger conduits can be placed, the incidence of reoperation resulting from growth of a paediatric patient should be less. (5) Postoperative sternal compression has not been a problem; (6) Transconduit gradients have been insignificant with pulmonary allograft reconstruction of the RVOT.

Although late follow-up is unavailable, early results are very encouraging, stimulating continued use of pulmonary valve allografts for reconstruction of the right ventricular outflow tract.

References

1. Agarwal KC, Edwards WD, Feldt RH, et al. (1981) Clinicopathological correlates of obstructed right-sided porcine valved extracardiac conduits. J Thorac Cardiovasc Surg 81: 591
2. Bailey WW, Kirklin JW, Bargeron LM Jr, et al. (1977) Late results with synthetic valved external conduits from venous ventricle to pulmonary arteries. Circulation 56: II-73
3. Kay PH, Ross DN (1985) Fifteen years', experience with the aortic homograft: the conduit of choice for right ventricular outflow tract reconstruction. Ann Thorac Surg 40: 360
4. Livi U, Abdulla AK, Parker R, et al. (1987) Viability and morphology of aortic and pulmonary homografts. J Thorac Cardiovasc Surg 93: 755
5. Miller DC, Stinson EB, Oyer PE, et al. (1982) The durability of porcine xenograft valves and conduits in children. Circulation 66: I-172
6. O'Brien MF, Stafford EG, Gardner MAH, et al. (1987) A comparison of aortic valve replacement with viable cryopreserved and fresh allograft valves with a note on chromosomal studies. J Thorac Cardiovasc Surg (in press)
7. Pacifico AD, Kirklin JW, Blackstone EH (1977) Surgical management of pulmonary stenosis in tetralogy of Fallot. J Thorac Cardiovasc Surg 74: 382
8. Ross D, Somerville J (1976) Homograft reconstruction of right ventricular outflow tract in pulmonary atresia: late results. Br Heart J 38: 316

Author's address:
David R. Clarke, M.D.
Chief, Cardiovascular and Thoracic Surgery
The Childrens Hospital
1056 East 19th Avenue
Denver, Colorado 80218
U.S.A.

Technique of inlay allografts into the RVOT to prevent pulmonary insufficiency*

H. Meisner, S. Hagl, F. Sebening

Clinic for Heart and Vascular Surgery, German Heart Center, Munich, F.R.G.

Pulmonary insufficiency presents a pathological condition which can occur after correction of congenital malformations of the right outflow tract. The aim of most surgical interventions of the right ventricular outflow tract concerns relief of pulmonary stenosis; if this is accomplished, normal lung perfusion is possible even in the absence of a pulmonary valve. Primary replacement of a pulmonary valve is recommended in cases of pulmonary atresia, truncus arteriosus or TGA, VSD and severe pulmonary stenosis. In tetralogy of Fallot, even with a severely distorted pulmonary valve or a necessary transanular patch at primary correction, valve replacement is generally avoided. It may, however, become necessary many years later (4, 5, 7). Here, in some instances, right heart failure has developed for a variety of reasons, e.g. presence of proximal or distal pulmonary valve or vascular stenosis, significant aortopulmonary collaterals and/or VSD-recurrency all resulting in an elevated pulmonary vascular resistance. These factors will present a high systolic and diastolic load on the right ventricle which ultimately leads to right heart failure with tricuspid insufficiency and its decisive sequelae (Table I). In these patients pulmonary valve replacement will become a necessity to increase life expectancy (1, 3, 4, 10, 21). An example is seen in Fig. 1: a 10-year-old boy who needed a transanular pulmonary outflow tract patch at correction 9 years ago, demonstrated the symptoms of severe right heart insufficiency. Now, 2 years after pulmonary allograft implantation, marked improvement is obvious.

In order to avoid these developments, some years ago the implantation of an outflow tract patch bearing single biological valve cusps was reported. The long-term beneficial function of these valve substitutes, however, could not be demonstrated (2, 18). Implantation of a xenograft prosthesis was common practice for some years until allografts were available (19). Today the increasing number of positive reports concerning long-term function of allografts favours their implantation for pulmonary valve incompetence (9, 14, 15, 20).

Materials and Methods

The methods of procurement, preparation and conservation of the allografts were copied from Ross and Yacoub (16, 17, 22). In cooperation with the Dept. of Forensic Medicine[1] aortic and pulmonary valve allografts were harvested from cadavers

---

* Dedicated to Prof. Dr. h. c. W. Brendel on his 65th birthday.
[1] Institute of Forensic Medicine, Univ. of München, Frauenlobstraße 7a, 8000 München; Director: Prof. Dr. W. Spann.

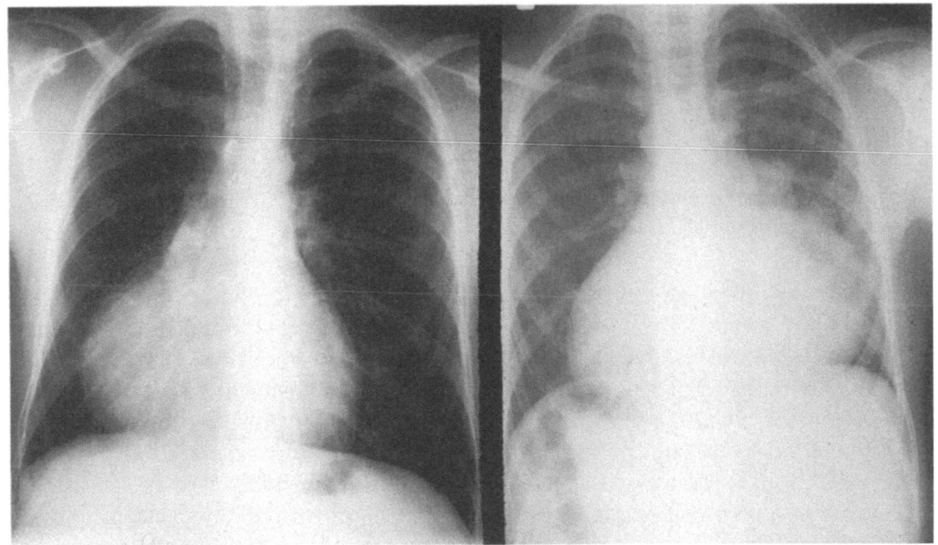

Fig. 1a. Preoperative X-ray of a 10-year-old boy with pulmonary incompetence, 9 years after TOF-correction using a transanular outflow tract pach because of severe pulmonary valve ring stenosis.

Fig. 1b. X-ray of the same patient 2 years after implantation of a pulmonary allograft. Significant improvement of right heart size and function was measured.

Table 1. Factors influencing pulmonary insufficiency after correction of e.g. Tetralogy of Fallot. The parameters can be relevant as a single event or in various combinations.

- VSD-recurrency
- valve/ring stenosis
- leaflet damage
- pulmonary vascular stenosis
- aorta-pulmonary collaterals

Table 2. Antibiotic solution used for preparation of allografts.

Substance	Dose
Cefaloridine	400 mg
Piperacillin-sodium	10 g
Polymyxin B-sulphate	0.5 g
Neo-mycin-sulphate	1.0 g
Nystatin	500 000 IE

After Yacoub (22)

within 24 h after death. Preparation of the allografts was standardised and described by Hagl (6). The tissue was sterilised and conserved in antibiotic solution (Table 2) for 9 days. Negative bacteriological swabs signaled availability for implantation during the following 3 weeks. They were then discarded. On average, the allografts were implanted in a period of 9—30 days, mean 20.4 days after conservation.

The age of the donors varied between 1 day and 35 years; mean 22 years. The time between declaration of death and explanation varied between 6 and 36 h, mean 21.6 ± 8.4 h.

Results

Between June 1982 and June 1987, 135 allografts were implanted exclusively in patients with congenital heart disease. Diagnoses of the malformation are summarized in Table 3. In most instances, the indication for operation was reconstruction of the right heart outflow tract. In 22 patients, a formerly implanted xenograft bearing conduit was exchanged for an allograft. On the left side of the heart, allografts were implanted in two patients only. A pulmonary allograft was used 11 times. Operative mortality was 7.4 % (10 out of 135) not connected at all to the conduit implanted. The postoperative course was mostly uncomplicated; in eight patients, a temperature rise was registered 6 to 14 days postoperatively without positive bacteriological findings or deterioration of the clinical conditions; no correlation of the allografts to age of donor or time after death or other factors was possible. Seven children died late: one 9-year-old boy with severe LV outflow tract stenosis who had received an apico-aortic allograft conduit 18 months earlier due to fatal LV-hae-

Table 3. Diagnosis of 135 patients operated on using pulmonary and aortic allografts between June 1982 and June 1987.

Diagnosis	n = 135
DOLV	3
DORV	4
TOF	28
PA	32
TGA + VSD + PS	12
SV	6
TrA	12
TAC	35
TS	1
AI + Marfan	1
AoVS	1

morrhage; two died suddenly, 1 and 3 years following a Rastelli and truncus operation; three died 3—9 months after truncus repair due to pulmonary complications; another died of intractable cardiac failure.

The age of our patients varied between 1 month and 29 years, mean 8 years, 2 months. The postoperative observation time varied from 1 to 60 months with a mean of 30 months. 95 % of our patients were followed closely in our paediatric outpatient department[2]. Up to now, no reoperation for allograft failure has been found necessary. 28 patients have lived with an allograft for more than 4 years, 31 for more than 3 years. Besides routine clinical examinations in 81 children, 1—60 months after allograft implantation, echocardiography was performed routinely. Sometimes it was difficult to demonstrate pulmonary stenosis by continuous wave Doppler because of anatomical determinants. For analysis of pulmonary incompetence, a pulsed Doppler was used. For these reasons, reproducible echocardiographic descriptions are not available for all survivors.

Overall, a stenosis of varying degrees was demonstrated in 30 %, valve insufficiency was found in 37 % (cf. Table 4). There were, however, a few cases of significant allograft stenosis or incompetence. In most patients this was present early after operation, suggesting distortion of the valve on implantation. 30 of the allograft conduits implanted showed calcification of the aortic wall on X-ray of varying degree without effect on valve function. Some were obvious as early as 6 months after implantation. From this experience, we have to discuss the operative technique applied, particularly in patients with heart failure, years after correction of tetralogy of Fallot due to severe pulmonary incompetence. In all cases secondary tricuspid valve incompetence was present, too. The indication for operation was given by clinical symptoms rather than catheter data (Table 5). All patients survived and were significantly improved; normalization, however, of right heart myocardial function was rarely achieved.

Table 4. Postoperative results of 81 patients 1 to 60 months after allograft implantation using clinical and echocardiographic evaluation (6/1982—6/1987).

pulmonary stenosis	n	pulmonary insufficiency	n
Δ p 10—20 mmHg	15	0—1 °	14
Δ p 25—35 mmHg	6	1 °	10
Δ p 40—50 mmHg	3	2 °	6

aortic wall calcification n = 30

Table 5. The indication for operative repair of pulmonary incompetence after tetralogy of Fallot correction is given if the parameters described are present.

- increased RVend > 15 mmHg
- decreased RV_{EF} < 0.50
- tricuspid incompetence
- cardiac enlargement

[2] Klinik für Herz- und Kreislauferkrankungen im Kindesalter, Deutsches Herzzentrum München, Lothstr. 11, 8000 München 2, Dir.: Prof. Dr. K. Bühlmeyer.

Operative technique and discussion

The implantation technique favours insertion of an allograft in the natural position of the pulmonary valve. Generally, the valve ring area is dilated due to extensive systolic and diastolic flow; thus, an "inlay technique" is practicable (11, 13). After institution of cardiopulmonary bypass, a longitudinal incision across the pulmonary valve ring permits good exposure and remnant leaflets or valve fragments can be excised. In cases with aorto-pulmonary collateral flow, both pulmonary branches are occluded temporarily, venting the left atrium. The horizontal diameter of the origin of the pulmonary vessel presents the basis for judgement of a suitable size of allograft; slight oversizing is recommended. The valve of choice is a pulmonary allograft because it accomodates best to the outflow tract, the valve ring and pulmonary vessel (8, 12). The muscular rim at the base of the allograft is trimmed as short as possible, the distal portion is cut obliquely to ensure optimal adaptation to the pulmonary vessel. Continuous polypropylene sutures are used for implantation, starting at the muscular base of the allograft. Usually closure of the natural valve ring over the conduit cannot be attained, the sutures ending on the upper end of the allograft (Fig. 2a). The allograft should be filled either by retrograde pulmonary flow or antegrade with a syringe, to demonstrate a competent valve in situ. Continuity to the right ventricle can be restored either by direct suture or using a patch avoiding distortion of the implanted and now distended valve (Figs. 2b and 3). If an aortic allograft has to be used for replacement, the base appears to be more bulky due to

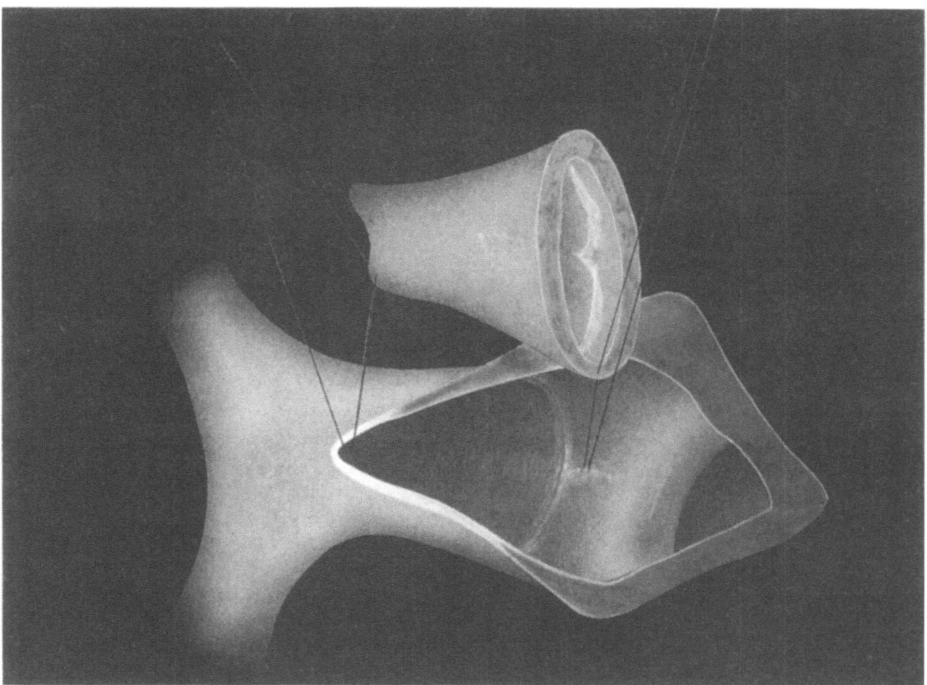

Fig. 2a. Demonstration of operative inlay technique for treatment of pulmonary incompetence.

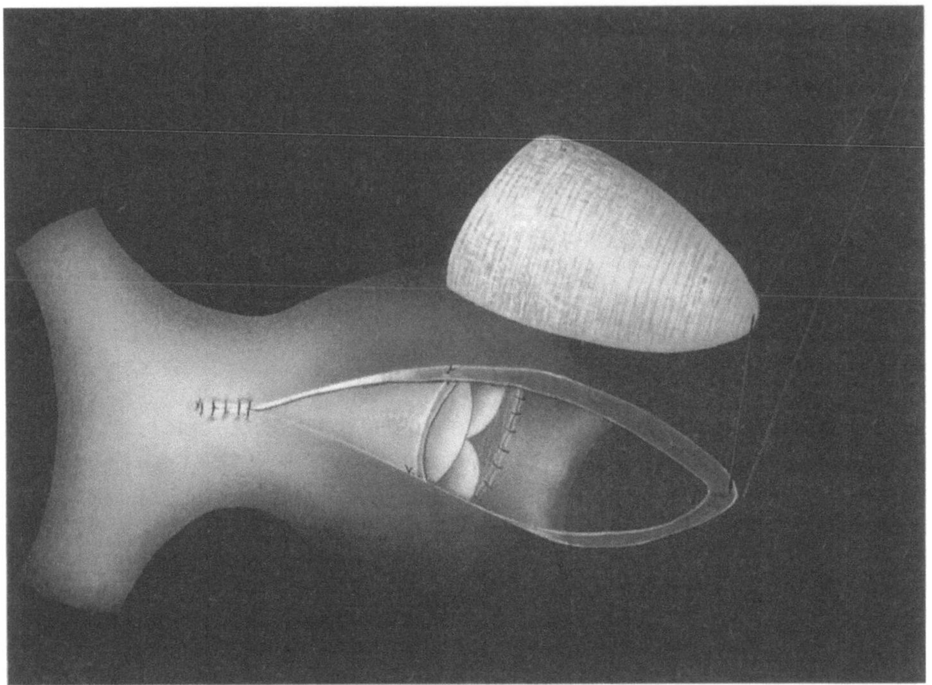

Fig. 2b. After implantation of the allograft with continuous sutures a patch is used for closing the gap to the right ventricle, thus avoiding traction on the valve.

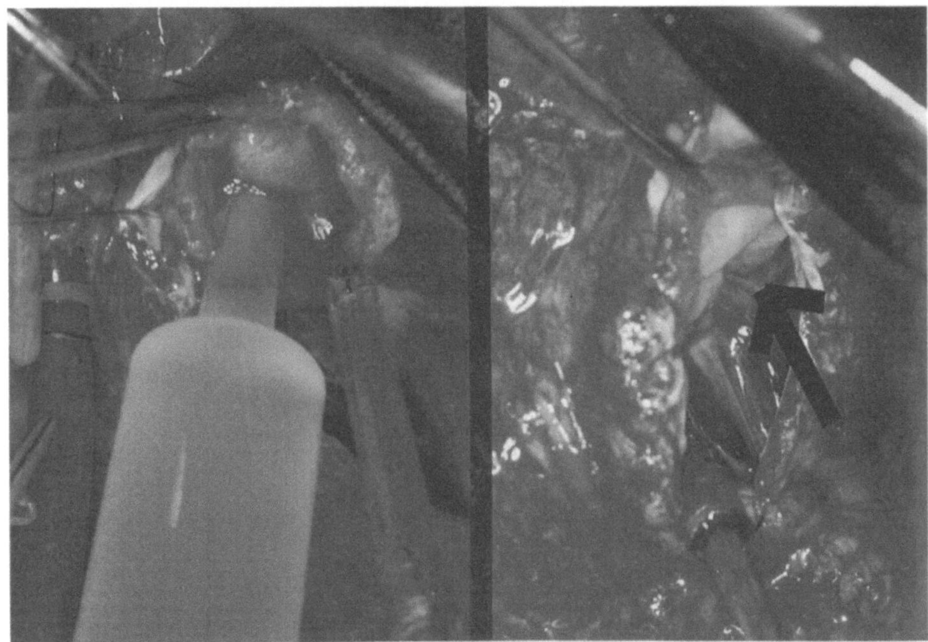

Fig. 3. Operative view: Filling of the allograft with saline in order to obtain optimal alignment to the right outflow tract (arrow marks expanded allograft in situ).

210

thicker muscular remnant of the aortic wall. Further on, the natural curve of the aorta has to be considered on implantation; on the other hand, parts of the mitral valve can be used for closure of the right ventricular incision.

In cases in which the common pulmonary vessel is absent or cannot be employed, an aortic allograft conduit is most suitable, presenting various options for connecting the pulmonary branches. Fig. 4 summarises some examples, e.g. if the common pulmonary trunk is missing, the branches can be implanted into a prepared allograft conduit. If the central pulmonary vessel is missing, unification with a ring Goretex graft and connection to the right ventricular outflow tract with an allograft is recommended.

For primary correction of pulmonary atresia, in infants, or truncus arteriosus, implantation of a valve bearing conduit into the right outflow tract is mandatory (13, 14). In these situations peripheral anastomoses with the pulmonary vessel end-to-end or end-to-side are done first, then the length of the conduit is adapted to the orifice of the right outflow tract. In order to assure proper connection to the right ventricle, extension of the allograft by a segment of artificial graft or a patch may become necessary. In all cases, filling of the allograft is essential in order to achieve optimal alignment of the implanted valve and avoid traction on the soft valve ring. In our opinion, an optimal implantation technique is fundamental for long-term allograft function. Besides possible immunological reactions (23, 24), flow disturbances and local turbulence may enhance leaflet structure deterioration and malfunction.

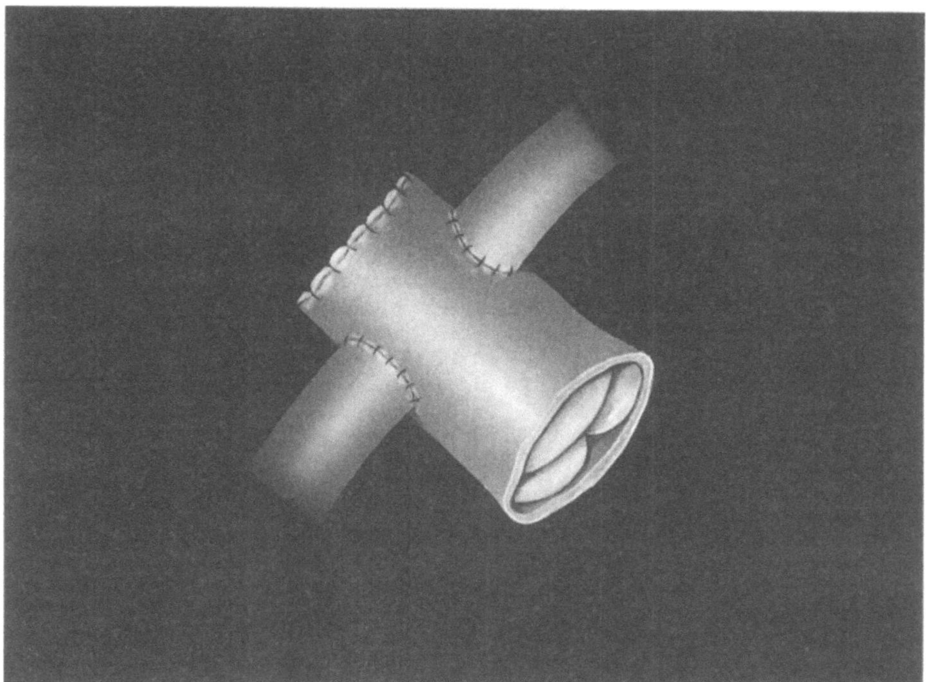

Fig. 4a

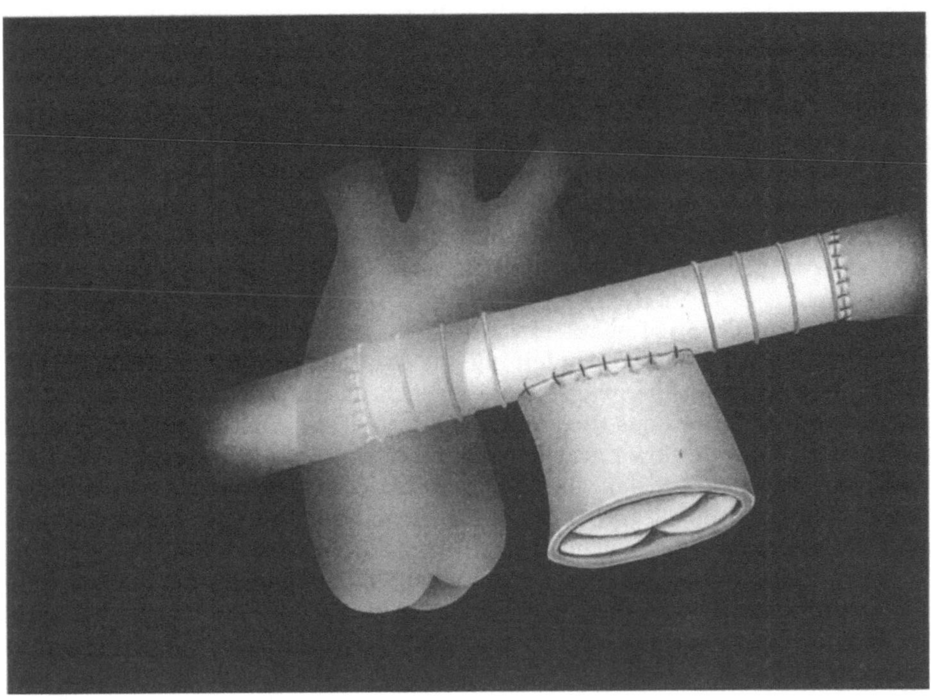

Fig. 4b
Fig. 4a and b. Implantation of an aortic allograft conduit in cases of absent common pulmonary artery. If the central pulmonary artery is missing, a ring Goretex graft is implanted for unification connecting it to the right ventricle with an allograft.

References

1. Asano K (1978) Long-term results of corrective surgery for the tetralogy of Fallot. Singapure Med J 14: 178
2. Bernhard A, Sievers HH (June 1977) Hemodynamic Results after Reconstruction of the Right Ventricular Outflow Tract in Tetralogy of Fallot. European Congress of Cardiovascular Surgery, Tel Aviv
3. Bristow JD, Kloster FE, Lees MH, Menaske VD, Griswald HE, Starr A (1979) Serial Cardiac Catheterizations and Exercise Hemodynamics after Correction of Tetralogy of Fallot: Average Follow-up 13 Months and 7 years after Operation. Circulation 41: 1057
4. Ebert PA (1982) Second operations for pulmonary stenosis or insufficiency after repair of tetralogy of Fallot. Am J Cardiol 50: 637
5. Fuster V, McGoon DC, Kennedy MA, Ritter DC, Kirklin JW (1980) Long-term Evaluation (12 to 22 Years) of Open Heart Surgery for Tetralogy of Fallot. Am J Cardiol 46: 635—642
6. Hagl S, Meisner H, Sebening F (1985) Die Rekonstruktion der rechtsventrikulären Ausflußbahn mit xenogenen und allogenen klappentragenden Conduits. Wiener Med Wschr 135: 478
7. Katz NM, Blackstone EH, Kirklin JW, Pacifico AD, Bargeron LM Jr (1982) Late Survival and Symptoms after Repair of Tetralogy of Fallot. Circulation 65: 403—410
8. Kay PH, Livi U, Robles A, Ross DN (1986) Pulmonary Homograft. In: Bodnar E, Yacoub M (eds) Biologic and Bioprosthetic Valves. Yorke Medical Books, p 58—63
9. Khagani A, Dhalla N, Penta A, Qureshi S, Theodoropoulos S, Esposito G, Yacoub M (1986) Patient status 10 years or more after aortic valve replacement using antibiotic sterilized homografts. In: Bodnar E, Yacoub M (eds) Biologic and Bioprosthetic Valves. Yorke Medical Books, p 38—46

10. Klinner W, Reichert B, Pfaller M, Hatz R (1984) Late results after Correction of Tetralogy of Fallot Necessitating Outflow Tract Reconstruction Comparison with Results after Correction without Outflow Tract Patch. Thorac Cardiovasc Surg 4: 244—249

11. Laks H, Hellenbrand WE, Kleinman CS, Stansel HC Jr, Talner NS (1981) Patch reconstruction of the right ventricular outflow tract with pulmonary valve insertion. Circulation 64 (Suppl II): II-154

12. McGrath LB, Gonsalez-Lavin L, Graf D (1987) Pulmonary Valve Homograft Implantation for Ventricular Outflow Tract Reconstruction: Early Phase Results. The Society of Thoracic Surgeons. 23rd Annual Meeting, Toronto, Ontario, Canada, September 21—23, p 54

13. Norwood WI, Bernhard WF, Freed MD, Roccini AP, Castaneda AR (1977) Experience right Valved Conduits for Repair of Congenital Cardiac Lesions. Ann Thorac Surg 24: 223

14. Rastelli GC, Davis PA, Kirklin JW (1965) Pulmonary atresia with coronary fistula. Mayo Clin Proc 40: 521

15. Ross DN, Somerville J (1966) Correction of pulmonary atresia with a homograft aortic valve. Lancet 2: 1446

16. Ross DN (1962) Homograft replacement of the aortic valve. Lancet 2: 487

17. Ross DN, Yacoub MH (1969) Homograft replacement of the aortic valve. A critical review. Prog Cardiovasc Dis 9: 275

18. Sievers HH, Lange PE, Regensburger D, Yankah CA, Onnasch DGW, Bursch J, Heintzen PH, Bernhard A (1983) Short-term hemodynamic results after right ventricular outflow tract reconstruction using a cusp-bearing transanular patch. J Thorac Cardiovasc Surg 86: 777

19. Stark J, de Leval M (1983) Surgery for Congenital Heart Defects. Grune & Stratton, London— New York—Paris—San Diego—San Francisco—Sao Paulo—Sydney—Tokyo—Toronto

20. Virdi IS, Munro JL, Ross JK (1986) Aortic valve replacements with antibiotic sterilized homografts valves: 11 year experience at Southampton. In: Bodnar E, Yacoub M (eds) Biologic and Bioprosthetic Valves. Yorke Medical Books, pp 29—37

21. Vogt J, Wesselhoeft H, Luig H, Schmitz L, de Vivie ER, Weber H, Beuren AJ (1984) The Preoperative and Postoperative Findings in 627 Patients with Tetralogy of Fallot. Thorac Cardiovasc Surg 4: 234—243

22. Yacoub M, Kittlen CF (1975) Sterilisation of valve homografts by antibiotic solution. Circulation 41, Suppl II: 29

23. Yacoub M, Snitters H, Khagani A, Rose M (1986) Localisation of major histocompatibility complex antigens in aortic homografts. In: Bodnar E, Yacoub M (eds) Biologic and Bioprosthetic Valves. Yorke Medical Books, pp 65—72

24. Yankah AC, Dreyer W, Wottge HU, Muller-Rucholtz W, Bernhard A (1986) Kinetics of Endothelial Cells of Preserved Aortic Valve Allografts Used for Heterotopic Transplantation in Inbred Rat Strains. In: Bodnar E, Yacoub M (eds) Biologic and Bioprosthetic Valves. Yorke Medical Books, pp 73—84

Authors' address:
Prof. Dr. H. Meisner
Klinik für Herz- und Gefäßchirurgie
Deutsches Herzzentrum München
Lothstraße 11
8000 München 2
F.R.G.

Allografts in the treatment of absent pulmonary valve syndrome and complex tetralogy of Fallot

M. J. Elliott, M. R. de Leval, J. Stark

Cardiothoracic Unit, The Hospital for Sick Children, London, U.K.

Introduction

The absent pulmonary valve syndrome comprises agenesis of the pulmonary valve, annular stenosis, pulmonary insufficiency, ventricular septal defect (VSD) and, usually, right ventricular (RV) hypertrophy. The pulmonary arteries (PA) are aneurysmal and usually compress the tracheobronchial tree. Several surgical techniques have been described, and many have been used in our unit (1). Our current policy is described in this short review.

Conduits may be required in the surgical treatment of tetralogy of Fallot for a number of reasons. For example, anomalous left coronary artery, repair to a single pulmonary artery, peripheral pulmonary stenoses or small pulmonary arteries or for post repair pulmonary incompetence or stenoses. This report concerns our experience with conduits in these circumstances.

Absent pulmonary valve syndrome

Between 1976 and 1987, 24 children (aged 5 days to 11 years) have been treated in our unit. As we have reported before (1) there were two clear modes of presentation; an infant group, with intractable respiratory symptoms caused by gross tracheobronchial compression, and an older group; with poor exercise tolerance, growth delay and recurrent respiratory infection. A variety of operative procedures have been employed and the types of procedures used until 1983 (when our data were previously reviewed) are shown in Table 1.

At the time of that review we formulated a policy, based on our experience, of closure of the VSD, plication of the pulmonary arteries and insertion of an aortic allograft RV-PA conduit irrespective of the age of the child. The technique of this procedure is shown in Fig. 1.

All 12 patients treated by this method either up to that time or subsequently have survived and done well. None of the conduits have required replacement.

We continue to utilise this policy. The frequent incidence of arborisation anomalies in the absent pulmonary valve syndrome necessitates, in our view, the insertion of a valved conduit, and the quality of the medium term results is very encouraging. The disadvantage of this approach is, of course, the likely need for conduit replacement in the future (see Elliott et al — Rastelli, this book).

Table 1. Operations for absent pulmonary valve syndrome at Great Ormond Street (1976—1983) (deaths/total patients).

Case No.	Operations	Infants < 1 yr old (mean = 15 wks)	Children > 1 yr old (mean = 5.7 yrs)	Total
1	VSD closure, PA resection, homograft valved conduit	0/2	0/5	0/7
2	VSD closure, PA resection, RVOT patch	0	0/1	0/1
3	VSD closure, PA resection, infundibular resection, Dacron xenograft valved conduit	1/1	0	1/1
4	VSD closure, PA resection, monocusp RVOT patch	0/2	0	0/2
5	VSD closure, PA resection, aortic valvuloplasty, homograft valved conduit	0	0/1	0/1
6	VSD closure, RVOT patch, xenograft valve	0	0/2	0/2
7	VSD closure, monocusp RVOT patch	3/3	0	3/3
8	VSD closure, infundibulectomy, RVOT patch		0/1	0/1
9	VSD closure	1/1	0	1/1
Total mortality		5/9 (55.6%)	0/10 (0%)	5/19 (26.3%)

VSD = ventricular septal defect; PA = pulmonary artery; RVOT = right ventricular outflow tract.
Reproduced with kind permission from ref. (1).

"Complex" tetralogy of Fallot

In our unit, since 1971, conduits have been inserted between RV and PA in 20 patients, with no operative deaths. The indications are shown in Table 2. The most frequent indication has been when the presence of peripheral pulmonary stenoses or diffusely small pulmonary arteries have been judged to be likely to result in a relatively high RV : LV pressure ratio at repair. Our usual policy is to perform lateralised shunts on young infants with Fallot's tetralogy and small pulmonary arteries. Thus residual small pulmonary arteries have been unusual in our experience.

The patient with Fallot and anomalous LAD (Fig. 2) can present a taxing problem. A variety of options have been tried:

1. Muscular resection and ventricular septal defect closure via the atrium to avoid ventriculotomy in appropriate patients;

216

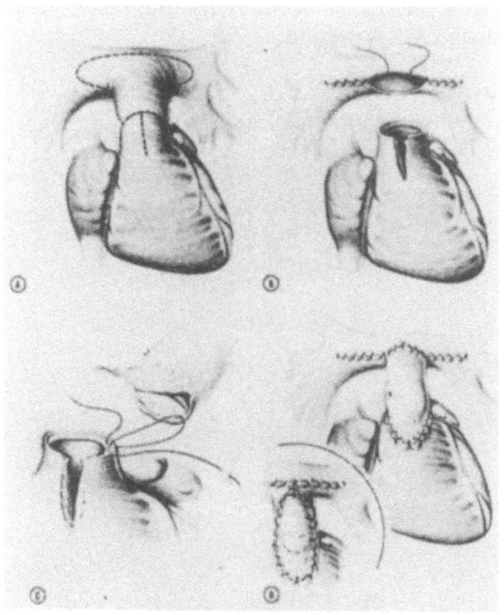

Fig. 1. (A) Line of resection of main pulmonary artery and anterior portion of main branches. Pulmonary artery is transected at anulus and an incision is made into RVOT. (B) Arterioplasty of right and left pulmonary artery branches reduces their calibre. (C) Aortic homograft is sutured to anulus. Anterior mitral leaflet of homograft is used as RVOT patch. (D) Completed repair using aortic homograft. When monocusp patch is used (inset) the posterior pulmonary artery wall is preserved. Reproduced with kind permission from ref. (1).

Table 2. Indications for conduit insertion in tetralogy of Fallot (Great Ormond Street, 1971–1986).

Indication	Number
Peripheral pulmonary stenosis or small pulmonary arteries	6
Anomalous left anterior descending coronary artery	5
Post repair pulmonary insuffiency	5
Post repair pulmonary stenosis	1
Repair to single pulmonary artery	3*

* = one after earlier "complete" repair.

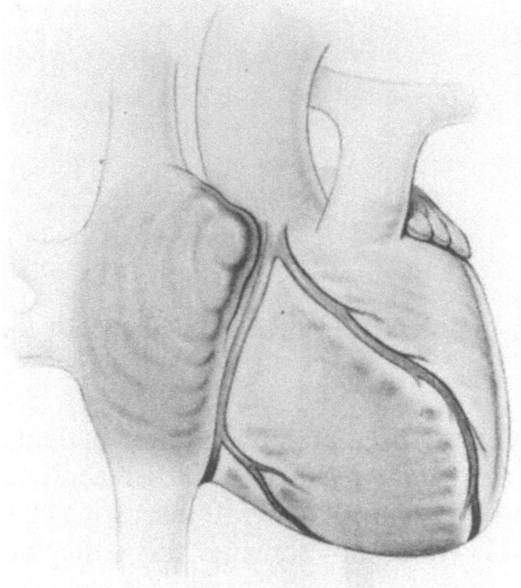

Fig. 2. Anomalous origin of the left anterior descending coronary artery from the right coronary artery.

217

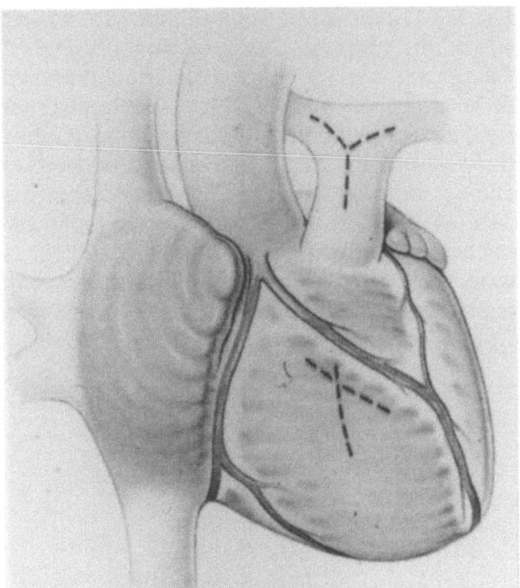

Fig. 3. Incisions for conduit insertion into anomalous LAD is present.

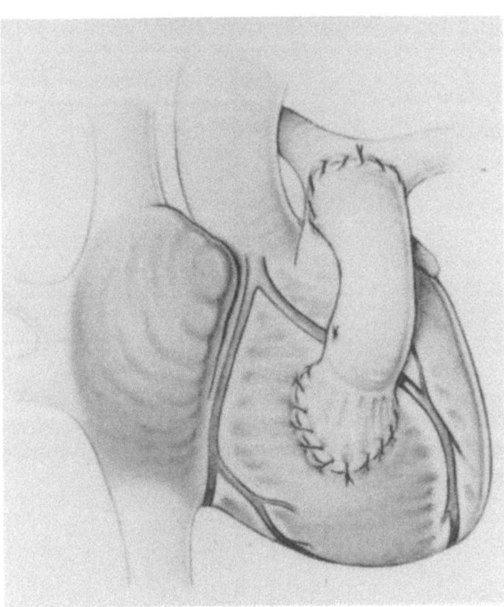

Fig. 4. Completed conduit insertion.

2. Coronary mobilisation, muscle resection and insertion of a patch beneath the mobilised artery;
3. Insertion of a conduit from RV-PA.

In our experience, transatrial repair has only rarely been possible in these patients, and the use of subcoronary patching has frequently resulted in either acute or chronic ischaemia. Thus, we have now adopted a policy of allograft insertion (Figs. 3 and 4) in all cases of truly anomalous LAD. We do not consider this policy necessary for a large conal artery.

218

Of the 20 patients who have had conduit insertion, the most recent six have had allografts. All obstructed xenografts in this group have also been replaced by allografts.

Conclusions

No allograft in either the absent pulmonary valve group or the Fallot group has yet required replacement. None have required Dacron extension. For these reasons they remain our conduit of first choice in reconstruction of the right ventricular outflow tract or pulmonary valve.

Acknowledgement

We would like to thank Mrs. Sarah Croot for her help in typing the manuscript.

References

1. Karl TR, Musumeci F, de Leval M, Pincott JR, Taylor JFN, Stark J (1986) J Thorac Cardiovasc Surg 91: 590—597

Authors' address:
M. J. Elliott
Cardiothoracic Unit
The Hospital for Sick Children
Great Ormond Street
London WC1N 3JH
U.K.

Technique of allograft repair of tetralogy of Fallot with pulmonary atresia

R. A. Jonas, J. E. Mayer, A. R. Castaneda

Department of Cardiac Surgery, Children's Hospital and Department of Surgery, Harvard Medical School, Boston, U.S.A.

Introduction and Methods

Following an analysis of the poor long-term performance of synthetic extracardiac conduits (1), we began, in February 1985, a program at the Children's Hospital, Boston, of insertion of aortic or pulmonary homografts as our extracardiac conduit of first choice. Between February 1985 and December 1986, 54 cryopreserved aortic homografts and 36 pulmonary homografts were inserted. The mean age of all patients was 52 months; there were 59 males and 31 females. Table 1 illustrates the anatomical diagnoses of patients who received homografts. There were 15 patients with tetralogy and pulmonary atresia, 8 males and 7 females. The mean age was 64 months, with a median age of 58 months. Children with hypoplastic left heart syndrome predominantly received a gusset of pulmonary artery homograft and patients with pulmonary artery stenoses generally received patch plasties of homograft artery wall. The remaining patients predominantly received complete conduits[a].

Results

By March 1987, no patient had required placement of a homograft for any reason. No patient had undergone balloon dilatation of a homograft valvar or anastomotic

Table 1. Anatomical diagnoses of patients who received homografts.

Hypoplastic left heart syndrome	22
Tetralogy, pulmonary atresia	15
Truncus	11
TGA, VSD, PS	9
Conduit change	8
Double outlet right ventricle	6
Tricuspid atresia or single ventricle	6
Pulmonary artery stenoses	6
Pulmonary regurgitation	3
Other	4
	90

[a] A videotape demonstration of the technique of insertion of a cryopreserved aortic homograft conduit between the right ventricle and pulmonary arteries in a patient with tetralogy and pulmonary atresia was presented. Copies of this videotape are available from the author.

stenosis. By March 1987, 15 of the total of 90 patients had undergone cardiac catheterisation. No gradient greater than 15 mm was detected. This finding was in marked contrast to the early performance of synthetic conduits, which regularly had initial gradients of 20—40 mm (1). Recently, one child with tetralogy and pulmonary atresia who had undergone placement of a 10-mm pulmonary homograft between the right ventricle and pulmonary artery at 8 months of age, developed a large aneurysm at the suture line between the roof of pericardium used to supplement the proximal anastomosis and the pulmonary valve. This child had severely hypoplastic pulmonary arteries and had systemic pulmonary artery pressure. The aneurysm appeared to be related to the muscle cuff below the pulmonary valve rather than in aneurysm of the pericardium itself. This emphasizes the importance of suturing any supplementary tissue roof to the pulmonary artery itself rather than the muscular infundibulum below the pulmonary valve.

Conclusion

The very short-term performance of cryopreserved aortic and pulmonary homografts applied to a wide range of clinical situations appears to be satisfactory.

Reference

1. Jonas RA, Freed MD, Mayer JE, Castaneda AR (1985) Long-term follow-up of synthetic right heart conduits. Circulation 72 (suppl II): 77—83

Authors' address:
Richard Jonas, M.D.
Department of Cardiac Surgery
Children's Hospital
300 Longwood Avenue
Boston, MA 02115
U.S.A.

The use of aortic allografts in the primary repair of truncus arteriosus in early infancy and replacement of previous conduits

K. Turley

University of California, San Francisco, U.S.A.

There has been a resurgence in the use of aortic allografts in the repair of congenital heart lesions. This has been due to the reports of excellent, long-term results of this technique and the advent of both cryopreservation and the effects of increased donor availability secondary to infant transplantation. Such cryopreserved aortic allografts have been used both in the primary repair of truncus arteriosus in the first 6 months of life and replacement of previously placed conduits at our institution. This report describes our experience with such repairs.

Truncus arteriosus is a rare congenital cardiac lesion occurring in less than 1% of infants born with congenital heart disease. It is a condition in which the main pulmonary truncus is not related to the right ventricle, but arises from a separate site on the aorta. The embryology of this lesion is important in understanding the approach to surgical repair and the possible anatomical configurations which may influence and complicate such repair. The development of the main pulmonary trunk is related to the development of the proximal portion of the 2nd—6th aortic arches. These arches form the right and left pulmonary arteries and, when they fuse, a transverse pulmonary artery and a ductus arteriosus are formed. As the truncus rotates in infancy, a spiral septum develops that separates the common trunk into the pulmonary and aortic components. If this does not occur, the main pulmonary artery does not separate, and no connection occurs between the transverse 6th arch and a separate main pulmonary artery. Thus, a transverse vessel connects directly to the pulmonary trunk (1). The natural history of truncus arteriosus, if unoperated, demonstrates that of 100 infants at birth, 75 die in the first year. Of the 25 remaining children, 35% become inoperable at age 4 due to pulmonary vascular disease. Of the 16 still operable at age 4 to 5, there is a 5% operative mortality. Of the 15 patients who survive the operation, 20% progress to late pulmonary vascular disease. Thus only 12 of the original 100 can be expected to live a relatively normal life.

Attempts at pulmonary artery banding have resulted in a natural history quite distinct from this, with, of 100 patients banded, 50% dying at the time of banding. Of those remaining, 10% die between 1 and 5 years of age, and of the 45 still alive, 9% die following band removal and repair. Finally, of the remaining 40 patients, 25% develop late pulmonary vascular disease, yielding only 30 relatively normal individuals (2).

Thus, an aggressive approach to early repair, in early infancy, has been undertaken since 1974 at the University of California, San Francisco. Initial medical management of infants with truncus is accomplished with the use of diuretics and digitalis and, on many occasions, ventilatory support. Tracheostomy should be avoided as it complicates the mediastinal surgical field and does not improve long-term results, as operative repair can be performed in early infancy, obviating the need for long-term respiratory support.

Since 1974, at our institution, the age of early correction has decreased from 6 months to approximately 6 weeks of age, in an attempt to preclude the problem of pulmonary vascular disease without increasing surgical mortality. Physiological correction of truncus arteriosus is performed through a median sternotomy incision. Under general anaesthetic, an arterial line is placed in the standard intravenous system attached to a peripheral vein. The purse-string sutures are placed high on the ascending aorta at the take-off of the inominate artery, in the right atrial appendage and a snare is placed about the pulmonary arterial trunk. Heparin is administered, and cardiopulmonary bypass is instituted. The snare about the pulmonary trunk is tightened, and the pulmonary arteries occluded. The oxygenated blood is precooled to 4—8 °C, and the body temperature rapidly cooled with bypass until the temperature reaches approximately 20 °C. The aorta is cross-clamped, and the pulmonary artery trunk separated from the underside of the aorta. The aortotomy is then closed, care being taken to avoid injury to the truncal valve or coronary arteries. The right ventricle is then opened near the truncal valve, the truncal valve inspected and made incompetent as the aortic clamp is released. The degree of truncal valve incompetence is then assessed. Rarely, severe truncal valve incompetence may be present, and a valve replacement may be necessary. The ventricular septal defect is then closed. If transseptal defect is present, care must be taken to avoid the conduction system, and a patch placed to the right side of the septum. If the usual truncal defect is present, a continuous suture technique is used. The perfusate is then rewarmed, and the distal anastomosis of the pulmonary arterial segment is performed. Finally, the proximal right ventricular to pulmonary anastomosis is performed. In the use of Dacron conduits in the past, actuarial survival of the 12 mm conduit placed in early infancy resulted in a 44 month, 50% survival. Further, the sites of significant obstruction in the 12 mm conduits were proximal anastomosis, 7; valve, 10; conduit, 12; distal anastomosis, 7; pulmonary artery, 7; and multiple sites, 11 (3). Although non-valve conduits were used initially in these patients, recurrent stenosis due to compression and pseudointemal proliferation within the nonvalve conduit has been demonstrated. Thus, an approach of early correction using an aortic homograft and subsequent replacement of previous Dacron or nonvalve conduits using the aortic homograft has been undertaken at our institution.

During the period 1986—87, 39 patients with right ventricular to pulmonary artery discontinuity underwent repair using a cryopreserved allograft at the University of California, San Francisco. There were ten primary repairs of patients less than six months of age with truncus arteriosus Type 1—2, and 16 patients in whom allograft replacements were placed (nine of whom had truncus arteriosus Type 1—2).

The placement of the allograft was typical of that previously described for truncus arteriosus Type 1—2. Significant in the placement was the use of the prior mitral valve as a right ventricular outflow tract patch, and placement of the septal muscular tissue approximately one third of the way within the right ventricular cavity, after the ventricular septal defect patch was closed using a Teflon felt pledget on the exterior of the right ventricular outflow tract patch, passing through the muscle and ventricular septal defect patch, with suture line tied within the ventricular cavity. The suture line then begins within the ventricular cavity, and is placed out to the

224

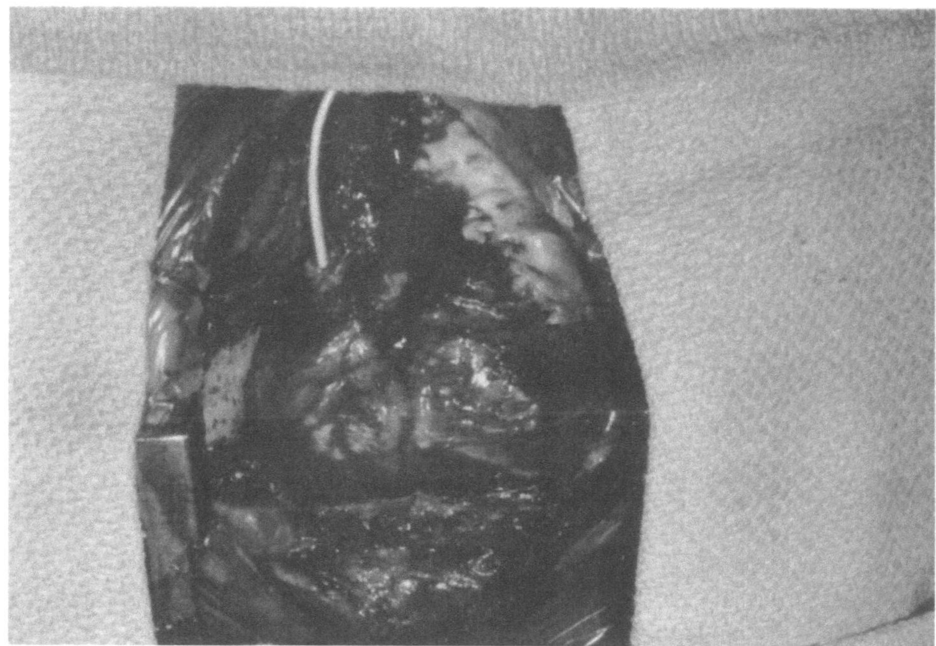

Fig. 1. An infant with truncus arteriosus repaired using an aortic allograft.

free ventricular wall. The previous mitral valve is then used as a patch with augmentation as necessary with pericardium (Fig. 1).

Among the ten patients with primary truncus repair, six were males and four females, and ages ranged from 1.9 to 5.3 months (mean 2.9 months). The sizes of the truncus ranged from 11 to 16 mm, with a mean of 13.8 mm (Table 1). Only one operative death occurred among the primary repair group — this patients was 2 days old with secondary to acute pulmonary hypertensive episode, refractory to attempts at resuscitation. Two patients experienced post-operative haemorrhage, neither from the allograft, significantly different from our previous experience with Dacron conduits in which 25—40% of patients required reoperation for haemorrhage from primary truncus repair, a significant incidence and reason for early mortality in the truncus group.

When early echocardiographic evaluation was performed, no patient demonstrated stenosis of the conduit in the primary truncus group (Fig. 2). Echocardiographic

Table 1. Results of primary repair.

#	10
Mortality	1
Haemorrhage (reop)	2
Echo stenosis	0
Echo insufficiency (mild)	4
Calcification	1
ABO incompatibility	4

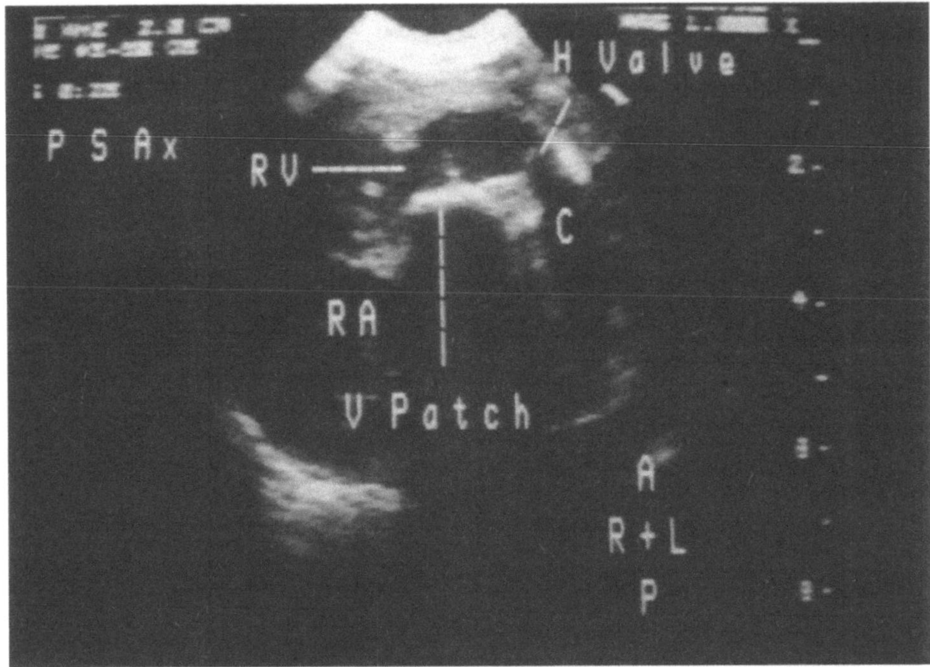

Fig. 2. Echocardiogram of an infant with truncus arteriosus repaired using an aortic allograft. RV, right ventricle; H-valve, allograft valve; RA, right atrium; V-patch, ventricular patch; C, allograft conduit.

evidence of insufficiency to a mild degree was noted in four of the ten patients. One patient was noted to develop calcification 8 months post-operatively without evidence of stenosis. Evaluation of ABO incompatibility among all ten patients revealed that four patients had such incompatibility, and yet none had developed the calcification or evidence of insufficiency. Continuing evaluation of this group for subsequent evidence of immunological degeneration of the grafts has been undertaken.

Replacement allografts have been placed in 16 patients, aged 4 to 16 years (mean 9 years), with a mean of 92 months post-operatively. Sizes ranged from 17 to 26 mm (mean 19.9 mm). Nine of these patients underwent replacement for truncus arteriosus Type 1—2, a mean of 63 months post-operatively (mean size 19.4 mm). There were no operative deaths in the replacement group. Post-operative haemorrhage occurred in two patients, one from the aortic allograft and one from diffuse mediastinal haemorrhage. Echocardiographic evidence of stenosis of the conduits was noted in five of seven patients with conduit replacement for non-truncus lesions in whom a tortuous conduit replacement was needed; however, none of these had valvar stenosis. None of the nine patients with truncus arteriosus Type 1-2 requiring replacement, using a allograft, had echocardiographic evidence of stenosis. Mild insufficiency was noted in one of the seven patients with truncus arteriosus, and in four of the nine patients in whom replacement with an allograft for truncus was accomplished. Further, calcification did occur in one patient in the non-truncus

Table 2. Results of replacement allografts.

	Total	Truncus
#	16	9
Mortality	0	0
Haemorrhage (reop)	2	0
Echo stenosis	5*	0
Echo insufficiency (mild)	5	4
Calcification	1	0
ABO incompatibility	3	1

* None Valvar (10—40 mmHg).

group. However, none of the truncus patients experienced such calcification of the allograft. ABO incompatibility was present in three of the total group, including only one of the truncus group. However, none of the patients in whom calcification or aortic insufficiency was noted were in the incompatibility group (Table 2). Thus the effects of ABO incompatibility on allograft transplantation remain unclear.

The use of aortic allografts have significantly increased the size of both the initial and replacement conduits in patients with truncus arteriosus Type 1—2, as well as patients with other congenital abnormalities without resulting in conduit compression while decreasing morbidity of post-operative haemorrhage and significant other morbidity. We believe the results of this study demonstrate that aortic allograft repair of truncus arteriosus in early infancy results in acceptable mortality and decreased morbidity. Longevity of the allograft may exceed that of the small tube or heterograft conduit with a larger initial conduit and the avoidance of pseudointimal proliferative obstruction, as seen in our previous conduit series. Replacement of prior conduits with aortic allografts of adult size greater than 188 mm may decrease the total number of replacements necessary in this unique group of patients in whom early repair of their significant inter-cardiac lesion may result in a normal lifespan if proper care is taken.

References

1. Van Praagh R, Van Praagh S (1965) The anatomy of common aorticopulmonary trunk (truncus arteriosus communis) and its embryologic implications: A study of fifty-seven necropsy cases. Am J Cardiol 16: 406
2. Oldham HN, Jr., Kakos GS, Jarmakani MM, Sabiston DC, Jr. (1972) Pulmonary artery banding in infants with complex congenital heart defects. Ann Thorac Surg 13: 342
3. Boyce SW, Turley K., Yee ES, Verrier ED, Ebert PA (1987) The fate of 12 mm porcine valve right ventricular to pulmonary artery conduit: A ten year experience. J Thorac Cardiovasc Surg, in press

Author's address:
K. Turley, M.D.
Cardiothoracic Surgery
University of California Medical Center
505 Parnassus Avenue
San Francisco, CA 94143
U.S.A.

Allografts in the Rastelli procedure: Techniques

M. J. Elliott, R. Almeida, R. K. H. Wyse, M. R. de Leval, J. Stark

Cardiothoracic Unit, The Hospital for Sick Children, London, U.K.

Introduction

Children with transposition of the great arteries (TGA) (VA discordance), ventricular septal defect (VSD) and anatomical left ventricular outflow tract obstruction (LVOTO) used to be treated by the Mustard operation, closure of the VSD and surgical relief of the obstruction. This carried out a mortality in excess of 50% (1, 2), largely due to the difficulty in relieving the LVOTO. The prognosis of children with this complex of disorders was improved by the application of the Rastelli operation (3). This operation consists in enlargement of the VSD, diversion of the LV outflow to the aorta by an intraventricular tunnel/patch and connection of right ventricle (RV) to pulmonary artery (PA) by an external valved conduit (Figs. 1—3). Details of the operative technique we use have been published elsewhere (4, 5).

Choice of conduit in the Rastelli operation

Most authorities gained early experience in the Rastelli procedure using heterograft valved conduits such as the Hancock. Our unit was no exception. Awareness that such conduits underwent calcific degeneration ± fibrin peel development meant that the introduction of the aortic allograft was greeted with enthusiam. In our unit, the fresh antibiotic-preserved aortic allograft has, over the years, become our conduit of choice.

Technical considerations

Because of the posterior position of the pulmonary arteries in most cases of TGA, the distance between RV and PA may be relatively large. Conduit compression can readily occur. Thus, in our experience, we have often found it necessary to extend the allograft by anastomosis with a Dacron tube (Fig. 4). The technique of insertion of such a composite conduit is illustrated in Fig. 5—8. Note the wide incision in the PA and distal placement of the allograft valve which was considered to be the best way of preventing valve dysfunction due to conduit compression. Note also the direct suturing of the VSD patch to the proximal end of the composite conduit after appropriate trimming.

229

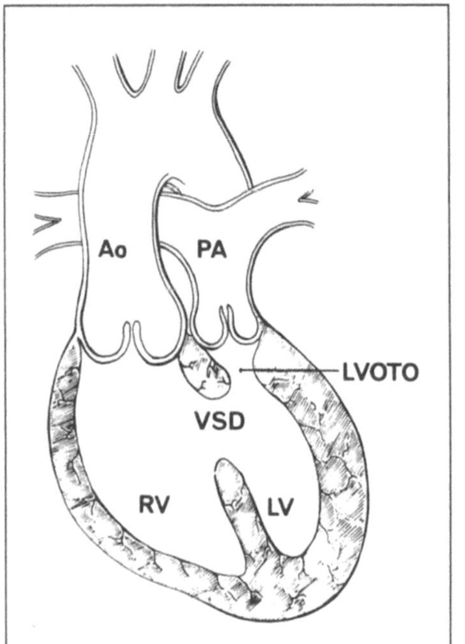

Fig. 1

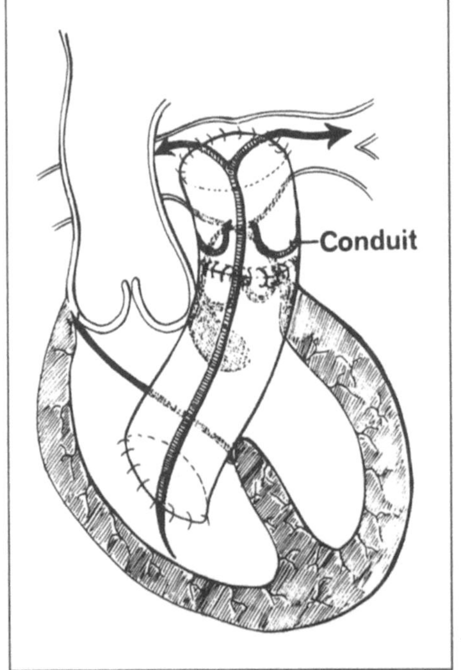

Fig. 3

Fig. 1–3. Diagrams to illustrate the principle of the Rastelli procedure. Reprinted with kind permission from ref. (5).

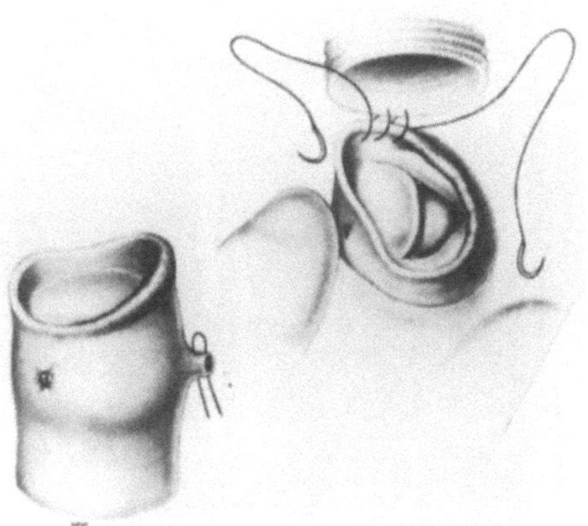

Fig. 4. The technique of extending an aortic allograft with a Dacron tube. Reprinted with kind permission from ref. (4).

Results

At The Hospital for Sick Children, Great Ormond Street, London, from 1971 to December 1986, 83 patients have undergone the Rastelli procedure. There were 13 hospital deaths (16%) and there have been 17 late deaths (20%). Total mortality was 36%. Actuarial survival (Fig. 9), including early deaths, was 78% at 1 year, 68% at 5 years and 50% at 10 years. Most of the early deaths relate to perioperative low cardiac output. The type of conduit used did not influence survival.

Of the 70 hospital survivors there have been 17 reoperations (24%). Eleven reoperations were indicated for valve or conduit change, and five to close a residual VSD.

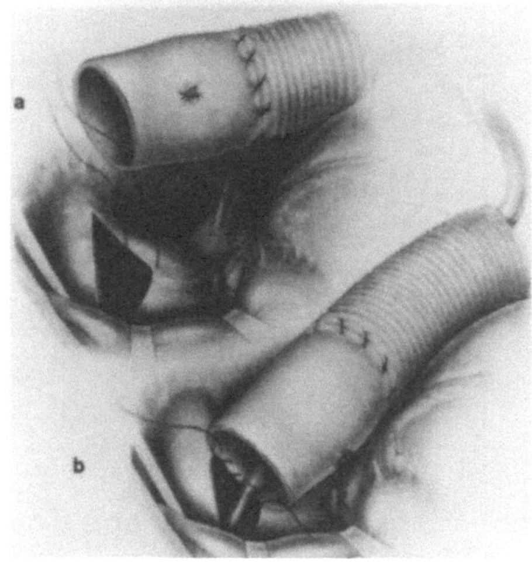

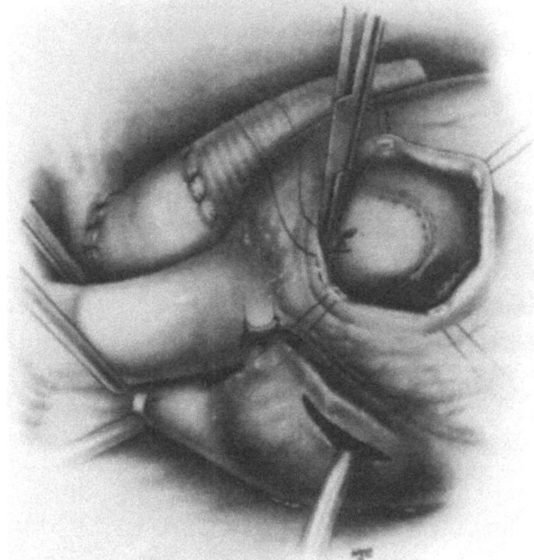

Fig. 5

Fig. 6

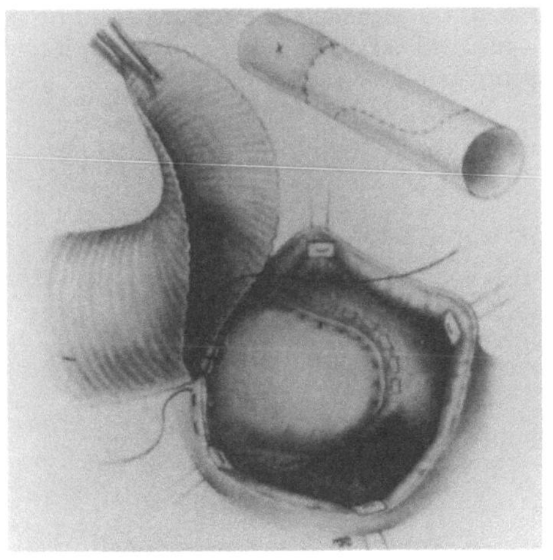

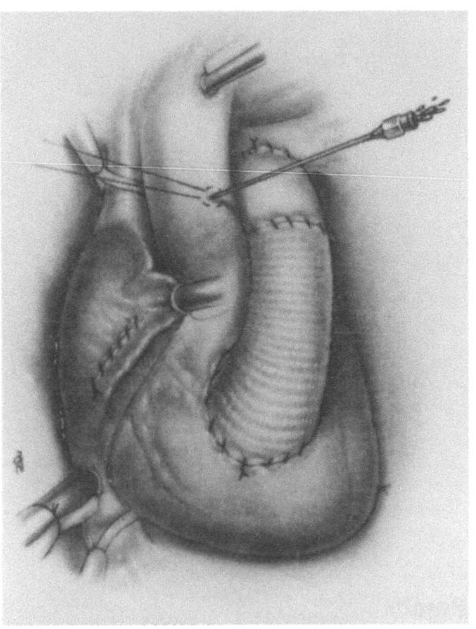

Fig. 7

Fig. 5–8. Diagram illustrating the technique of insertion of a composite allograft in the Rastelli procedure. Reprinted with kind permission from (4).

Fig. 8.

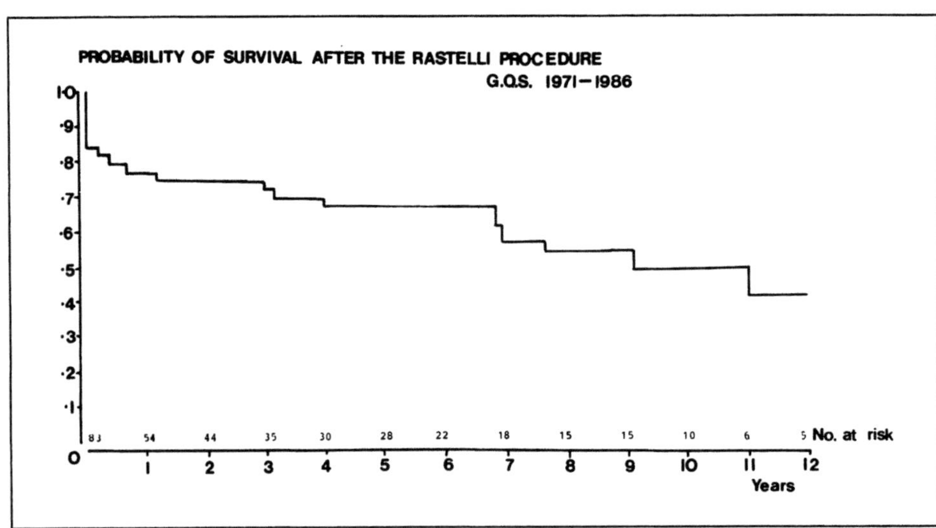

Fig. 9. Actuarial survival after the Rastelli procedure.

Conduit performance

The results of conduit insertion for the Rastelli procedure do not differ from those in other procedures in our unit. From 1971 to December 1986, 338 conduits have been inserted in our unit. They were made up as follows:

232

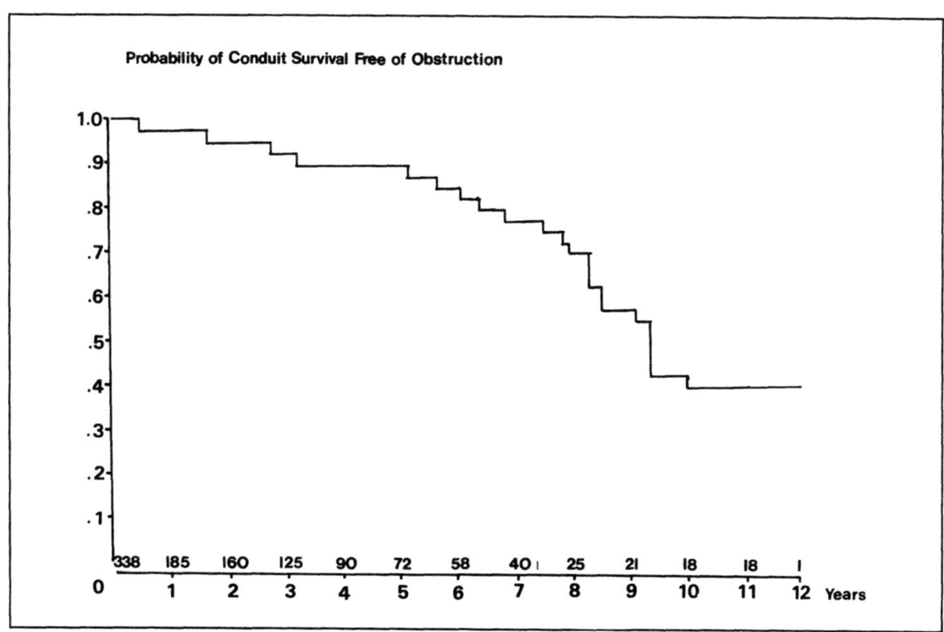

Fig. 10. Actuarial freedom from obstruction (all conduits). Great Ormond Street 1971–1986. Courtesy of Almeida (in press).

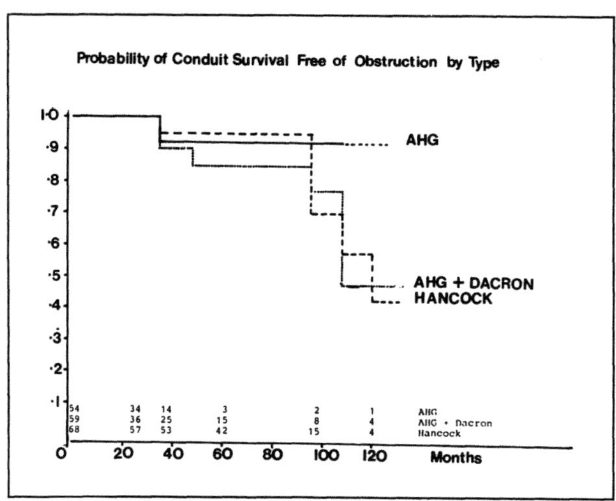

Fig. 11. Comparison of actuarial freedom from obstruction between allografts with and without extension and Hancock xenografts. Courtesy of Almeida (in press).

Aortic allografts	84
Aortic allografts with Dacron extension	76
Aortic allografts in Dacron tube	16
Hancock xenografts	97
Carpentier-Edwards	13
Ross	25
Other	27

233

Taking these conduits and considering their actuarial freedom from obstruction (ignoring death as an event) (Fig. 10), there was no significant difference in conduit "survival" between allografts alone, allografts with Dacron tube extension or other varieties (Fig. 11). However, the trend suggests that the homograft without extension has performed best, but its follow-up is too short to allow statistical comparison or definitive conclusion.

Comment

Our data support the view that the Rastelli procedure has improved the prognosis of patients with TGA, VSD and LVOTO. The incidence of late mortality is disappointing, however, reflecting the severity of the disorder, persistent decreased LV function (6), and the risk associated with frequent reoperations.

Conduits replacement has been the major indication for such procedures and thus conduit durability must be a significant risk factor for morbidity and mortality in the long-term. We have been disappointed by the failure of the allografts to meet their initial promise in our hands. We could not detect a significant difference in conduit survival free of obstruction between the allografts and Hancock valved conduits.

There may be a number of reasons for this poor performance:

Dacron tube extension was thought to be a major factor because of the frequent occurence of fibrin peel within the tube. However, the differentiation between the performance of the composite graft and the allograft alone has not been as clear as anticipated.

The interval between harvesting of the allograft and implantation may also be relevant. Preliminary data (Almeida et al., unpublished observations) suggest that this interval is a significant ($p = 0.02$) risk factor for the development of later obstruction. The technique of preservation must be an important modulator of later performance. Rapid usage or early cryopreservation may thus perhaps be indicated, but more detailed analysis is required to confirm this.

Our current policy is to use antibiotic-preserved aortic allografts of as short a storage age as possible and to avoid extension with Dacron if possible. If unavoidable, we now extend the allograft with knitted rather than woven Dacron, and preseal it with Tisseel fibrin glue (Immuno, Sevenoaks, Kent, U.K.) to try to reduce the risk of peel formation. The long-term results of this intervention are not known. Clearly, greater understanding of the factors influencing allograft survival will assist our choice of conduit for the Rastelli procedure.

Acknowledgement

The authors would like to thank Mrs. Sarah Croot for her help in typing the manuscript.

References

1. Danielson GK, Tabry IF, Mair DD, Fulton RE (1978) Great-vessel switch operation with coronary relocation for transposition of great arteries. Mayo Clin Proc 53: 675—682
2. Breckenridge IM, Oelert H, Stark J, Graham GR, Bonham-Carter RE, Waterston DJ (1972) Mustard's operation for transposition of the great arteries. Review of 200 cases. Lancet 1: 1140—1142
3. Rastelli GC (1969) A new approach to "anatomic" repair of transposition of the great arteries. Mayo Clin Proc 44: 1—12
4. Stark J (1983) Concordant transposition and left ventricular outflow tract obstruction. In: Stark J, de Leval M (eds) Surgery for Congenital Heart Defects, Grune and Stratton, London, p 361—373
5. Stark J (1986) Transposition of the great arteries with left ventricular outflow tract obstruction. In: Jamieson SW, Shumway NE (eds) Rob and Smith's Operative Surgery — Cardiac Surgery. Butterworths, London, 319—327
6. Graham TP, Jr, Franklin RCG, Wyse RKH, Gooch V, Danfield JE (1987) Left ventricular wall stress and contractile function in transposition of the great arteries after the Rastelli operation. J Thorac Cardiovasc Surg 92: 775—784

Authors' address:
M. J. Elliott
Cardiothoracic Unit
The Hospital for Sick Children
Great Ormond Street
London WC1N 3JH
U.K.

Allograft conduit for Fontan procedure

G. Fernandez, C. Deville, A. Ebner, Ch. Doutremepuich, F. Fontan

Clinique Chirurgicale des Maladies Cardiaques Hôpital Cardiologique du Haut-Lévêque, Pessac-Bordeaux, France

Introduction

The use of an extracardiac conduit in the treatment of complex congenital heart disease was first reported by Rastelli in 1965 (1) and by Ross and Somerville in 1966 (2) with an aortic valve allograft. Irradiated aortic allografts were abandoned early (3, 4). The use of a conduit containing a porcine aortic valve was first reported by Planche (5), but late complications in some series (6, 7) led to the discontinuation of their use. If non-valved conduits and direct cardiopulmonary anastomosis, first described by Lillehei (8), are often advocated, the use of aortic valve allografts is frequently favored by several groups: Shabbo (9) and Radley-Smith (10).
We reported our results with the aortic valve allograft in 1984 (11). Since then, five reoperations for conduit obstruction were performed in patients with aortic valve allografts used as extracardiac conduit in the Fontan procedure.
We have analysed our results to determine the influence of this surgical procedure on immediate and late results.

Patients and Methods

Among the 154 patients who underwent surgical repair using Fontan procedure from April 1968 to July 1987, 73 received aortic valve allografts. There were 39 males and 34 females with a mean age of 11 years 4 months (ranging from 2 years 2 months to 36 years). The most common cardiac malformation was tricuspid atresia, n = 42. The malformations are listed in Table I. 51 patients had undergone 61 previous palliative surgical procedures: one procedure in 42 patients, two procedures in 8 patients and 3 in one patient (Table 2). The indication for operation included, in all cases, increasing cyanosis and dyspnoea at rest and/or on exertion at the time of surgical repair (mean haemoglobin value: 21.4 g/100 ml; arterial oxygen saturation: 78.5%).

Operation

All interventions were done through a median sternotomy with standard methods of cardiopulmonary bypass and varying degrees of hypothermia (25 ° to 28 °C). Pericardial cooling and cold cardioplegia have been accomplished since 1976 for myocardial protection during the ischaemic period of aortic cross-clamping. The pre-

237

Table 1. Preoperative diagnoses

Cardiac malformations	Patients
Tricuspid atresia	42
Double inlet univentricular heart	26
Hypoplastic right heart	2
Criss-cross heart	1
Mitral atresia	1
Double outlet left atrium	1
Total	73

Table 2. Previous palliative surgery in 51 patients.

Surgical procedure	N
Blalock Taussig	33
Waterston	7
Glenn anastomosis	10
Pulmonary artery banding	9
Blalock Hanlon	1
Davidson	1
Total	61

vious surgically created aorto-pulmonary shunts were controlled and repaired; Glenn anastomoses were left in place. The intracardiac defects were repaired: atrial septal defect was closed with a direct continuous suture or with a patch, and ventricular septal defect was closed with a dacron patch. Atriopulmonary or atrioventricular continuity was established with an aortic valve allograft, as previously described for the correction of tricuspid atresia (12, 13). Additional procedures were performed in three patients: mitral valvuloplasty and mitral valve replacement in two cases of mitral valve incompetence, pulmonary commissurotomy for valve stenosis in one case.

The postoperative mean right atrial pressure (3 h p.o.) was available in 58 patients. The 52 survivors who had undergone operation were evaluated by direct examination, or direct contact with their cardiologist or physician. The follow-up period ranged from 2 years 1 month to 19 years 3 months (average 7 years 6 months). The date of enquiry or examination for the 44 actual surviving patients was June—July 1987. Exercise tests were performed on a cycle ergometer or a treadmill in 26 patients and expressed as a percentage of normal value for age, sex, weight and height. Postoperative control cardiac catheterisations were available in 37 patients at a mean age of 3 years 7 months (range: 1 month to 14 years 6 months), 16 patients had serial control catheterisations. The following pressures were studied in 37 patients: right atrial, right ventricular and pulmonary artery pressure. Postoperative right angiocardiograms were available in all these patients.

Data in proportional form are presented with 70% confidence limits. Variables tested were: anatomical type, mode of surgical repair, immediate postoperative right atrial pressures, late postoperative, right ventricular, pulmonary artery pressures and exercise capacity parameters. Actuarial survival curves were constructed by the Kaplan and Meier method.

Aortic valve allograft

A total of 85 aortic valve allografts were used, either as an outlet valve: 68 (atrio-pulmonary connection 52, atrioventricular connection: 16) or as an inlet valve: 15 (in the inferior caval vein 14, in the superior caval vein 1). Allografts were used for replacement of an obstructed aortic valve allograft in two patients.

Since 1971, all aortic valves allografts were collected under sterile conditions within 24 h of death. The different techniques of sterilisation and storage are indicated in Table 3. Since 1982, 19 cryopreserved aortic valve allografts have been used. ABO Rh compatibility of blood groups was taken into account in the selection of the aortic valve allograft whenever possible since 1979.

Results
Early mortality

Early mortality was considered within the first 6 months, since hospital mortality is rarely representative of the early risk of death, particularly in this surgery.
29 of the 73 patients died within 6 months after operation. In the group of 42 patients with tricuspid atresia there were 11 deaths (26%). Six patients died in the first 48 h, four of them from pulmonary vascular disease, one from cardiac and renal failure and, the last from atrial dysrhythmia and cardiac failure. One patient died 5 days after surgery from disseminated intravascular coagulation. Four patients died within 3 months postoperatively, three of them from cardiac failure and the fourth patient from pulmonary embolism. In the group of 26 patients with double inlet univentricular heart, there were eight deaths (31%). One patient died 5 months

Table 3. Preparation of aortic valve allograft (85 aortic valve allografts).

Sterilisation	Storage		
	Medium	+ 4 °C N	−196 °C N
Betapropiolactone (1968—1970)	Hank TC 199	5 52	
Antibiotic (1971—1982)	Trowell	9	
Antibiotic (1982—1987)	TC 199 DMSO		19

DMSO = dimethyl sulphoxide; TC 199 = tissue culture 199.

after surgery from cardiac failure, possibly related to some degree of pulmonary vascular disease. All other deaths occurred in the postoperative period, due to cardiac failure in two patients, and in the others due to atrial dysrhythmia, renal failure, pulmonary vascular disease, neurological complications and tracheal bleeding, respectively.

In the group of five patients with other complex cardiac malformation, two patients (40%) died from cardiac failure, one of them had hypoplastic right heart and the other had mitral atresia.

Postoperative mean right atrial pressure (3 h postoperatively)

The different types of correction or operations are shown in Table 4. In Table 5, the postoperative right atrial pressures in the group with direct anastomosis and with aortic valve allograft connection are shown.

Reoperations

In the immediate postoperative period, 13 patients required reoperations: five for bleeding, three for a dehiscent tricuspid patch, three for atrioventricular block (necessitating pace-maker implantation). In two other patients, cardiac failure 24 h postoperatively was the indication for reoperation; in one of them a Glenn proce-

Table 4. Mean right atrial pressure (3 h post operatively) in 58 patients.

Type of Connection	RAP Survivors			RAP Deaths		
	Patients	Mean	Range	Patients	Mean	Range
RA–PA	25	16	10—22	12	20	14—29
RA–RV	10	17	12—24	2	22	20—23
RA–PA + AVA in ICV	4	20	18—22	2	21	19—22
Direct anast. + AVA in ICV	2	18	15—20	1	18	
Total	41	16	10—24	17	20	14—29

RAP = right atrial pressure; RA = right atrium; PA = pulmonary artery; AVA = aortic valve allograft; ICV = inferior caval vein; RV = right ventricle.

Table 5. Post-operative mean right atrial pressure.

Type of connection	Patients	Mean RA pressure	
AVA	58	18	
			$0.01 < p < 0.02$
Direct anastomosis	66	16	

AVA = aortic valve allograft; RA = right atrial.

Table 6. Late reoperations non AVA-related.

Dg.	Procedures	Delay	Results
DIUH	Pericardial drainage	6.5 months	Dead
	VSD closure + Glenn	2 years	Good
TA	VSD enlargement	3 years 2 months	Good
	AVA in ICV	3 years 4 months	Good*

* This patient was reoperated for AVA obstruction 4 years 5 months after this procedure.
DIUH = double inlet univentricular heart; TA = tricuspid atresia; AVA = aortic valve allograft;
ICV = inferior caval vein; VSD = ventricular septal defect.

dure had been performed previously, and in the second patient, reopening of the atrial and ventricular septal defects was necessary. There were four late reoperations not related to aortic valve allograft (Table 6).

Five patients were reoperated for aortic valve allograft obstruction (9.6% of the 52 survivors). A 19-year-old patient with tricuspid atresia corrected 3 years 7 months before, had mild obstruction of the aortic valve allograft. At the last follow-up; he was waiting for reoperation using direct anastomosis.

Actuarial rate of aortic valve allograft obstruction is 11.5% from 2 years 10 months to 14 years 8 months (average 8 years 9 months) after operation. The results of the patients with reoperations and additional procedures are listed in Table 7. Second aortic valve allografts were used in the first two patients and direct anastomosis was performed in three others. There were two early deaths, one patient with tricuspid atresia, died 5 days after reoperation from cardiac failure, and another patient with double inlet univentricular heart died 14 days after reoperation from cardiac and renal failure. The oldest patient (51 years) with tricuspid atresia died 7 months after reoperation in progressive right cardiac failure. One of the two survivors had a excellent result 6 months after reoperation. The other, a 16-year-old girl, after a good initial result 1 year 2 months after reoperation, had dyspnoea and hepatic pains at full exercise. Her exercise test tolerance was very low (25% of normal). Angiography showed a very important right ventricular to right atrium regurgitation. This patient is awaiting reoperation: exclusion of the right ventricle and direct anastomosis between right atrium and pulmonary artery are scheduled. This reoperation was recently performed with excellent results.

Pathological anatomy

Explanted aortic valve allografts were studied by electron microscopy and results in three patients showed a sclero-hyaline degeneration with calcification of the aortic valve allograft.

Late mortality

Eight patients died between 1 year 4 months and 15 years 3 months postoperatively. The actuarial survival rate of patients is shown in Fig. 1. The causes of late deaths

Table 7. Reoperations for aortic valve allograft obstruction.

Patients Age/Date	Diag-nosis	Connection Type AVA	Time inter-val 1st and 2nd operation	Type of reoperation	Additional procedure	Result	Deaths early 6 m.	late 6 m.
36 y. 4-1-1970	TA	RA—PA ICV	14 y. 8 m.	AVA RA—PA	Mitral valvuloplasty Atrial shunt closure	±		7 months
27 y. 14-3-1978	DIUH	RA—PA	6 y. 10 m.	AVA RA—PA	Tricuspid valve closure	—	14th day	
9 y. 6 m. 2-5-1974	TA	RA—PA	12 y. 10 m.	Direct anastomosis	Tricuspid valve closure	+ + +		
11 y. 4 m. 16-3-1978	TA	RA—PA	7 y. 9 m.	Direct anastomosis RA—PA	RA thrombectomy VSD enlargement Pacemaker	—	5th day	
11 y. 8 m. 12-7-1983	TA	RA—RV	2 y. 10 m.	Direct anastomosis RA—RV		+ +		

AVA = aortic valve allograft; RA = right atrium; PA = pulmonary artery; RV = right ventricle; ICV = inferior caval vein; DIUV = double inlet univentricular heart; TA = tricuspid atresia; VSD = ventricular septal defect; y. = years; n. = months.

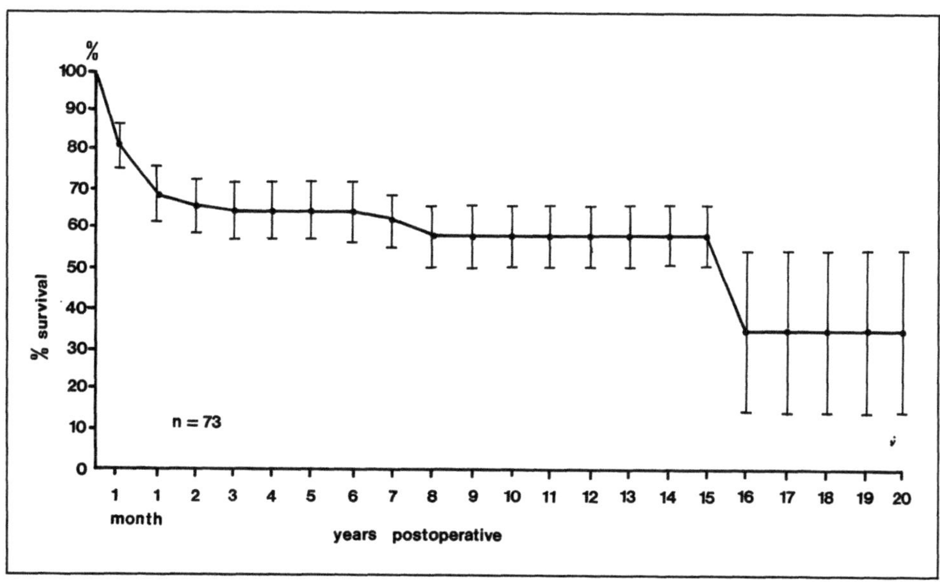

Fig. 1. Actuarial overall survival of patients, extending to 19 years postoperatively.

are reported in Table 8. Three of the patients who died had had reoperation for aortic valve obstruction.

The overall survival was 60% extending up to 19 years in this series of 73 patients. This was lower in complex cardiac malformations (40%) and in double inlet univentricular heart (54%) and higher in tricuspid atresia (67%).

Table 8. Late deaths (8 patients).

Cause	Patients	Delay	Malformation
Ventricular arrhythmia	1	1 year 4 months	TA
Heart failure	4	6 years 3 months	DIUH
		7 years 8 months	DIUH*
		7 years 9 months	TA*
		15 years 3 months	TA*
Adeno carcinoma (liver)	1	8 months	HRH
Reoperation (drainage)	1	6.5 months	DIUH
Cerebrovascular Accident	1	2 years 8 months	DIUH
Total	8		

TA = tricuspid atresia; DIUH = double inlet univentricular heart; HRH = hypoplastic right heart.
* These patients had had reoperation for aortic valve allograft replacement.

Functional status of the 42 survivors (two patients were reoperated for aortic valve allograft obstruction and underwent a direct anastomosis and were excluded) according to the New York Heart Association (NYHA) Classification are summarized in Table 9: 95% of patients belong to class I or II. Two patients are in class III: one of the two patients in class III, a 19-year-old boy with tricuspid atresia corrected 3 years 7 months ago, received another aortic valve allograft for his obstructed graft: the second patient a 19-year-old boy with criss-cross heart has pulmonary valve insufficiency. The percentage of patients in class I or II is higher in the atrioventricular connection group (100%) than in the group with atriopulmonary connections (92%). Among the three patients with allograft pulmonary connections and inferior vena cava inflow allograft valves, 2 are in class I and the third is in class II, with a follow-up of 6 years to 13 years 4 months (mean 8 years 4 months). Three other patients with exclusive inferior vena cava inflow allograft valves are in class I with a follow-up of 6 years to 19 years 6 months (mean: 13 years 2 months).

Exercise capacity

The exercise tolerance was identical in patients with atrioventricular connections (mean: 79% of normal), in patients with direct connections and inferior vena cava

Table 9. Functional results in 42 patients*.

NYHA Class	Patients	
	N	%
I	25	60
II	15	35
III	2	5
Total	42	100

* Two patients of 44 survivors, reoperated with aortic valve allograft for obstruction underwent a direct anastomosis.

Table 10. Exercise tolerance in 25 patients*.

Connection	Number of patients	% of normal	
		Mean	Range
RA—PA	16	73	30—100
RA—RV	7	79	70—100
Direct anastomosis + AVA in ICV	2	78	55—100
Total	25	75	30—100

* Excluded one patient with AVA obstruction who must have a reoperation in some weeks.
RA = right atrium; PA = pulmonary artery; RV = right ventricle; AVA = aortic valve allograft; ICV = inferior caval vein.

inflow valves (mean: 78%) and slightly lower in patients with atriopulmonary connections (73%) (Table 10).

Post-operative catheterisation data

A 4—9 mm Hg gradient was observed in six patients. The gradient never exceeded 10 mm Hg in the 37 patients with available data. These results confirm our previous report (11). However, we must point out that in patients with stenosis and calcified allograft walls, the analysis of the catheterisation data did not reveal pressure gradient higher than 2 mm Hg at the last check-ups. Among the six patients with aortic valve obstruction, five had serial catheterisation. The data are shown in Fig. 2.

Discussion

In our previous report (11) there were no reoperations for aortic valve allograft obstruction in atriopulmonary or atrioventricular connections within a 10-15-year follow-up and we were encouraged to continue the use of aortic valve allografts. Since 1984, six of the 52 survivors (11.5%) of these series, had an aortic valve allograft obstruction at a mean time of 8 years. Five of them were reoperated at a mean time of 8 years 9 months. This complication demonstrates a real risk of reoperation in aortic valve allograft conduits. This complication therefore seems to occur later and more rarely than with other types of valved conduits (14, 15) except

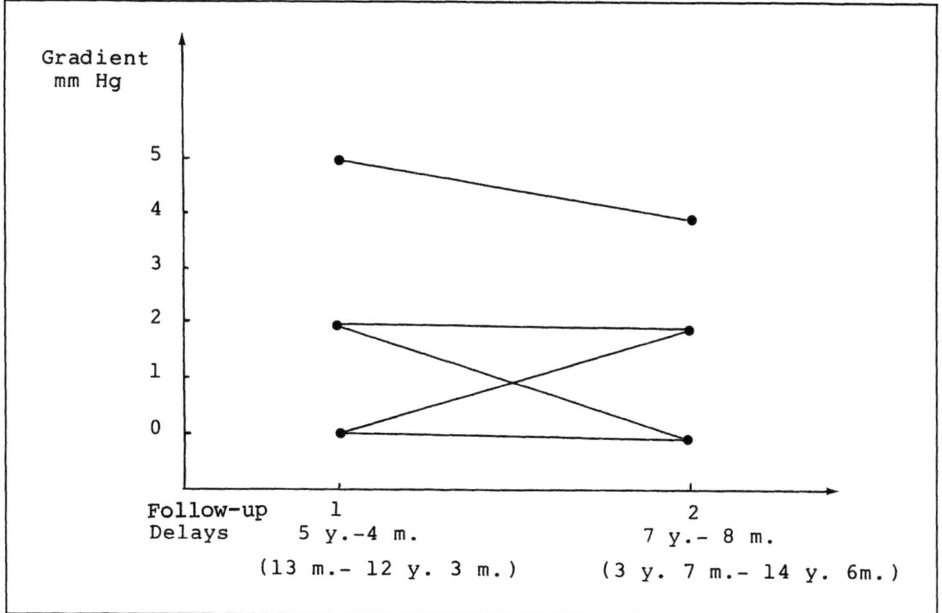

Fig. 2. Gradient at the site of aortic valve allograft in 5 patients with aortic valve allograft obstruction. Y = years; m = months.

in a recent report by Bull (16) in which no difference was observed according to the type of the valved conduit. The diagnosis of aortic valve allograft obstruction was made on clinical (NYHA class III) and angiographic data: the angiocardiogram could show valve obstruction. Neither right atrial pressure nor transvalvular gradient led to the diagnosis. Like others (16), we think that the gradient following obstruction across an atriopulmonary valved connection is less informative than in ventriculo-pulmonary valve connections. In the removed aortic valve allografts, sclero-hyaline degeneration with calcifications were found and the aortic valves had lost their normal structure. The type of antibiotic sterilisation and storage did not seem to influence the valve degeneration in our results. Mean right atrial postoperative pressure (3 h p.o.) was higher (20 mm Hg) in patients who died than in survivors (16 mm Hg) (Table 4). This predictive factor is more specific in patients with right atrium-pulmonary artery allograft valve connection (16 mm Hg in survivors − 20 mm Hg in dead patients, $p < 0.01$) than in patients with inferior vena cava inlet valve with an outlet allograft (20 mm Hg in survivors, 21 mm Hg in dead patients) or without outlet allograft (18 mm Hg in both groups). When comparing this factor in patients with aortic valve allograft connection and in patients with direct anastomosis connection, the mean right atrial pressure is significantly higher ($p < 0.02$) in patients with allograft connection (18 mm Hg) than in patients with direct connection (16 mm Hg) (Table 5). The overall mortality was significantly lower (21%) in direct atriopulmonary or atrioventricular connections than when an outlet aortic valve allograft was used (40%) ($0.01 < p < 0.02$). Among the 42 patients still bearing an aortic valve allograft, 25 (60%) are in class I of the NYHA, 15 (35%) are in class II and two (5%) in class III. Among the five patients who received an aortic valve allograft exclusively in the inferior caval vein, there was an early death from pulmonary vascular disease. There was one late death after 1 year 4 months due to ventricular arrhythmia. The three survivors are in class I with a mean follow-up of 13 years 2 months. Aortic valve allograft as inlet valve in inferior vena caval position seems to provide good results.

Conclusion

This experience shows that the use of an aortic valve allograft as an outlet valve in this type of surgery introduces a risk of reoperation which is lower in our series than in others using a different type of valved conduits (17, 18).

However, direct anastomosis should be the technique of choice in the Fontan procedure. Aortic valve allograft still may have a place as inlet valve in inferior caval vein, particularly in patients with hypoplastic or absent eustachian valve, also in case of atrioventricular connection when a well-developed right ventricular trabecular chamber is to be kept in circuit, or in patients presenting heart failure with or without protein-losing enteropathy due to reflux from right ventricle to right atrium as an option to trabecular chamber exclusion.

References

1. Rastelli GC, Ongley PA, Davis GD, Kirklin JW (1965) Surgical repair for pulmonary valve atresia with coronary pulmonary artery fistula. Report of case. Mayo Clin Proc 40: 521

2. Ross DN, Somerville J (1966) Correction of pulmonary atresia with a homograft aortic valve. Lancet 2: 1446
3. Park SC, Neches WH, Lenox CC, Zuberbumler JR, Bahnson HT (1973) Massive calcification and obstruction in a homograft after the Rastelli procedure for transposition of the great arteries. Am J Cardiol 32: 860—864
4. Moodie DS, Mair DD, Fulton RE, Wallace RB, Danielson GK, McGoon DC (1976) Aortic homograft obstruction. J Thorac Cardiovasc Surg 72: 553—561
5. Planche C, Binet JP, Langlois J, Conso JF (1972) Reconstruction de la voie d'éjection du ventricule droit à l'aide de tubes valves. Nouv. Presse Méd. 1: 541
6. Norwood WI, Freed MD, Rocchini AP, Bernhard WF, Castagneda AR (1977) Experience with valved conduits for repair of congenital cardiac lesions. Ann Thorac Surg 24: 223
7. Bailey WW, Kirklin JW, Bargeron LM, Pacifico HD, Kouchoukos NT (1977) Late results with synthetic valved external conduits from venous ventricle to pulmonary arteries. Circulation 56, Suppl. 2: 73
8. Lillehei CW, Cohen M, Warden HE, Read RC, Aust JB, Dewer RA, Varco Rl (1955) Direct vision inracardiac surgical correction of the tetralogy of Fallot, pentalogy of Fallot and pulmonary atresia defects: Report of first ten cases. Ann Surg 142: 418
9. Shabbo FP, Wain WH, Ross DN (1980) Right ventricular outflow tract reconstruction with aortic homograft conduit: analysis of long-term results. Thorac Cardiovasc Surg 28: 21—25
10. Radley-Smith RIC, Yacoub M (1980) The late results of reconstruction of the right ventricular outflow tract using a complete aortic homograft. Congress of the European Society of Cardiology, Paris, France
11. Fontan F, Choussat A, Deville C, Doutremepuich C, Coupillaud J, Vosa C (1984) Aortic valve homografts in the surgical treatment of complex cardiac malformations. J Thorac Cardiovasc Surg 87, 5: 649
12. Fontan F, Mounicot FB, Baudet E, Simonneau J, Gordo J, Gouffrant JM (1971) Correction de l'atrésie tricuspidienne, rapport de 2 cas corrigés par l'utilisation d'une technique chirurgicale nouvelle. Ann Chir Thorac Cardiovasc 10: 39
13. Fontan F, Baudet E (1971) Surgical repair of tricuspid atresia. Thorax 26: 240
14. McGoon DC, Danielson GK, Puga FJ, Ritter DG, Mair DD, Ilstrup DM (1982) Late results after extracardiac conduit repair for congenital cardiac defects. Am J Cardiol 49: 1741—1749
15. Tatooles CJ, Ardekani RG, Miller RA, Seratto M (1976) Operative repair for tricuspid atresia. Ann Thorac Surg 21, 6: 499
16. Bull C, McCartney FJ, Horvath P, Almeida R, Merril W, Douglas J, Taylor JFN, de Leval MR, Stark J (1987) Evaluation of long term results of homograft and heterograft valves in extracadiac conduit. J Thorac Cardiovasc Surg 94: 12-9
17. Ciaravella JM, McGoon DC, Danielson GK, Wallace RB, Mair DD (1979) Experience with extracardiac conduits. J Thorac Cardiovasc Surg 78, 6: 920
18. Castaneda AR, Norwood W (1982) Valved conduits, a panacea for complex congenital heart defects? In: Cohn LH, Galluci V (eds) Cardiac bioprosthesis. Proceeding of the 2nd International Symposium. Yorke Medica Books, New York

Authors' address:
Prof. F. Fontan, M.D.
Clinique Chirurgicale des Maladies Cardiaques
Hôpital Cardiologique du Haut-Lévêque
33604 Pessac-Bordeaux
France

Late results of homograft function used for right ventricular outflow obstruction

J. Somerville

Paediatric and Adolescent Unit, National Heart Hospital, Westmoreland Street, London, U.K.

Introduction

The concept of using a homograft aortic valve and length of aorta as a conduit to reconstruct the right ventricular outflow tract (RVOTR) was introduced in 1966 by Ross (1) in the National Heart Hospital, London. The patient, a 9-year-old with complex pulmonary atresia now, 21 years later, works as a garage mechanic and is the father of three healthy children. The original valve was replaced after 9 years. The technique has been modified successfully to repair other congenital cyanotic anomalies. It was quickly tried by several centres in the U.S.A. but condemned because of rapid degeneration of the valve due to destructive sterilisation methods. We have continued the use of the aortic homograft for RVOTR since 1966, only using something else when there was none available. As there is now a renaissance in use of the commercially prepared homografts in America, it would seem appropriate to examine the longterm results, paying attention to the fate of the homograft rather than the patient. In order to reduce the influence of natural history of the basic lesion, only patients with Fallot, pulmonary atresia and ventricular septal defect, and absent pulmonary valve are included.

Table 1. Aortic homograft right ventricular outflow tract reconstruction: RV extension of homograft and outcome in 58 patients.

RV extension of homograft			Re-op. Obstr.	Re-op. Homo.	Re-op. Other	Deaths
Dacron tube		−20	3	2	6	8
Teflon tube		− 2	0	0	0	0
Gusset		−33				
Dacron or Teflon	(13)		1	1	1	1
Pericardium	(10)		0	0	1	1
Mitral leaflet	(7)		0	1	1	1
Mitral leaflet + Dacron	(1)		0	0	0	0
Mitral leaflet + Pericardium	(2)		0	1	0	0
Nothing		− 3	0	0	1	1
Total		58	4	5	10	12

Abbreviations: Homo.: homograft; Obstr. = obstruction; Re-op. = Reoperation; RV = right ventricular.

Materials

From the period 1966—1984, 58 patients left hospital after reconstruction of the right ventricular outflow tract using a cadaver aortic homograft with various extensions (Table 1). The anatomical diagnosis was pulmonary atresia with subaortic ventricular septal defect (33), extreme Fallot (23), and Fallot with absent pulmonary valve (2). The data relating to age, method of valve sterilisation, and year of operation are shown in Figs. 1 and 2.

Attention was routinely given to audibility of aortic homograft closure (P_2); when clear, it was assumed the cusps were pliable.

Necropsy examination was performed in 11 of the 12 deaths and the specimen inspected by the author. At reoperation the state of the homograft was inspected when possible and when the operation was for other reasons.

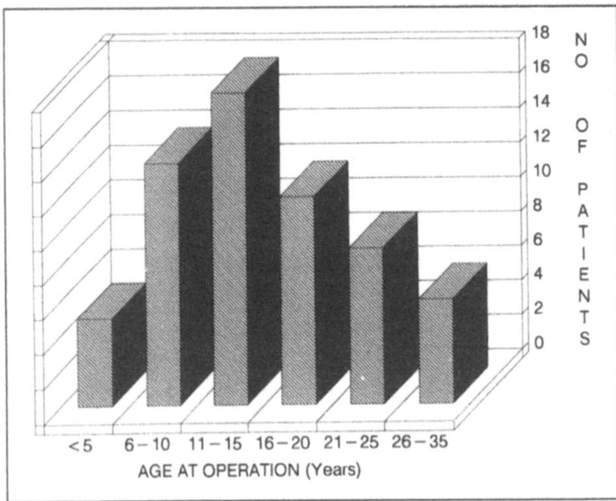

Fig. 1. The age at operation of 58 patients who left hospital between 1966 and 1984 having undergone reconstruction of the right ventricular outflow tract using an aortic homograft.

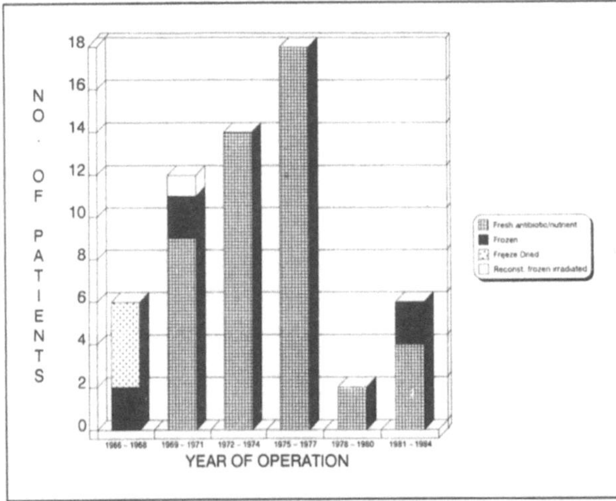

Fig. 2. Diagram to show the year of operation of 58 patients who left hospital after reconstruction of the right ventricular outflow tract using an aortic homograft. The method of valve sterilisation is also shown.

250

Results

Deaths

Twelve patients died (21%), 2 months to 19 years after the procedure. Causes of death and state of the homograft are summarized (Tables 2 and 3). Two patients died aged 29 and 55 years from coronary artery disease, 8 and 19 years after homograft implantation. The cusps were pliable in these. Only one died from a complication directly related to the homograft; the original aortic homograft was replaced 10 years later with a pulmonary homograft and she died from uncontrolled Staph. Aureus infection, probably in the valve. No patient died at reoperation for a homograft replacement.

Reoperation

Four patients died in relation to the second or subsequent reoperation (Table 4); two with severe obstruction in Dacron conduits, one with aortic regurgitation, and one hypoxic from ligation of systemic collaterals.
What is known about the state of the homograft is shown (Table 3).

Table 2. Aortic homograft reconstruction of the right ventricular outflow tract in 58 patients: late deaths in 12 of 58 patients.

Cause of death	Number of patients	Time Post-op.
"Sudden" (1, VT, 1 LVF)	5	2 months — 19 years
Reoperation	4	1—14 years
Ventricular failure	2	5—9 years
Reoperation — Infected homograft	1*	10 years
Total	12 (21%)	2 months — 19 years

Abbreviations: LVF: left ventricular failure; Post-op.: post-operatively; VT: ventricular tachycardia.
* Only 1 death related to homograft.

Table 3. Aortic homograft right ventricular outflow tract reconstruction: state of aortic homografts examined in 15 patients.

Place of examination	No. of patients	Ca + + wall	Cusps thin	Cusps Ca + +	Time Post-op.
Reoperation	8	8	3	5	5—16 years
Necropsy	7	6	7	0	2 months—19 years
Total	15	14	10	5	2 months—19 years

Abbreviations: Ca + +: calcified; No.: number; Post-op.: post-operatively.

Table 4. Aortic homograft reconstruction of the right ventricular outflow tract in 58 patients: re-operations in 19 of 58 patients.

Reason for reoperation	Time postoperatively	Number of patients	Number of deaths at Re-op.
Obstruction	2—13 years	4	2
Aortic regurgitation	10 months—14 years	4	1
Valve obstruction	9—16 years	5	0
Reclosure V.S.D.	6 months—5 years	4	0
Hypoxic, shunt	1 year	1	1
Ligation collateral	1 year	1	0
Total	6 months—16 years	19	4

Abbreviations: Re-op.: reoperation; V.S.D.: ventricular septal defect.

Other complications

Infective endocarditis occurred in four patients (7%), introduced in one (see Deaths), in 688 patient-years. The incidence, excluding the one where it was probably introduced at the time of valve replacement, is low (5%). In two the infection was on the patient's own aortic valve, occurring 9 months and 6 years respectively after the insertion of the homograft, which was not involved in the infection. One occurred 5 years later and was successfully treated with antibiotics. 10 years after operation he shows progressive right ventricular dysfunction with gross pulmonary regurgitation with one cusp destroyed and pulmonary hypertension. He has developed pulmonary artery aneurysms in the left lung (Fig. 3), probably due to infection. Whether this could have been in the original valve is unproven but the possibility exists.

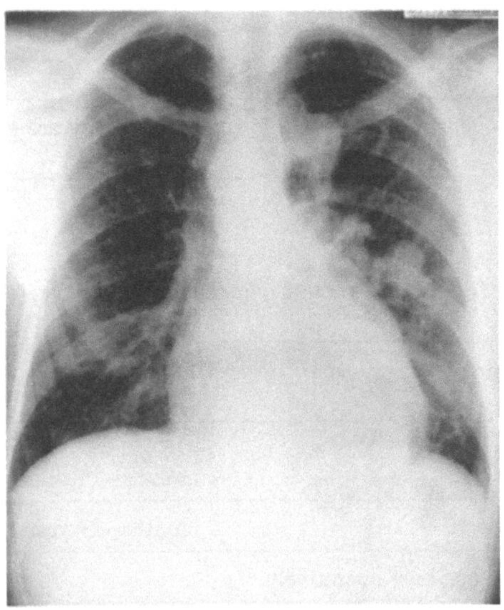

Fig. 3. Chest X-ray showing mycotic aneurysms in the left lung which developed probably in relation to an infected homograft, valve organism satellite streptococcus. No aneurysm is seen on the right side, probably because of right pulmonary artery stenosis in relation to closure of Waterston anastomosis.

Rhythm problems were documented in 19 patients (33%) (Table 5). Sudden death occurred in five patients aged from 18 to 55 years, one of these known to be due to ventricular tachycardia initiated by a blow on the chest. His homograft cusps looked thin and pliable and the aortic wall was calcified.
The overall complications for the entire series are summarized in Table 6.

Table 5. Aortic homograft reconstruction of the right ventricular outflow tract: rhythm disorders in 19 of 58 patients.

Arrhythmia	No. of patients	Age at onset (years)
Sudden death (1 V.T.)	5	18—55
Fast atrial	6	8—34
Multiple V.E.	5	16—31
Nodal rhythm	2	9—20
C.H.B. paced (died)	1	13
Total	19 (33%)	8—55

Abbreviations: C.H.B.: complete heart block; V.E.: ventricular ectopics; V.T.: ventricular tachycardia.

Table 6. Aortic homograft right ventricular outflow tract reconstruction: late complications in 33 of 58 patients (57%) over 688 patient-years.

Complication	No. of patients	%
Inf. endocarditis	4	7
Re-op. valve	5	9
Re-op. other	14	24
Arrhythmias	14	24
Sudden death	5	9
Total deaths	12	21

Abbreviations: Inf.: infective; Re-op.: reoperation.

Pregnancy

21 pregnancies occurred in ten patients. One mother died suddenly during pregnancy at the 37th week from a coronary thrombosis shown at necropsy; the pathologist noted calcium in the right outflow but did not comment on any abnormality of the pulmonary valve! She had previously delivered a child with congenital heart disease (exact diagnosis unknown). Another died one year after her second successful delivery having shown evidence of deteriorating left ventricular function a few months earlier; she had had a left coronary artery supplying the pulmonary arteries and it is suspected that myocardial flow was compromised prior to and probably after bypass.

Examination of homografts

It was possible to examine the homograft in 15 instances. Eight were examined at reoperation (five of which were replaced), while seven were seen at autopsy. Calcification of the aortic wall had occurred in 14 patients, but the leaflets were thin and mobile in ten of these. One patient who died suddenly after 2 months had a normal valve and normal aortic wall. Calcification of the leaflet causing obstruction and rigidity occurred in five valves, implanted 9 to 16 years previously (Table 7). With one exception, "pulmonary" valve closure (P_2) is clear, and sometimes loud (Fig. 4). In the survivors who have not required reoperation, systolic gradients greater than 25 mm Hg across Dacron conduits and suture lines are present in 14. Reoperation will not be recommended until there is evidence of homograft failure, deterioration in right ventricular function, or increasing size of the heart.

Summary of results

The results are summarized in the actuarial curves prepared by Dr. John Kirklin (Figs. 5—7). The ability index (2) of the group is summarized (Fig. 8).

Sterilisation

As can be seen from Table 8, the method of valve sterilisation did not influence the fate of the valve. However, there are too small numbers of freeze dried and frozen to be certain that they compare favourably with "fresh" homograft.

Table 7. Aortic homograft right ventricular outflow tract reconstruction: findings at reoperation for homograft in 5 of 58 patients (9%).

Years after RVOTR	Findings	Valve replacement	Outcome/time Post re-op.
9	2 cusps pliable, 1 Ca^{++}	Aortic homograft	Well, 12 yrs.
10	Wall & cusps Ca^{++}, Cusps largely destroyed	Pericardial xenograft	Well, 6 yrs.
10	Wall Ca^{++}, Cusps retracted, lightly Ca^{++}	Pulmonary homograft	Well, 2 yrs.
10	Wall Ca^{++}, Cusps disappeared	Pulmonary homograft	Died 6 months, infected
16	Wall Ca^{++}, 2 cusps Ca^{++}, 3rd pliable	Pulonary homograft	Well, 2 yrs.

Abbreviations: re-op.: reoperation; RVOTR: right ventricular outflow tract reconstruction using an aortic homograft; yrs.: years; Ca^{++}: calcified.

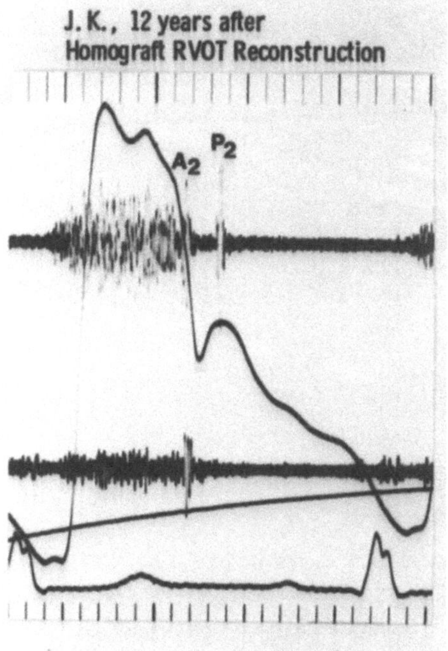

Fig. 4. Phonocardiogram showing loud pulmonary valve closure (P_2).

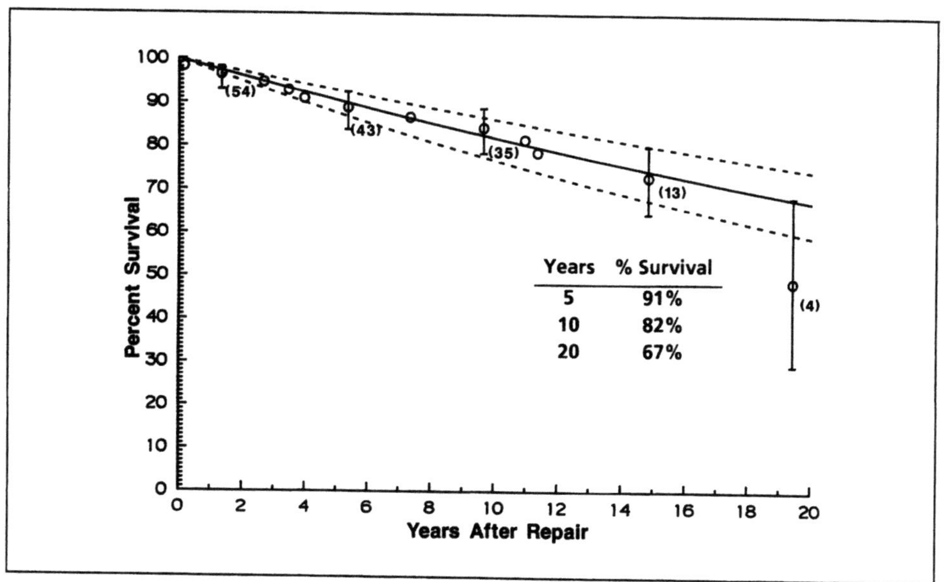

Fig. 5. Actuarial survival curve of 58 patients who left hospital after right ventricualr outflow tract reconstruction using an aortic homograft between 1966 and 1984.

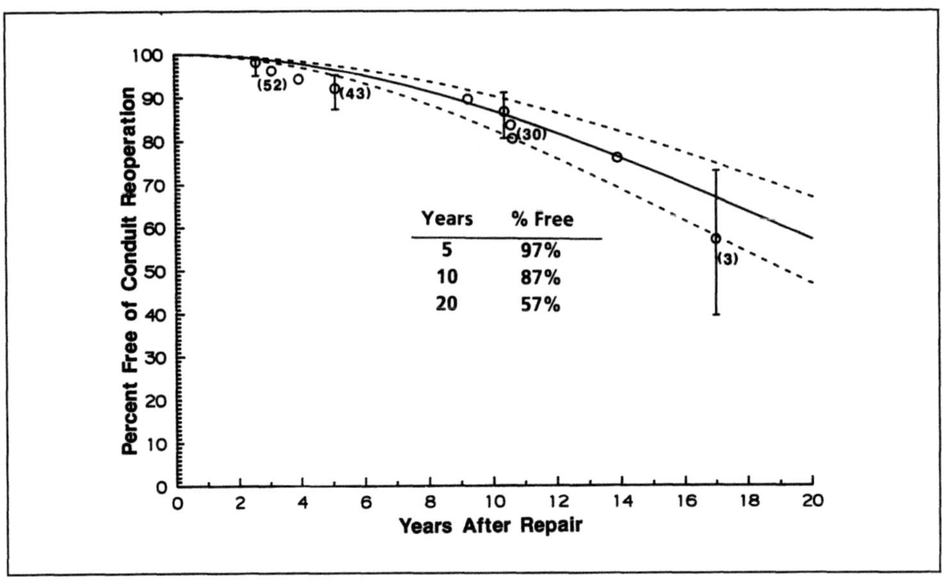

Fig. 6. Freedom from conduit reoperation in a time-related manner in 58 patients who left hospital after right ventricular outflow tract reconstruction using an aortic homograft between 1966 and 1984.

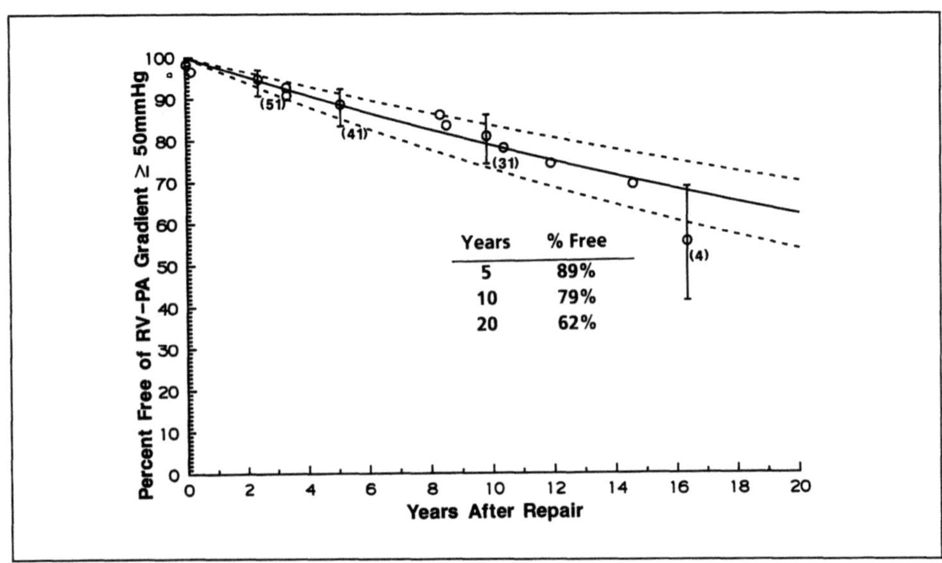

Fig. 7. Percent freedom from an evident right ventricular-pulmonary artery gradient $\geq$ 50 mmHg in a time-related manner in 58 patients who left hospital after right ventricular outflow tract reconstruction using an aortic homograft between 1966 and 1984.

256

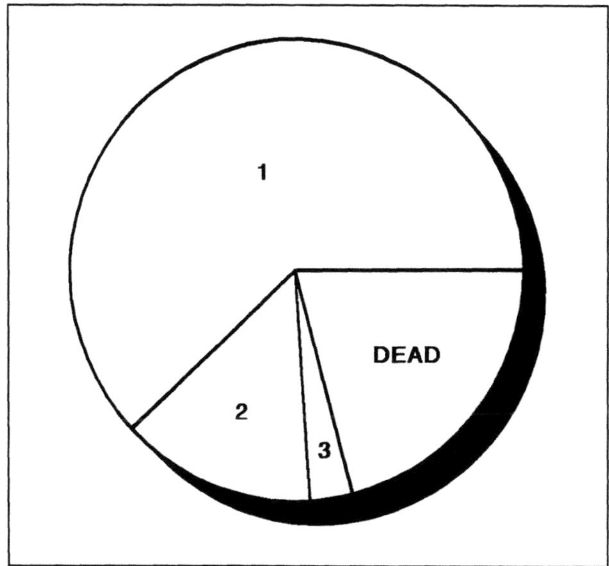

Fig. 8. Ability index of 58 patients who left hospital after RVOTR using an aortic homograft.

Table 8. Aortic homograft reconstruction of the right ventricular outflow tract: relationship of sterilisation method to valve function in 58 patients.

Method of sterilisation	No.	Good	Bad
Freeze dried	4	3	1 (10 yrs.)
Frozen	6	4	2 (9, 16 yrs.)
γ Irradiated	1	1	0
Antibiotic	47	45	2 (10 yrs.)

Abbreviations: No.: number; yrs.: years.

Conclusion

Although 12 (21%) patients died during this long follow-up and 19 (33%) required reoperation, obstructive degeneration of the homograft valve occurred in only five. This was not found before the ninth postoperative year, despite constant searching and calcification in the aortic wall which was usually evident by the end of the first year.

Dacron tubes used as extensions in 20 patients (Table 1) caused more problems than the homograft. Thus, more attention is needed to this aspect of technique. Presently, pericardium is used for extensions if the homograft is not long enough.

The major cause of death was myocardial failure or "sudden". We suspect this is in relation to extensive myocardial fibrosis consequent upon lack of myocardial protection, long periods of ischaemia and resultant myocardial damage. It is possible that some of the late myocardial damage was in part related to the late age when reparative surgery was performed. It remains to be seen if earlier operation will result in longer survival or whether newer techniques of graft preservation will result in longer durability of valve function.

In this group we would not favour repairing with homografts before age 5—6 years as after this an adult sized graft can be used. Certainly these grafts do not grow and in the first patient where a small graft was used, because he was a small boy, no growth of the graft (1.5 cm) was the major cause of the obstruction in the boy who grew to 175 cm.

Pulmonary regurgitation, by auscultation and now Doppler, was common after the first 1 to 2 years but only progressive at the end of the 8—9 years enough to embarrass the right ventricle in two from residual pulmonary hypertension. Without pulmonary hypertension, progressive homograft valve dysfunction causing pulmonary regurgitation is unlikely to cause problems. Unfortunately, pulmonary artery hypertension from pulmonary artery stenoses, sometimes acquired, or progressive pulmonary arteriolar disease, are not rare with pulmonary atresia, particularly in the complex with congenital systemic collaterals.

Methods of sterilisation are important in graft durability. The early reports (3—4) damning the use of the homograft because of rapid calcific degeneration failed to mention the disastrous effects of their chosen method of sterilisation, namely irradiation. Although this series cannot demonstrate any difference in long-term function related to sterilisation, only one, placed in 1969 and known to be still functioning, had some gamma irradiation. It is important that valve tissues are not damaged when the valve is being rendered sterile. The valves examined had no living cells in them and we have no evidence of viability influenced durability as there is no sign of viability. It is possible that viability may stimulate immune reaction and that there will be less problems with dead but not damaged tissues.

Pulmonary hypertension predisposes to earlier valve deterioration and failure, as does graft compression. Rather than concentrate on viability it may be better to study means of preventing calcium deposition. Rupture and dehiscence is not a problem in the right sided grafts. Thus, it can be appreciated that the future of the valve, just as the future of the host patient, are profoundly influenced by the underlying condition for which the operation has been performed. Even in this series, chosen deliberately for similarity of anatomy, there are differences in prognosis between those with complex pulmonary atresia (systemic collaterals, abnormal pulmonary arteries and branches) and those with Fallot or pulmonary atresia and no collaterals.

Other types of valve have been tried by choice or need. None have the durability or number of problem-free years given by the aortic homograft. It remains to be seen if the pulmonary valve homograft is as good or better. Whether the use of valveless conduits has a place requires evaluation. They predispose to early failure with chronic and progressive right ventricular distension and damage, particularly with pulmonary hypertension from peripheral or central pulmonary arterial disease or damage. If a homograft is available we would never consider this option now.

For the present we consider these results justify the continued use of the homograft for right ventricular outflow reconstruction. There is a low infection rate of the homograft valve, no haemolysis, no thrombosis, a reasonable guarantee of 10 or

258

more trouble-free years from problems with the homograft, and no problems for pregnancy. It is doubtful if grafts will last more than 20 years. For those who wish to adopt the technique, good surgery, good laws (to allow harvesting), and good sterilisation are required for a successful outcome and long maintained result.

Acknowledgements

We acknowledge with admiration and appreciation the work of Mr. Donald Ross. We thank Dr. John Kirklin, Dr. Eugene Blackstone and Dr. Nitu Mandke with their help and interest in the preparation of statistics which authenticate the results. We thank the anonymous donor who supports Susan Stone, Research Assistant, enabling us to maintain up-to-date data and statistics.

References

1. Ross DN, Somerville J (1966) Correction of pulmonary atresia with a homograft aortic valve. Lancet 2: 1446—1447
2. Warnes CA, Somerville J (1986) Tricuspid atresia in adolescents and adults: Current state and late complications. Br Heart J 56: 535—543
3. Moodie DS, Mair DD, Fulton, RE, Wallace RB, Danielson GK, McGoon DC (1976) Aortic homograft obstruction. J Thorac Cardiovasc Surg 72: 553—561
4. Norwood WI, Freed MD, Rocchini AP, Bernhard WF, Castaneda AR (1977) Experience with valved conduits for repair of congenital cardiac lesions. Ann Thorac Surg 24: 223—232
5. McGoon DC, Danielson GK, Puga, FJ, Ritter DG, Mair DD, Ilstrup DM (1982) Late results after extracardiac conduit repair for congenital cardiac defects. Am J Cardiol 49: 1741—1749

Author's address:
J. Somerville
Paediatric & Adolescent Unit
National Heart Hospital
Westmoreland Street,
London,
U. K.

Pulmonary autografts, viable and non-viable aortic homografts in the subcoronary position: A comparative study

E. Bodnar

Cardiothoracic Institute and National Heart Hospital, London, UK

Introduction

Aortic homografts in the subcoronary position have been in clinical use since 1962 and pulmonary autografts for aortic valve replacement since 1967. Both operations were first performed and published by Donald Ross who subsequently extended the surgical applicability of these valves to insertions into the mitral, right ventricular outflow and tricuspid position and eventually completed the replacement of the entire aortic root and valve with an aortic homograft (1—5).

Aortic valve replacement, however, has remained the most common indication for using homografts or pulmonary autografts over the years. Therefore, these valves have been selected for the current study to investigate problems related to sterilisation, preservation, cellular viability and immunology. As pulmonary autografts are sterile but not sterilised, are not preserved, have unimpaired cellular viability and do not provoke immunological reaction, it seemed logical to compare experiences with the different groups of homografts not only to each other but to those with autografts.

Clinical materials and methods of assessment

780 consecutive hospital survivors after aortic valve replacement have been selected for the study. The selection criteria were: isolated, free hand aortic valve replacement with a homograft or an autograft, one surgeon performing the operation (DNR) and, for homografts, that all valves were processed and inserted at the National Heart Hospital, London. The follow-up period was 1—20 years, the total follow-up information 4025 patient-years with a mean of 5.3 patient-years.

The surgical technique of the insertion of homografts and autografts has been published recently and has remained unchanged over the years, the only exception being a limited period during the 1970s when the proximal suture line was completed with a continuously running suture (6).

The pulmonary autografts were kept in the patient's own blood in the pericardial cavity during the short interval between excision and insertion. All homografts were harvested as mortuary material within 48 h after routine hospital or forensic autopsies. Details of the individual methods of sterilisation and preservation have been published elsewhere (7).

Statistical assessment was carried out using the standard life table method and the follow-up experience was expressed as a single or multiple decrement, as appropriate (8). The standard error of the difference between two survival proportions at any given cut-off point was calculated as defined earlier (8). Student's t-test was used to ascertain the significance of the difference.

Valve function and/or malfunction was defined in stringent and comprehensive terms as proposed previously by us and by the Stanford group (8, 9). The ultimate failure of the valve was defined as death due to valve failure or surgical removal of the failed valve at reoperation. The hospital mortality after reoperation was considered as valve-related death.

Statistical comparisons between the methods of homograft preservation were performed by applying a 10-year frame to each group. This period was considered long enough to provide a fair base for comparison yet the significance levels were not undermined by the (subsequently) decreasing numbers at risk.

Results

The actuarial proportions of freedom from valve-related death, primary tissue failure, subacute bacterial endocarditis and all complications (including valve-related death and technical failure) were assessed in each group and the results were as shown in Tables 1—4.

The freeze-dried group of homografts suffered a higher percentage of valve-related death than any other group and primary tissue failure (Tables 1, 2) and all complications were significantly less with pulmonary autografts than with any type of the homografts valves. No other statistically significant differences could be found.

Table 1. Valve-related deaths.

	5 years (%)	SE	10 years (%)	SE
Pulmonary autograft	100.0	0.0	89.8	3.7
Freeze-dried homograft	88.9	2.7	83.2	3.5*
Frozen homograft	93.8	3.5	91.5	4.1
Hank's/antibiotics homograft	96.8	2.2	96.8	2.2
Nutrient/antibiotics homograft	96.7	1.6	89.5	4.4

* denotes statistically significant differences.

Table 2. Primary tissue failure.

	5 years (%)	SE	10 years (%)	SE
Pulmonary autograft	99.5	0.5	91.0	3.4*
Freeze-dried homograft	87.9	4.6	59.1	5.0
Frozen homograft	93.5	3.6	59.5	8.0
Hank's/antibiotics homograft	89.2	4.6	60.5	9.2
Nutrient/antibiotics homograft	87.0	3.4	49.5	6.7

* denotes statistically significant differences.

Table 3. Subacute bacterial endocarditis.

	5 years (%)	SE	10 years (%)	SE
Pulmonary autograft	96.1	1.6	87.8	3.9
Freeze-dried homograft	94.4	2.1	85.8	3.9
Frozen homograft	94.1	3.3	94.1	3.3
Hank's/antibiotics homograft	94.7	3.0	86.5	6.3
Nutrient/antibiotics homograft	95.0	2.1	91.3	3.3

Table 4. Valve related death and/or all complications.

	5 years (%)	SE	10 years (%)	SE
Pulmonary autograft	86.0	2.9	68.2	5.0*
Freeze-dried homograft	76.3	3.6	45.7	4.6
Frozen homograft	84.7	5.0	50.4	7.5
Hank's/antibiotics homograft	76.3	5.8	47.3	8.3
Nutrient/antibiotics homograft	76.8	3.9	41.1	5.9

* denotes statistically significant differences.

Discussion

This assessment of long-term clinical performance failed to reveal any difference caused by, or related to, the method of homograft preservation. The high proportion of valve-related death with freeze-dried valves is not the direct consequence of any particular mode of failure characteristic of this group; as these valves were the earliest among the four clinical series, both reoperation and bacterial endocarditis carried a higher mortality than experienced during the subsequent time frames.

Cellular viability does not seem to have any effect on the longevity of homografts in the subcoronary position. This is apparent from the lack of difference between the freeze-dried and the nutrient/antibiotics preserved or frozen valves. The instantaneous rate of primary tissue failure increased after 7 years with all types of valves assessed. This observation is a strong argument against the theoretically important immunological factors.

The superiority of the pulmonary autografts is obvious from the results but it cannot be related to one single factor. It is the combination of the perfect immunological environment, full cellular viability, structural integrity and lack of any chemical treatment which contribute to the unparalleled good results.

In conclusion, it is suggested that all methods proposed for homograft preservation provide an acceptable level of long-term valve performance. The only advantage of cryopreservation seems to be the unlimited storage period. However, it has to be balanced against the problems in transportation. The best solution might be to store valves at 4 °C if the date of insertion will certainly be within 3 weeks or to cryopreserve them if the date of insertion is unknown.

References

1. Ross, DN (1962) Homograft replacement of the aortic valve. Lancet 2: 487
2. Ross DN (1967) Replacement of aortic and mitral valve with a pulmonary autograft. Lancet 2: 959
3. Ross DN, Somerville J (1966) Correction of pulmonary atresia with a homograft aortic valve. Lancet 2: 1446
4. Somerville J, Ross DN, Ross JK (1972) Mitral valve replacement with stored, inverted pulmonary homograft valve. Thorax 27: 583
5. Lao GKH, Robles A, Cherian A, Ross DN (1984) Surgical treatment of prosthetic endocarditis. J Thorac Cardiovasc Surg 87: 712
6. Ross DN (1968) Homograft replacement of the aortic valve surgical technique. Surgery 63: 382
7. Ross DN, Martelli V, Wain WH (1979) Allograft and autograft valves used for aortic valve replacement. In: Ionescu M (ed) Tissue heart valves. Butterworths, London, p 127
8. Bodnar E, Wain WH, Habermann S (1982) Assessment and comparison of the performance of cardiac valves. Ann Thorac Surg 34: 146
9. Miller DC, Oyer PE, Mitchell RS, Stinson EB, Jamieson SW, Baldwin JC, Shumway NE (1984) Performance characteristics of the Starr-Edwards model 1260 aortic valve prosthesis beyond ten cears. J Thorac Cardiovasc Surg 88: 193

Author's address:
E. Bodnar, M.D.
Cardiothoracic Institute
and National Heart Hospital
Westmoreland Street
London, W.1.,
U.K.

Long-term results of antibiotic-treated aortic allografts in subcoronary position

R. Radley-Smith, M. H. Yacoub

Harefield Hospital, Thoracic and Cardiac Surgical Unit, Harefield, Uxbridge, UK

Introduction

Methods of sterilisation and storage are known to have a profound effect on the long-term performance of aortic allograft valves. This type of valve substitute has been preferred for aortic valve replacement at Harefield Hospital since 1969.
In this report we analyse the long-term follow-up of antibiotic-sterilised aortic allografts with particular reference to the pattern of survival and valve-related complications and their possible predictors over a period of 15—18 years.

Patients and Methods

Between September 1969 and September 1972, 199 patients underwent allograft replacement of the aortic valve at Harefield Hospital. Of these patients, 124 consecutive patients who underwent isolated elective aortic valve replacement have been followed up a minimum of 15 (mean: 16.2) years. The age of the patients was between 12—76 (mean: 52) years (Fig. 1). There were 87 males and 37 females. Indications for operation were a bicuspid, predominantly stenotic valve, in 86 (69%), rheumatic heart disease, mainly regurgitant, in 32 (26%), previous endocarditis in five and a syphilitic valve in one patient.

Technique

Valves were obtained from cadavers aged between 21—76 (mean: 56) years at routine post mortem examination. They were dissected within 48 h of death, sterilised in antibiotic solution for 24 h and then stored in tissue culture medium at 4 °C. The valves were inserted in the subcoronary position, without stents using a 2 suture line technique. 80% of valves were implanted within 2 weeks and all within 40 days.

Follow-up

All patients in this series have been followed up annually at Harefield Hospital with a clinical, radiographic, electrocardiographic and, for the past 10 years, echocardiographic examination. Routine anticoagulation has not been used.

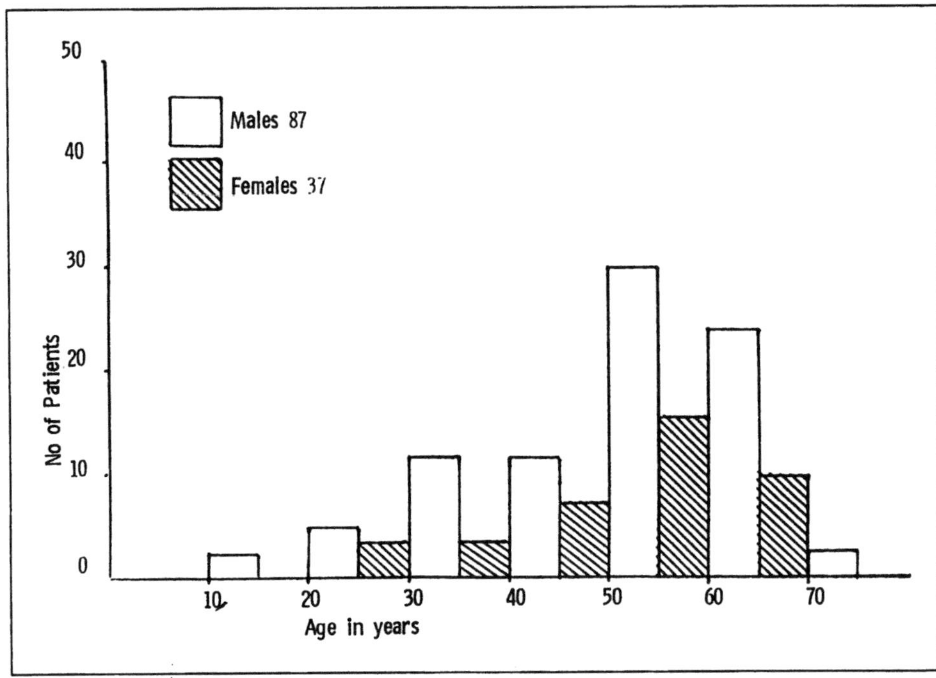

Fig. 1. Age and sex of patients.

Valve failure was defined as dysfunction, either requiring re-operation or causing death. The presence of a diastolic murmur did not signify valve failure unless there was a wide pulse pressure (>50 mm), in which case re-operation was indicated. Technical failure was defined as dysfunction due to distortion (generally cusp prolapse) caused by a mismatch between valve and aortic root. Degeneration occurred with cusp thinning, rupture or calcification in the absence of endocarditis.
Actuarial analysis of survival, Cox's regression model and step-wise logistic regression analysis were used for multivariant analysis to determine predictors of survival and valve failure.

Results

Early mortality

There were two early deaths. One patient died of left ventricular failure and the other of a myocardial infarction.

Late mortality

With a follow-up of between 15—18 (mean: 16.2) years, there have been 60 late deaths. 44 (42%) deaths were due to cardiac causes and 16 (13%) non-cardiac. Of

266

the cardiac deaths, 15 were valve-related — seven occurring before and eight after re-operation for valve failure or endocarditis. The 29 (23%) non-valve-related cardiac deaths were due to myocardial dysfunction, myocardial infarction, arrhythmia and sudden death.

Actuarial survival was 83% at 5 years, 67% at 10 years and 52% at 15 years (Fig. 2).

Predictors of survival

Of several patient-related variables submitted for analysis, the older age of the patient and the development of post-operative left bundle branch block were the only factors found to be statistically significant (Table 1).

Valve failure

Valve failure occurred in 42 (34%) patients. Valvar degeneration, 4—15 years after operation occurred in 32 patients. Technical failure occurred in three patients 6 weeks to 3 years after valve replacement. Seven patients with valve degeneration early in the series died before re-operation because of late re-referral.

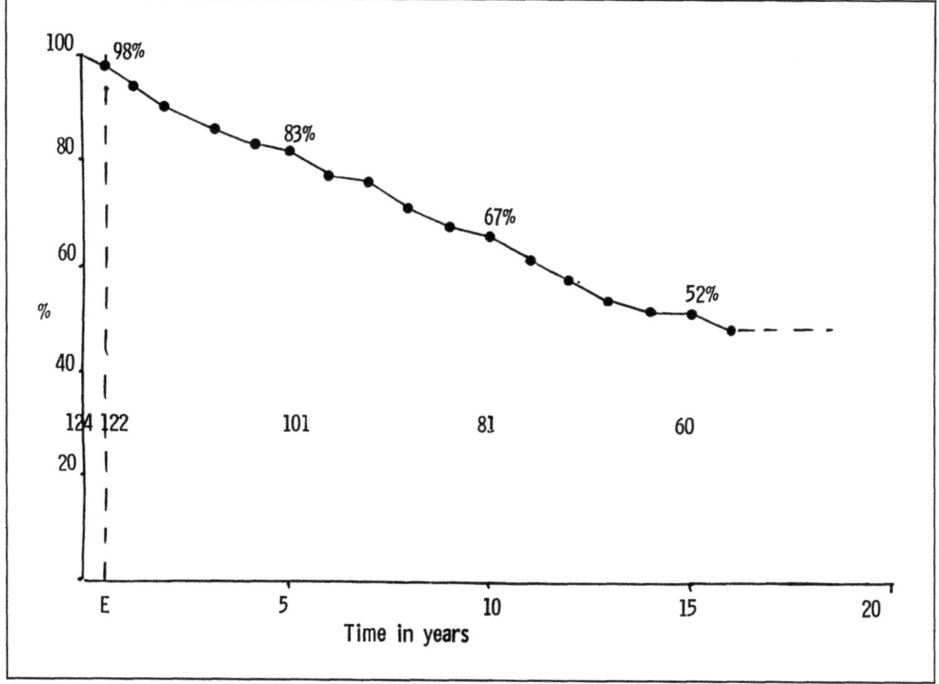

Fig. 2. Actuarial survival.

Table 1. Predictors of patient survival.

Variable	p value
Patient age	<0.01
Post-op LBBB	<0.05
Patient sex	N.S.
Pre-op CTR	N.S.
Pre-op LBBB	N.S.
Ejection fraction	N.S.
A. R.	
Diagnosis	N.S.
A. S.	

$p > 0.05$: N.S. (not significant).

Degeneration

Valve failure due to degeneration occurred in 32 (26%) patients between 4 and 15 years after operation. The incidence of valve failure increased after the seventh post-operative year. Cusp thinning causing regurgitation was the cause of this in 25. Freedom from valve failure, excluding endocarditis, was 90% at 5 years, 72% at 10 years and 61% at 15 years (Fig. 3).

Endocarditis

This occurred in seven (5.6%) patients, 2 months to 13 years after operation, the highest incidence occurring in the first 5 years. In two patients, both early after operation, the causative organism was Candida albicans. Three patients had bacterial endocarditis — Streptococcus viridans in two and S. faecalis in one. In two patients, no organism was isolated. The probability of developing endocarditis was 3.2% at 5 years, 4.8% at 10 years and 5.6% at 15 years (Fig. 4).

Re-operation

35 patients required re-operation. There was valve degeneration in 26, endocarditis in six and technical failure in three. In the majority of cases, another aortic allograft was used. There were eight operative deaths, all early in the series. A contributing factor to this mortality was the late re-referral.

Predictors of valve failure

Table 2 lists the patient and allograft variables analysed. The risk of valve failure was significantly higher in older patients, the female sex and with increasing interval between death and dissection of the valve. There was also a higher incidence with aortic stenosis.

268

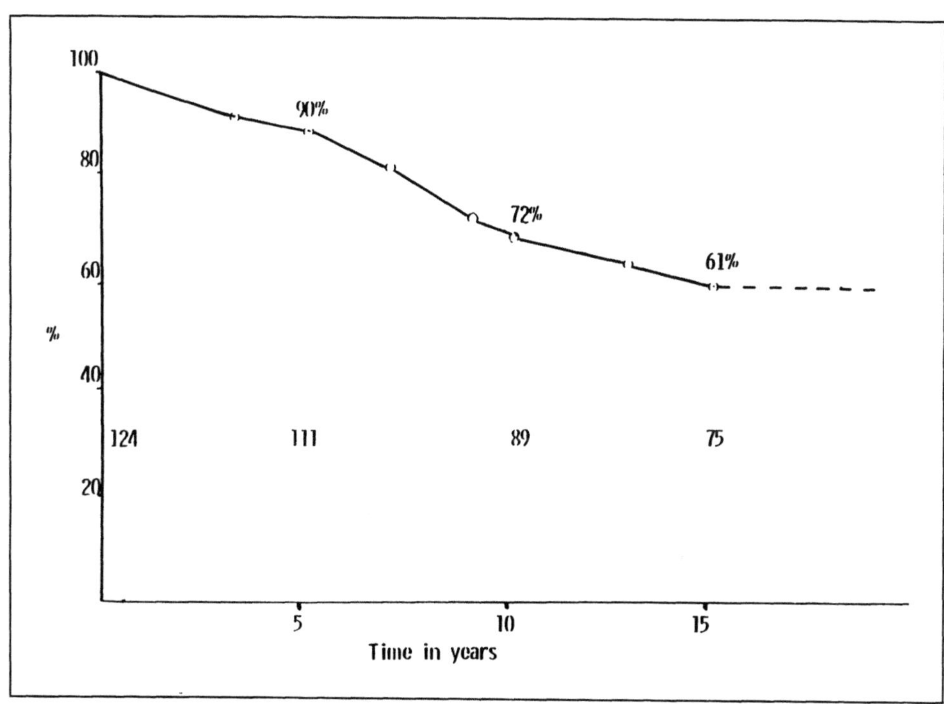

Fig. 3. Freedom from valve failure (excluding endocarditis).

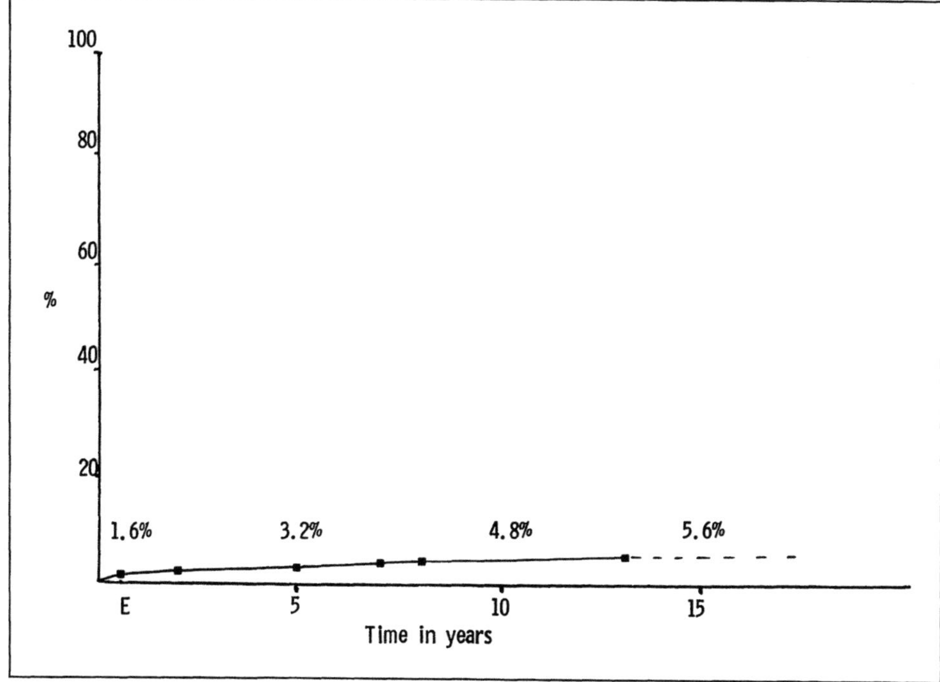

Fig. 4. Probability of developing endocarditis.

Table 2. Predictors of valve failure.

Variable	p value
Patient age	<0.01
Patient sex	<0.01
A. R.	N.S.
Diagnosis	
A. S.	<0.05
Death to dissection	<0.01
Donor age	N.S.
Donor sex	N.S.
Dissection to insertion	N.S.

p > 0.05: N.S. (not significant).

Thromboembolism

Early or late systemic emboli were not encountered in spite of the fact that routine anticoagulation was not used.

Patient status

With a follow-up of 15—18 (mean 16.2) years, 37 (30%) of the surviving patients retain their original allograft.

Discussion

The choice of a valve substitute for aortic valve replacement, should ideally suit each individual's requirement. Although insertion of an allograft valve is technically more difficult, the risk of operation in this series is no greater than with other forms of valve replacement. Late survival and freedom from valve failure compare favourably with other biological valve substitutes, and in our study the younger age of the recipients was not associated with either accelerated calcification or the valve degeneration seen with porcine valves.

Endocarditis has been relatively common, but the incidence of fungal endocarditis has markedly decreased since the addition of amphotericin B and nystatin to the antibiotic solution.

It is hoped that analysing data in this manner, will help in improving the long-term results of unstented aortic allografts.

References

1. Barratt-Boyes BG (1965) Method for preparing and inserting a homograft aortic valve. Br J Surg 52: 847
2. Bjork VO, Henze A (1979) Ten year experience with Bjork-Shiley tilting disc valve. J Thorac Cardiovasc Surg 78: 331
3. Craver JM, Jones EL, McKeown P, Bone DK, Hatcher CR Jr, Kandrach M (1982) Porcine cardiac xenograft valves: Analysis of survival, valve failure and explanation. Ann Thorac Surg 34: 16

  4. Dunn JM (1981) Porcine valve durability in children. Ann Thorac Surg 32: 357
  5. Engelman L (1983) Stepwise logistic regression. In: Dixon WJ (ed) BMDP Statistical Software. University of California Press, Berkeley, p 330
  6. Hopkins A (1983) Survival analysis with co-variates-Cox models. In: Dixon WJ (ed) BMDP Statistical Software. University of California Press, Berkeley, p 576
  7. Janusz MT, Jamieson WRE, Allen P, Munro AI, Tutassura H, Burr LH, Gerein AN, Tyers GFO (1982) Experience with the Carpentier-Edwards porcine valve prosthesis in 700 patients. Ann Thorac Surg 34: 625
  8. Longmore DB, Lockey E, Ross DN, Pickering BN (1966) Preparation of aortic valve homografts. Lancet 2: 463
  9. Penta A, Qureshi S, Radley-Smith R, Yacoub MH (1984) Patient status 10 or more years after 'fresh' homograft replacement of the aortic valve. Circulation 70 (Suppl 1): 182
 10. Ross DN, Yacoub MH (1969) Homograft replacement of the aortic valve. A critical review. Prog Cardiovasc Dis 9: 275
 11. Teply JF, Grunkemeier GL, D'Arcy Sutherland H, Lambert LE, Johnson VA, Starr A (1981) The ultimate prognosis after valve replacement. Ann Thorac Surg 32: 111
 12. Yacoub MH, Kittle F (1970) Sterilisation of valve homograft by antibiotic solution. Circulation 41 (Suppl 11): 11

Author's address:
Rosemary Radley-Smith, M.D.
Consultant Cardiologist
Harefield Hospital
Thoracic and Cardiosurgical Unit
Harefield, Uxbridge
Middlesex UB9 6JH,
U.K.

Survival of aortic allografts containing living cells

W. W. Angell, J. H. Oury, J. A. Koziol, M. H. Dussault

Department of Cardiac Surgery Research, Scripps Clinic and Research
Foundation, La Jolla, California, U.S.A.

Introduction

There is agreement among investigators that the "in vivo reaction" to the implanted
allograft is complex and variably related to (1) donor age; (2) procurement and
processing methods; (3) implantation position and technique; and (4) immunogenic
reaction within the valve cusps (1, 2, 3). Many human and animal experiments have
been performed to determine the nature of the donor and host reaction after implantation, and there is disagreement as to whether the transplanted donor cells
remain viable. Our findings, as well as O'Brien's remain opposed to those of Brian
Barrett-Boyes and Ross on this issue (4, 5, 6, 7). We believe that donor cells remain
viable for extended periods, and that long-term valve function is related to the presence of viable cells in the donor graft (Fig. 1). If viable donor cells are not present,
then long-term function is secondary to the basic tissue integrity of the functional
valve cusp and not due to repopulation by host cells. It is proven that viable fibroblasts in valve cusps can be detected histologically and by tissue culture after explantation. Our data suggests that these are living donor fibroblasts, and there is
limited host invasion into and onto the functional valve cusps after implantation
(5, 8, 9). Morphology of both experimental and clinical valve explants indicate that
donor cell hyperplasia and host overgrowth or pannus can be advantageous or deleterious depending upon the location and intensity of collagen deposition (Fig. 2).
Explant morphology also clearly identifies non-viable valve segments which may
function for extended periods or deteriorate by elongation and prolapse with resultant valvular insufficiency (Figs. 3A, B). Calcification, although less common
than with xenografts, does occur with shortening, stiffening, and stenosis or insufficiency. Some of these reactions are not dissimilar to those observed in the native
valve which may stiffen, thicken, shrink and calcify secondary to turbulence or inflammation.
Much of the early homograft experience was with the utilisation of sterilisation or
storage methods which rendered the valves non-viable. Long-term survival of the
valves was thus dependent upon the integrity of the original donor collagen stroma
and/or support of the donor leaflets by host pannus over the base of the cusps. The
subsequent techniques of physiological antibiotic sterilisation with storage at 4 °C
resulted in destruction of some, but not all of the collagen producing fibroblasts so
that valves implanted a few days after procurement were "partially viable" (3) (Fig.
4).

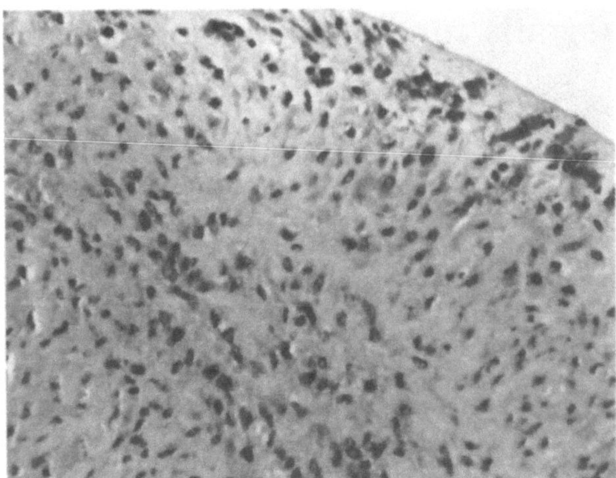

Fig. 1. A demonstration of the marked hypercellularity and collagen deposition that occurs within 30 days after allograft transplantation in an experimental animal.

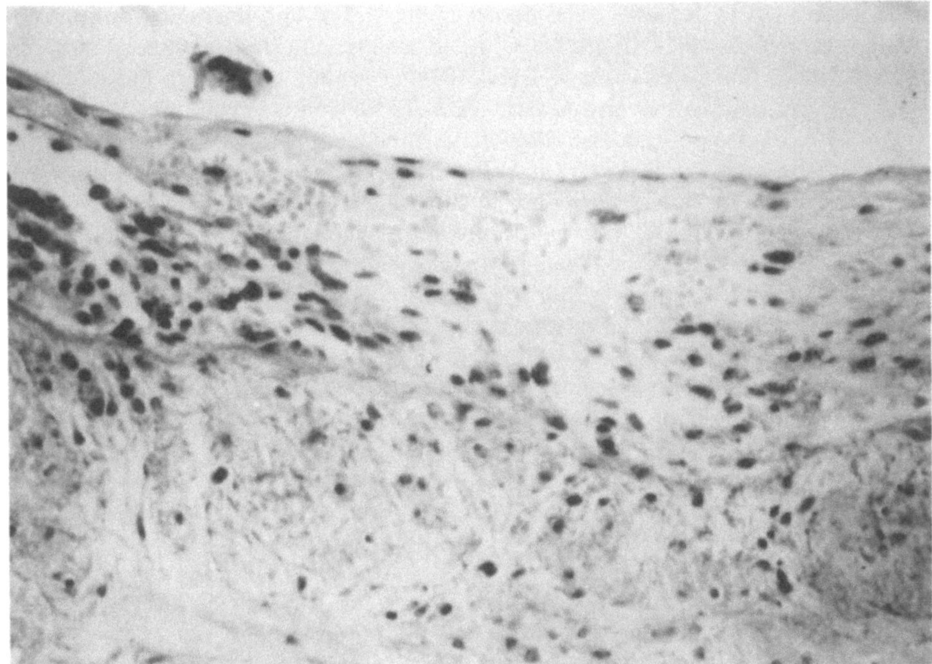

Fig. 2. Pannus formation growing over a viable segment of allograft cusp. There are clearly living fibroblasts from the donor below and from the recipient above. The pannus also contains numerous inflammatory and trapped haematogenous cell elements.

Most of these findings were of academic interest only to a handful of surgeons until frozen human allograft valve banks became established. The stimulus for this is

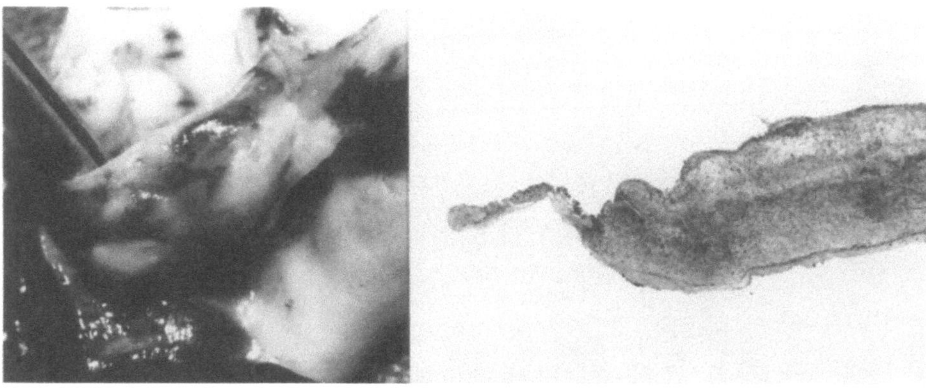

Fig. 3A.

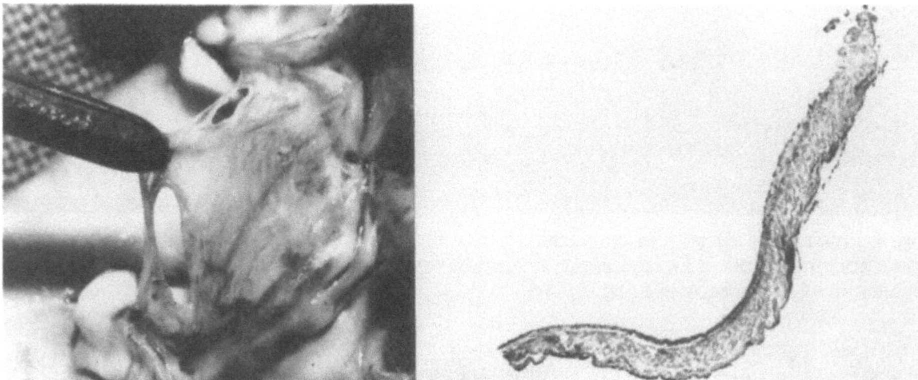

Fig. 3B.

Fig. 3A. Experimental viable valve with an acellular tip of the cusp which was not viable at the time of implantation. This demonstrates the marked collagen deposition and thickening of the viable portions of the allograft cusp.
B. Nonviable beta-proprylactone sterilised experimental valve, thinned and fenestrated with no living cells.

based upon proven graft viability after storage in the frozen state as well as the observation that the intrinsic valve failure rate of allografts is lower than with glutaraldehyde treated porcine xenografts in children and young adults (10). Human aortic valves are made available in much the same way that commericial blood banks make blood available to hospitals that do not provide their own donors. Allografts can now be used by nearly any surgeon who wishes and can be procured and processed in a manner that will guarantee viability of the fibroblast in the functional stroma portion of the allograft leaflet. It is accepted by all investigators that if viability can be maintained at least up until the time of implantation it will be an advantage to long-term function. Therefore, either frozen viable storage with antibiotic sterilisation or immediate sterile transplantation have become the preferred methods of handling allograft valves.

275

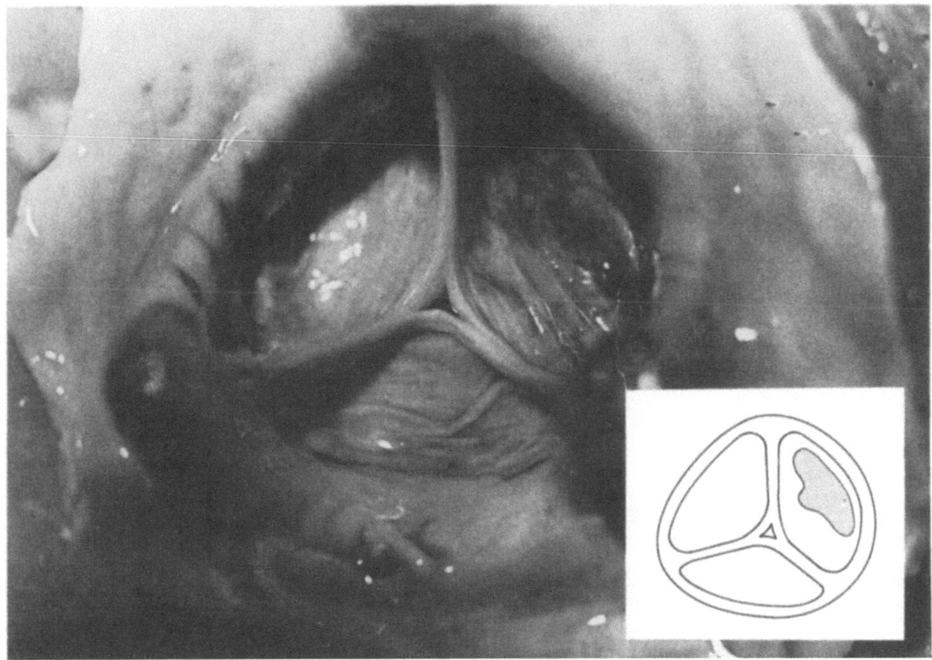

Fig. 4. Premounted allograft in the mitral position obtained at autopsy from a 48-year-old woman 1 year after implantation. Death was due to cardiomyopathy. The shaded area represents a nonviable segment in what is otherwise a viable valve.

Clinical data base

Over a 20-year period from 1968 to 1987, 577 allografts were inserted. Our data base is unique in that the early valves* were cleanly procured by surgeons, antibiotic sterilised with physiological doses of antibiotics and stored at either 4 °C or frozen with tissue culture controls. Valves stored at 4 °C were variably viable depending upon the length of storage. In no case were harsh methods of processing employed. Included in our data base is the oldest series of frozen allografts, comprising 33 patients. Seven frozen valves were premounted on support rings and 26 were inserted with the traditional free-hand graft method.

The objective of this analysis is a comparison of valve failure rates among nonrandom unmatched consecutive patient series with different methods of valve preparation. The focus is predominantly on the four groups as given in Table 1, excluding the allografts that were used for right ventricular outflow tract obstruction or tricuspid replacement as well as all allografts for which follow-up information was unavailable. Our primary endpoint is time to valve failure for the four groups.

Endocarditis is taken to be a censoring event and not a treatment failure for the purposes of our analysis.

---

* 1968—1974

276

Table 1. Comparison of valve failure rates among non-random unmatched consecutive patient series with different methods of valve preparation.

Group	Frozen Free Aortic valves	Fresh Free Aortic valves	Fresh Mounted Aortic valves	Fresh Mounted Mitral valves
N (sample size)	25	103	79	185
Average age at time of first allograft	46.4	49.0	54.6	46.5
Percent female	59.3	72.3	83.7	47.1
Median time to valve failure (years)	12.1	12.5	6.6	8.6

Results

This is a prospective cohort study involving all patients entered into this clinical data base over the past 20 years. No attempt was made to randomize or match patient series with different methods of valve preparation. Comparison of the proportions of males to females in the four groups, as in Table 1, was statistically significant: $X^2_3 = 41.6$, $p < 0.001$. In particular, the fresh mounted mitral valve group is comprised disproportionately of males relative to the other groups. Comparison of the four groups in terms of age at the time of initial allograft was also statistically significant: $F_{3, 251} = 3.38$, $p < 0.02$, with a one-way analysis of variance procedure. By means of a subsequent Newman-Keuls multiple comparison procedure, those patients receiving fresh mounted aortic valves were found to be significantly older on average than patients in other groups.

Next are the comparisons of time to valve failure for the four groups. From Table 1, it is apparent that the two groups receiving unmounted aortic valves experienced comparable levels of median time to valve failure and that these levels are substantially higher than those for the groups receiving mounted valves. Though this comparison is useful, a more sensitive analysis of valve failure rates is the examination of the product-limit valve survival curves for the four groups with log rank statistics. Figure 5 depicts the valve survival curves for the four groups.

Table 2 contains the relevant log rank statistics for group comparisons. The explanation is clear: the overall difference in valve survival among the four groups is readily explained by a dichotomisation in which the free allograft groups do not differ significantly; the mounted allograft groups do not differ significantly, but the free groups are characterized by significantly longer valve survival than the mounted groups. We also undertook a stratified analysis, adjusting for the age-sex differences across groups; results were qualitatively identical to those reported in Table 2.

Figure 6 is the cumulative hazard function for the four groups. The hazard functions are mathematically defined as minus the logarithm of the corresponding survival functions from Fig. 5, and describe the ways in which the instantaneous probabilities of valve failure for individuals in each group change with time. The concave upward

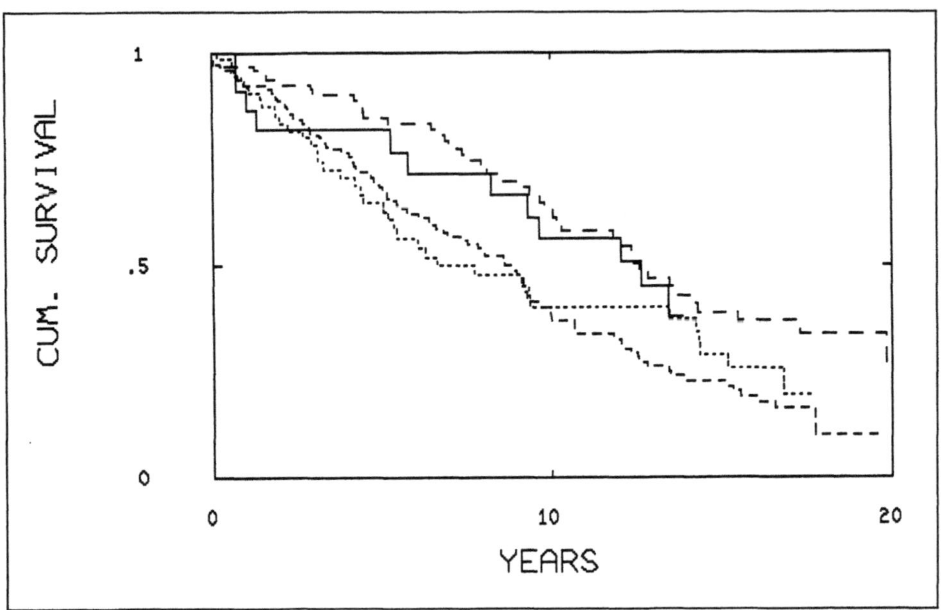

Fig. 5. Cumulative distribution functions of post-operative survival until valve failure versus time (in years) for the four groups. The group codes are: (——) Frozen free aortic valves; (— — —) fresh free aortic valves; (··········) fresh mounted aortic valves; (- - - - - -) fresh mounted mitral valves.

Table 2. Log rank statistics for comparison of times to valve failure.

Comparison	Log rank statistic	Degrees of freedom	p value
All 4 groups	14.12	3	0.0027
Frozen vs fresh, free AoV	0.281	1	0.596
Fresh mounted AoV vs mitral	0.049	1	0.824
Free groups vs mounted groups	13.61	1	0.0002

curvatures of the hazard functions for the two free aortic valve groups are indicative of increasing hazards, or risks of valve failure, with time. This tendency is also apparent with the mounted aortic valve group, but the mounted mitral valve group appears to exhibit a more constant hazard over time.

Discussion

Analysis of long-term follow-up of valve replacement patients is the most informative method of assessing valve failure rates. In grafts treated with caustic, destructive methods of sterilisation and/or storage, experimental and clinical valve failure occurs earlier and is associated with cusp tearing, perforation, and rupture. The character of valve failure was not different quantitatively or qualitatively between

278

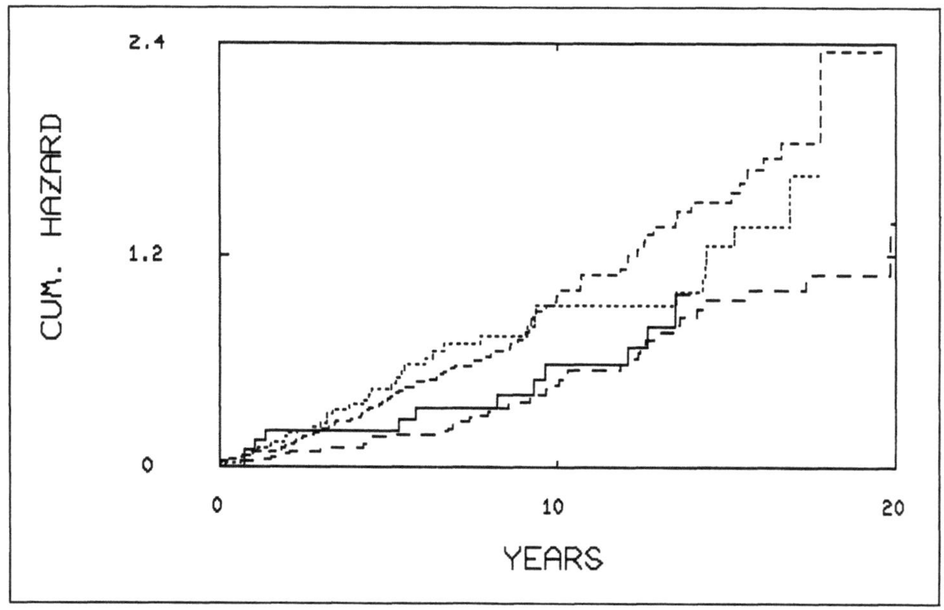

Fig. 6. Cumulative hazard functions of post-operative failure rates versus time in years for the four groups. Group codes are as in Fig. 5.

fresh and frozen valves. One might expect that frozen valves are more likely to be viable at implantation and thus to have a greater likelihood of postimplantation fibroblast activity, with thickening of leaflets from increased collagen deposition and a resultant lower risk of cusp rupture. However, our analysis of valve failure rates does not support this contention, and the incidence of cusp rupture was not greater for fresh valves. It should be emphasized that there were definite proven donor valve fibroblasts seen in frozen valves up to 14 years after implantation.

With our patient data base, valve failure rates are significantly greater for mounted than for unmounted valves. Modes of failure were also different for mounted versus unmounted valves. Mounted grafts were more likely to fibrose·and calcify and also to fenestrate and rupture, presumably due to turbulent blood flow patterns around the stent. Curiously, the mean time to valve failure was longer for mounted valves despite greater mitral pressure against the valve leaflets; this suggests that high velocity and turbulent flow in the aortic position is more significant than a higher valve closing pressure. The character of tissue destruction is not clearly different between groups.

The age difference between mounted and unmounted fresh aortic grafts is easily explained by our tendency to use the unmounted grafts in younger patients with smaller diameter aortic roots.

The survival analysis we have performed is an objective and informative statistical technique for assessing valve failure. In tissue valve replacement, the issue of primary concern to the patient, physician, and surgeon is recommending a particular valve type and understanding the intrinsic risks and failure rate of that choice. Our responsibility is to find and report not only the more readily apparent short-term

279

morbidity and mortality, but also the long-term incidence of valve failure. Responsibility for this lies heavily on accurate and meaningful analysis of the available early clinical series.

Conclusion

Our prior experience and clinical data support the concept that viable fibroblasts contribute to long-term allograft function: This analysis of freedom from valve failure in frozen and fresh antibiotic sterilised grafts supports the concept that fibroblast valves in the early interim after implant results in increased collagen deposition which contributes to decreased incidence of leaflet rupture. Allografts with viable fibroblasts did not function longer as frozen viable grafts. Although the frozen viable graft is the method of choice it did not result in prolonged valve survival when compared to fresh grafts. Mounting of allografts resulted in a striking increase in the rate of valve failure of both aortic and mitral valve replacements.

References

1. Barratt-Boyes BG (1979) Cardiothoracic surgery in the antipodes: including a report of a randomized trial of medical and surgical treatment of asymptomatic patients with severe coronary artery disease; a long-term follow-up of both fresh and antibiotic-treated homograft valves; and some observations on glutaraldehyde-preserved valve tissue. J Thorac Cardiovasc Surg 78 (6): 804—822
2. Bodnar E, Wain WH, Martelli V, Ross DN (1979) Long-term performance of 580 homograft and autograft valves used for aortic valve replacement. Thorac Cardiovasc Surg 27 (1): 31—38
3. Buch WS, Kosek JC, Angell WW (1971) The role of rejection and mechanical trauma on valve graft viability. J Thorac Cardiovasc Surg 62: 423
4. Barratt-Boyes BG, Roche AH, Subramanyan R, Pemberton JR, Whitlock RM (1987) Long-term follow-up of patients with the antibiotic-sterilized aortic homograft valve inserted freehand in the aortic position. Circulation 75 (4): 768—777
5. Angell WW, Pillsbury RC, Shumway NE (1969) Storage and function of the canine aortic homograft. Arch Surg 99: 92
6. O'Brien MF, Stafford EG, Gardner MAH, Pohlner PG, McGiffin DC. A comparison of aortic valve replacement with viable cryopreserved and fresh allograft valves with a note on chromosomal studies. J Thorac Cardiovasc Surg, in press
7. Khanna SK, Ross JK, Monro JL (1981) Homograft aortic valve replacement; seven years' experience with antibiotic-treated valves. Thorax 36 (5): 330—337
8. Kosek JC, Iben AB, Shumway NE, Angell WW (1969) Morphology of fresh heart valve homografts. Surg 66: 269
9. Angell WW, Buch WS, Shumway NE (1972) The viable aortic homograft. In: Ionescu MI (ed) Biologial tissue in heart valve replacement. London, Butterworth and Co., p 383
10. Kay PH, Ross DN (1985) Fifteen years' experience with the aortic homograft: the conduit of choice for right ventricular outflow tract reconstruction. Ann Thorac Surg 40 (4): 360—364

Authors' address:
William W. Angell, M.D.
8008 Frost Street, Suite 403
San Diego, California 92123
U.S.A.

Short-term results after allograft transplantation in the pulmonary position following previous repair of tetralogy of Fallot

P. E. Lange, A. Wessel, H. H. Sievers*, A. C. Yankah, D. G. W. Onnasch,
J. H. Bürsch, A. Bernhard*, P. H. Heintzen

Departments of Paediatric Cardiology and Cardiovascular Surgery*,
University of Kiel, F.R.G.

Introduction

Commonly employed methods for the relief of the right ventricular outflow tract stenosis in tetralogy of Fallot are not ideal. In particular, pulmonary insufficiency cannot be prevented in most instances. For reconstruction, pulmonary and aortic allografts have been utilised (2, 5, 6, 9, 10, 14, 15, 19, 20), especially since newer methods of preservation (1, 3, 6, 10, 13, 16, 19, 22) justify the hope that longevity of the allograft may increase. Pulmonary insufficiency of unknown degree and small gradients post-transplantation have been reported (5, 6, 10, 15, 19, 20). The cause of these residual abnormalities have not been clarified, but may, however, be related to the surgical technique. Thus we have studied our patients shortly after transplantation.

Patients and Methods

Patients

14 patients had a typical tetralogy of Fallot (TF) with a hypoplastic right ventricular outflow tract (RVOT), an overriding aorta, and a large ventricular septal defect. One patient (No. 8, Table 1) had infundibular and valvular pulmonary stenosis and an atrial septal defect.

During corrective surgery in the patients with TF, a transannular patch was used to relieve the RVOT stenosis, while in the patient with the pulmonary stenosis commissurotomy and infundibulectomy were performed. The age at corrective surgery was 5.5 years (min: 3 months, max: 8.8 years) and at allograft transplantation 14 years (min: 6 years, max: 18.8 years). The indications for transplantation (Tables 2, 3) were volume overload (n = 9), pressure and volume overload (n = 3) and pressure overload (n = 2). Routine cardiac catheterization was performed in nine patients, 17 days to 2.9 years (mean: 10 months) post-transplantation (Table 1). None of the patients was clinically symptomatic before and after transplantation.

In all patients, the inlay technique was used (14, 17), the residual myocardial tissue of the allograft being used as the posterior sewing ring at the level of the pulmonary annulus. Five patients received a pulmonary and nine an aortic allograft (Table 1).

Table 1. Vital statistics pre- and post-allograft implantation (days).

No.	symb.	AL	ACS	CS-CC	CC-AL	AL-CC	CS-AL	AAL	ACCpreA	ACCpoA
1.	○	Ao	1243	904	40	396	944	2188	2147	2583
2.	◇	PA	2709	12	126	295	4305	7014	6888	7309
3.	✢	PA	1988	24	72	19	3875	5862	5791	5882
4.	◆	Ao	2973	18	141	1054	3490	6463	6322	7517
5.	▲	Ao	2062	22	99	19	4083	6144	6045	6164
6.	□	Ao	2314	61	727	17	4510	6824	6098	6841
7.	●	PA	1467	21	15	34	1658	3125	3110	3159
8.	△	Ao	2195	918	377	569	4388	6583	6205	7152
9.	■	PA	3215	26	449	405	3649	6864	6357	7269
Mean: (n=9)			2241	223	227	312	3434	5674	5440	5986
Min:			1243	12	15	17	944	2188	2147	2583
Max.:			3215	918	727	1054	4510	7014	6888	7517
SD:			652	390	240	348	1267	1764	1639	1852
10.	○	Ao	2661	278	3285		3379	6039	5946	
11.	○	Ao	2450	46	1112		1223	3673	3562	
12.	○	Ao	90	121	121		2302	2392	2231	
13.	○	Ao	2617	578	2345		2364	5080	4961	
14.	○	PA	223	495	1913		3100	3323	2136	
Mean: (n=14)			2014	252	773		3091	5112	4843	
Min:			90	12	15		944	2188	2136	
Max:			3215	918	3285		4510	7014	6888	
SD:			951	334	1028		1197	1782	1792	

Abbreviations: No.: patient identification number; symb.: identification symbols shown in figures; AL: type of allograft; Ao: aortic allograft; PA: pulmonary allograft; ACS: age at corrective surgery; CS-CC: time between corrective surgery and postoperative cardiac catheterization; CC-AL: time between cardiac catheterization and allograft transplantation; AL-CC: time between allograft transplantation and postoperative cardiac catheterization; CS-AL: time between corrective surgery and allograft transplantation; ACCpreA: age at cardiac catheterization pre-allograft transplantation; ACCpoA: age at cardiac catheterization post-allograft transplantation; Mean, Min, Max: mean, minimal, maximal values; SD: standard deviation.

In the case of an aortic allograft, the medial mitral leaflet was utilised for closing the anterior right ventricular gap, and in a pulmonary allograft, glutaraldehyde fixed calf pericardium was used.

Methods

During cardiac catheterization, the patients were in a fasting state, studied in the supine position, having received Luminal (acidum phenylbarbituricum) (10 mg/kg, maximum 200 mg), Dolantin (pethidine) (1—1.5 mg/kg), and atropin (0.01—0.015 mg/kg) as premedication 1 hour before cardiac catheterization. Before the first cineangiocardiogram was taken, arterial oxygen saturation was determined and left and right ventricular pressures were recorded using a side-hole catheter connected to an external pressure transducer (Statham Instruments, Oxnard, California). Zero pressure was referenced to the level of the vena cava in the lateral projection.

282

Table 2. Haemodynamic data pre- and post-allograft implantation.

No.	symb.	RVPmaxpr (mm Hg)	RVPmaxpo (mm Hg)	RVEDPpr (mm Hg)	RVEDPpo (mm Hg)	PAPmaxpr (mm Hg)	PAPmaxpo (mm Hg)	GRDvalpr (mm Hg)	GRDvalpo (mm Hg)	GRDsubpr (mm Hg)	GRDsubpo (mm Hg)	GRDsuppr (mm Hg)	GRDsuppo (mm Hg)
1.	○	22	63	1	4	18	23	4	16	0	24	0	0
2.	◇	71	31	12	11	46	29	0	0	0	0	25	15
3.	⊹	30	26	8	4	23	23	0	0	0	0	10	0
4.	◆	86	60	6	8	23	20	60	32	0	8	0	0
5.	▲	38	36	9	8	34	26	8	10	0	0	0	0
6.	□	94	48	11	21	29	42	40	8	20	0	0	8
7.	●	76	40	9	9	20	38	55	3	0	0	0	0
8.	△	30	40	13	10	24	33	5	10	0	0	0	0
9.	■	49	45	19	8	42	20	0	0	5	25	0	0
Mean: (n=9)		55	43	10	9	29	28	19	9	3	6	4	3
Min:		22	26	1	4	18	20	0	0	0	0	0	0
Max:		94	63	19	21	46	42	60	32	20	25	25	15
SD:		27	12	5	5	10	8	25	10	7	11	9	5
10.	○	43		6		34		0		9		0	
11.	○	54		8		52		0		0		0	
12.	○	30		8		32		0		0		0	
13.	○	104		8		25		80		0		0	
14.	○	30		12		26		3		0		0	
Mean: (n=14)		54		9		31		18		2		3	
Min:		22		1		18		0		0		0	
Max:		104		19		52		80		25		25	
SD:		27		4		10		28		6		7	

Abbreviations: No.: patient identification number; symb.: identification symbols shown in figures; RV: right ventricle; PA: pulmonary artery; valv: valvular; sub: subvalvular; sup: supravalvular; pre: pre-allograft transplantation; po: post-allograft transplantation; Pmax: maximal pressure; EDP: end-diastolic pressure; GRD: maximal pressure gradient; Mean, Min, Max: mean, minimal, maximal values; SD: standard deviation.

Table 3. Haemodynamic data pre- and post-allograft implantation.

No.	symb.	EDVpr (ml)	EDVpo (ml)	ESVpr (ml)	ESVpo (ml)	EFpr	EFpo	RGFpr (%)	RGFpo (%)	SHpr (%)	SHpo (%)	VLpr (%)	VLpo (%)
1.	○	111	117	49	52	0.560	0.560	78	23	0	0	355	34
2.	◇	146	123	76	67	0.480	0.450	50	5	10	0	120	5
3.	✢	105	86	61	39	0.420	0.520	50	10	0	0	100	10
4.	◆	81	71	37	45	0.540	0.370	15	15	0	0	20	20
5.	▲	86	94	46	40	0.470	0.570	52	0	0	0	120	0
6.	□	60	48	33	23	0.460	0.510	8	0	0	0	10	0
7.	●	185	106	138	55	0.420	0.480	0	0	0	0	0	0
8.	△	54	57	19	27	0.650	0.520	52	0	10	20	120	20
9.	■	116	79	57	44	0.510	0.450	47	65	0	0	100	230
Mean: (n=9)		105	87	57	44	0.501	0.492	39	13	2	2	105	35
Min:		55	48	19	23	0.420	0.370	0	0	0	0	0	0
Max:		186	123	139	67	0.650	0.578	65	10	10	20	355	230
SD:		42	26	35	14	0.070	0.060	26	21	4	7	106	74
10.	○	144		80		0.440		55		10		140	
11.	○	127		64		0.500		60		0		150	
12.	○	186		95		0.490		53		0		100	
13.	○	88		44		0.500		40		0		70	
14.	○	145		75		0.480		50		0		100	
Mean: (n=14)		117		62		0.494		44		2		111	
Min:		55		19		0.420		0		0		0	
Max:		186		139		0.650		78		10		400	
SD:		41		30		0.060		21		4		96	

Abbreviations: No.: patient identification number (Table 1); symb.: identification symbols shown in figures; pre: pre-allograft transplantation; po: post-allograft transplantation; EDV: end-diastolic volume; ESV: end-systolic volume; EF: ejection fraction; RGF: regurgitant fraction; SH: left-to-right shunt; VL: volume load.

Volumes of the right ventricle (RV) were obtained on the basis of biplane videoangiographic projections (posterior-anterior and lateral), recorded with 50 frames/s side by side in one video-field on magnetic tape, after the selective injection of 76% Urografin (Schering, Berlin) into the RV (1.5 ml/kg body weight). For calibration purposes, a steel sphere of known diameter was filmed at the location the ventricles occupied during angiocardiography (18). The bordes of the biplane projections (steel sphere and ventricles in sinus rhythm) and "anatomical landmarks" (18) were manually marked with an x/y coder. The largest ventricular projection was assumed to represent end-diastole and the smallest end-systole. Model volumes were calculated with the multiple slice method (18). All values were corrected with factors appropriate for spatial orientation and cardiac phase (11).

Results

In six out of nine patients studied post-transplantation, the transvalvular pressure gradient was less than 10 mm Hg and pulmonary insufficiency less than 10% of the stroke volume (Fig. 1, Tables 2, 3). In both patients (Nos. 1 + 9) with a predominant pulmonary insufficiency (Fig. 1, Table 3) a short pulmonary trunk and a suballograft stenosis were found (Fig. 4), the latter being mainly due to posterior residual myocardial tissue of the allograft sewn to the original pulmonary annulus. Patient No. 9 had an additional narrowing at the site of the insertion of glutaraldehyde preserved calf pericardium which probably shrank. In the patient (No. 4, Table 2) with a predominant valvular stenosis, marked kinking of the RVOT was seen (Figs. 2, 5). The patient (No. 2, Table 2) with the supravalvular stenosis (Fig. 2) had a narrowing of the pulmonary trunk.
End-diastolic and end-systolic volumes, as well as ejection fraction and end-diastolic pressure before and after transplantation, did not change significantly (Tables 2, 3).

Discussion

Relief of obstruction secondary to a hypoplastic right ventricular outflow tract in tetralogy of Fallot, by means of inserting a transannular patch, is common practice. It leads inadvertedly to a postoperative pulmonary insufficiency, however.
Experimental work on the effect of pulmonary incompetence on right ventricular function has shown that despite the lack of overt right heart failure in experimental animals, there is an increase in right ventricular end-diastolic volume and a decrease in cardiac output and ejection fraction (4). Similar results have been reported in patients following previous repair, on the basis of invasive (7, 8, 12) examination and non-invasive exercise (21) studies. On exercise, a decreased working capacity (21) and by quantitative angiocardiography a diminished right ventricular ejection fraction in patients with postoperative pulmonary insufficiency have been disclosed. The majority of these patients were clinically asymptomatic (7, 8, 12, 21). Thus treatment is discussed controversially.
Studies supporting the view that surgically induced significant pulmonary valvular insufficiency is not deleterious in the long run, base their conclusion on the assess-

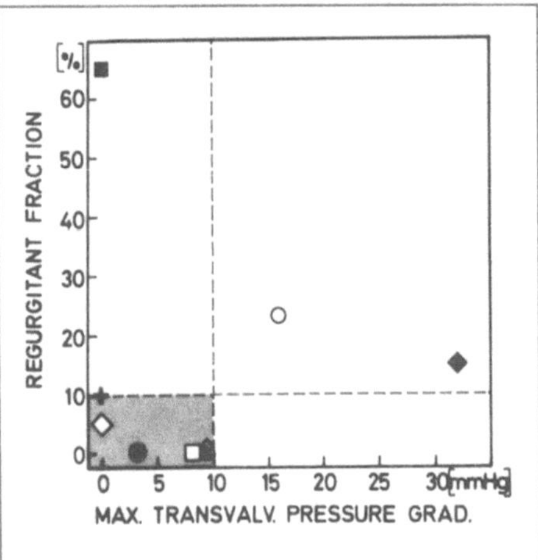

Fig. 1. Function of the allograft valve as determined by the degree of pulmonary insufficiency (regurgitant fraction) and transvalvular pressure gradient was satisfactory in 6 out of 9 patients studied postoperatively. The poor results seem to be related to an unfavorable preoperative anatomy and residual myocardial tissue used as a posterior sewing ring at the level of the original annulus (Fig. 4). Modification of the utilized inlay technique should prevent these abnormalities. Symbols: identification of the patients (see Tables 2, 3).

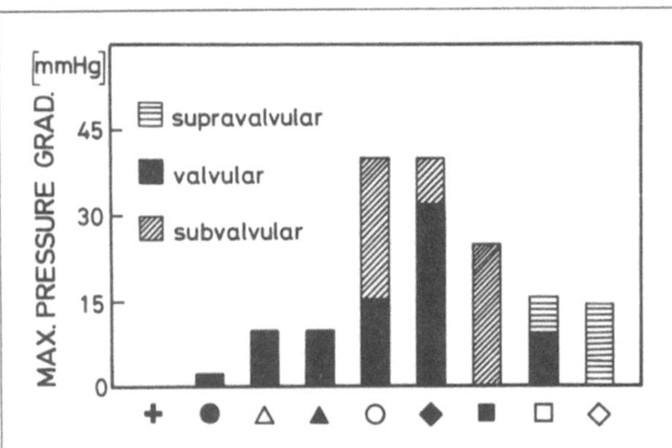

Fig. 2. Type of residual stenosis of the right ventricular outflow tract. The only significant valvular stenosis (No. 4 ◆; Table 2) is related to kinking of the outflow tract. The subvalvular stenoses (No. 1 ○ + 9 ■; Table 2) are mainly caused by residual myocardial tissue, used as a posterior sewing ring at the level of the original annulus (Fig. 4). The supravalvular stenosis (No. 2 ◇; Table 2) is caused by residual narrowing of the main pulmonary artery. Symbols: identification of the patients (see Table 2).

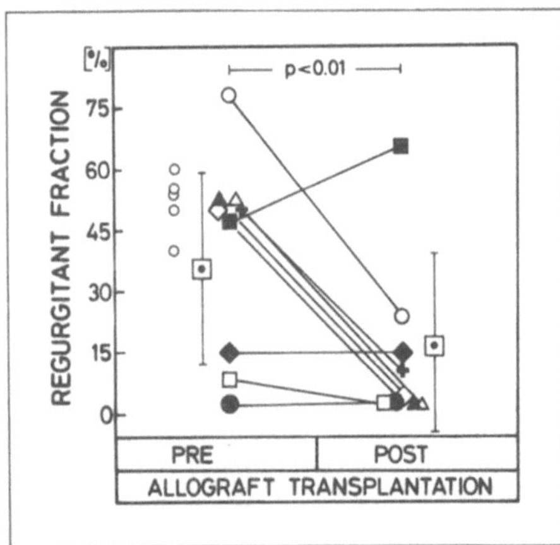

Fig. 3. Significant pulmonary insufficiency (regurgitant fraction) was observed in three out of nine patients. This is probably related to traction of the allograft with subsequent distortion of the valve geometry, caused by an unfavorable preoperative anatomy and residual myocardial tissue used as posterior sewing ring at the level of the original pulmonary annulus (Fig. 4). Modifications of the utilized inlay technique should prevent these abnormalities. Symbols: identification of the patients (see Table 3).

286

ment of the clinical status of the patient and on the assumption that lack of symptoms reflects normal overall cardiac performance. Such assumptions, however, have not been substantiated by objective data during rest or exercise (8). Since 1985, we have adopted the policy of considering asymptomatic patients for allograft 'transplantation, who, on routine cardiac catheterization after previous repair of tetralogy of Fallot, were found to have either a predominant RVOT stenosis, with a maximal pressure gradient of more than 55 mm Hg (n = 3) (Table 2), or a pulmonary insufficiency with a regurgitant fraction of more than 40% (n = 11) of the stroke volume (Table 3, Fig. 3) and concomitantly a right ventricular ejection fraction (Table 3) of less than 80% of normal. The mean volume load secondary to a pure pulmonary insufficiency was 141% of the stroke volume (n = 9), which corresponds, in terms of a left-to-right shunt, to a QP to QS of 2.4 to 1. A shunt of that magnitude secondary to a residual ventricular septal defect would be an indication for reoperation in most centers. In all instances we used the inlay technique (14, 17). Two of the patients restudied postoperatively had a significant pulmonary insufficiency. Preoperatively, both had a right ventricular outflow tract with a short pulmonary trunk

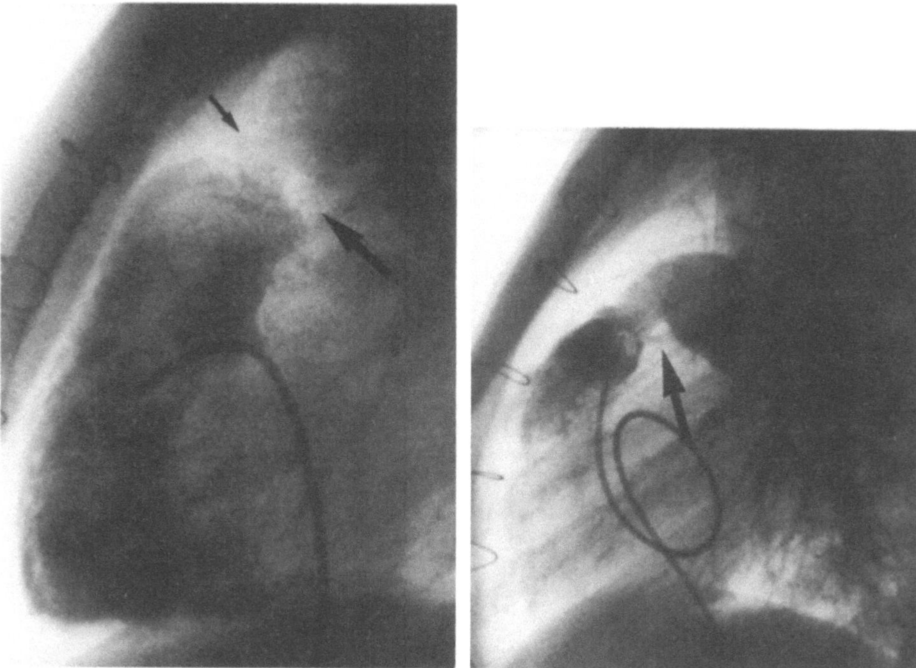

Fig. 4. Lateral angiocardiographic projections of the right ventricular outflow tract of patients No. 9 (left) and No. 1 (right) with significant pulmonary insufficiency and subvalvular stenosis. The posterior subvalvular narrowing (large arrow) is related to residual myocardial tissue used as a sewing ring at the level of the original pulmonary annulus. The anterior narrowing (small arrow) is probably secondary to shrinkage of glutaraldehyde-preserved calf pericardium. The combination of a preoperative short pulmonary trunk and the posterior myocardial tissue, acting as hypomochlion, causes traction and subsequent distortion of the valve geometry leading to pulmonary inusfficiency. Modifications of the utilised inlay technique should prevent these abnormalities (see Tables 2, 3).

taking a distinct course in the sagittal plane from anterior to posterior. Utilising the inlay technique, the combination of a short pulmonary trunk, together with posterior allograft myocardial tissue (Fig. 4) acting as a hypomochlion, may cause traction and subsequently distortion of the normal valve geometry and pulmonary insufficiency. Kinking of the right ventricular outflow tract (Fig. 5, left panel) represents another type of unfavourable anatomy for the inlay technique, being the probable cause of the only significant valvular stenosis (Fig. 5, Table 2). Thus it appears indicated that the inlay technique should be modified if a smooth curvature of the reconstructed right ventricular outflow tract (Fig. 6) cannot be expected on the basis of the preoperative anatomy.

A suballograft stenosis, found in two patients (Fig. 2) is probably related to the residual myocardial tissue of the allograft sewn to the original pulmonary annulus, thus causing the posterior narrowing (Fig. 4). An additional anterior narrowing in one patient (Fig. 4) may be caused by shrunken glutaraldehyde-preserved calf pericardium, utilized to close the anterior myocardial gap. These abnormalities can be prevented by sewing the myocardial tissue proximal to the original pulmonary annulus or by keeping it anterior. Material which may shrink should not be used.

The optimal timing of an allograft transplantation in children is difficult to determine at present. The ideal would be to implant a growing valve during infancy which functions for ever. On the other hand, one does not want to wait until the right

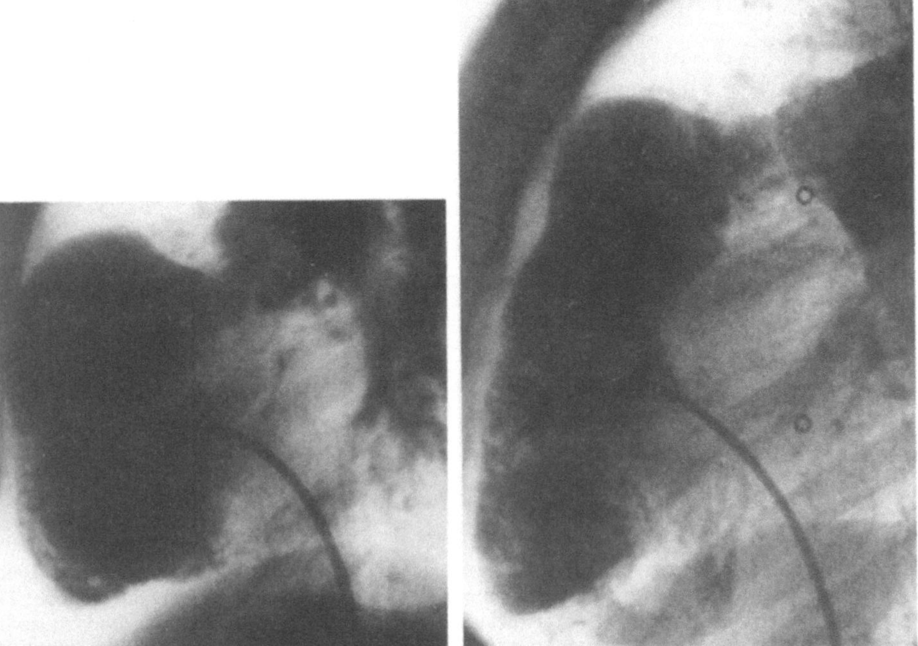

Fig. 5. Lateral angiocardiographic projections of the right ventricular outflow tract in patient No. 4 (Table 2) pre-(left) and post-(right) implantation of an allograft. The preoperative unfavorable anatomy seems to be the cause of the valvular stenosis. Modification of the inlay technique used should prevent postoperative kinking.

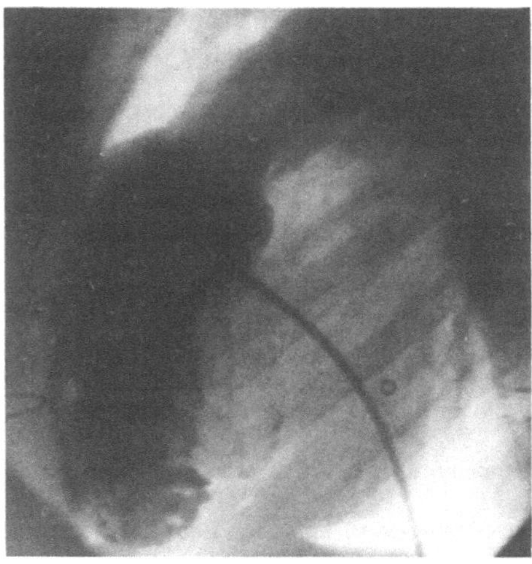

Fig. 6. Lateral angiocardiographic projection of the right ventricular outflow tract in a patient without pulmonary insufficiency or stenosis (No. 5; Tables 2, 3). The curvature of the outflow tract is smooth.

ventricular myocardium is irreversibly damaged. The latter may well be the case in most of our restudied patients, since in none of them did right ventricular ejection fraction return to normal within 10 months (min: 17 days, max: 2.9 years) post-transplantation (Table 3). According to the findings of Ilbawi et al. (8), however, an improvement of global right ventricular function can be expected if insertion of a pulmonary valve is performed within 2 years following surgical repair. This, in turn, would certainly mean that every effort should be undertaken to identify patients with impaired right ventricular function during this period.

References

1. Barratt-Boyes BG, Roche AHG, Subramanyan R, Pemberton JR, Whitlock RML (1987) Long-term follow-up of patients with the antibiotic-sterilized aortic homograft valve inserted freehand in the aortic position. Circulation 75: 768—777
2. Barratt-Boyes BG (1988) 25 years clinical experience of allograft surgery — a time for reflection. This volume
3. Baust J, May R (1988) Cryobiology of tissues. This volume
4. Burnell RH, Woodson RH, Less MH, Starr A (1969) Right ventricular performance in dogs following pulmonary valvectomy. Surgery 65: 952—957
5. Clarke D (1988) Experience with the use of pulmonary allografts for reconstruction of RVOT. This volume
6. Di Carlo D, de Leval MR, Stark J (1984) "Fresh", antibiotic sterilized aortic homografts in extracardiac valved conduits: long-term results. J Thorac Cardiovasc Surg 32: 10—14
7. Graham TP, Cordell D, Atwood GF, Boucek RJ Jr, Boerth RC, Bender HW, Nelson JH, Vaughn WK (1976) Right ventricular volume characteristics before and after palliative and reparative operation in tetralogy of Fallot. Circulation 54: 417—423
8. Ilbawi MN, Idriss FS, DeLeon SY, Muster AJ, Gidding SS, Berry TE, Paul MH (1987) Factors that exaggerate the deleterious effects of pulmonary insufficiency on the right ventricle after tetralogy repair. J Thorac Cardiovasc Surg 93: 36—44
9. Jonas R, Castaneda A (1988) Allograft repair of tetralogy of Fallot in infancy. This volume
10. Kay PH, Ross DN (1985) Fifteen years' experience with the aortic homograft: the conduit of choice for right ventricular outflow tract reconstruction. Ann Thorac Surg 40: 360—364

11. Lange PE, Onnasch DGW, Farr F, Heintzen PH (1978) Angiocardiographic right ventricular volume determination. Accuracy, as determined from human casts, and clinical application. Eur J Cardiol 8: 477—501
12. Lange PE, Onnasch DGW, Bernhard A, Heintzen PH (1982) Left and right ventricular adaptation to right ventricular overload before and after surgical repair of tetralogy of Fallot. Am J Cardiol 50: 786—794
13. Livi U, Abdulla D, Parker R, Olsen E, Path FRC, Ross DN (1987) Viability and morphology of aortic and pulmonary homografts. A comparative study. J Thorac Cardiovasc Surg 93: 755—760
14. Meisner H (1988) Technique of inlay allografts into the RVOT to prevent pulmonary insufficiency. This volume
15. Moore CH, Marteli V, Ross DN (1976) Reconstruction of right ventricular outflow tract with a valved conduit in 75 cases of congenital heart disease. J Thorac Cardiovasc Surg 71: 11—19
16. O'Brien MF et al. (1988) Cryopreserved viable allograft aortic valves. This volume, pp 311—322
17. Ross DN, Somerville J (1966) Correction of pulmonary atresia with a homograft aortic valve. Lancet 2: 1446—1447
18. Onnasch DGW (1985) Computerized geometric evaluation of angio- and echocardiographic images. Herz 10: 228—237
19. Shabbo FP, Wain WH, Ross DN (1980) Right ventricular outflow reconstruction with aortic homograft conduit: analysis of the long-term results. Thorac Cardiovasc Surg 28: 21—25
20. Somerville J (1988) Fate of the aortic allograft used for reconstruction of the RVOT. This volume
21. Wessel HU, Cunningham WJ, Paul MH, Bastanier CK, Muster AJ, Idriss FS (1980) Exercise performance in tetralogy of Fallot after intracardiac repair. J Thorac Cardiovasc Surg 80: 582—593
22. Yankah AC, Hetzer R (1987) Derzeitige und zukünftige Trends der Transplantation allogener Herzklappen. Z Herz-, Thorax-, Gefäßchir 1: 12—19

Authors' address:
Priv.-Doz. Dr. P. E. Lange
Universitätskinderklinik
Abt. Kinderkardiologie
Schwanenweg 20
2300 Kiel
F.R.G.

Intermediate-term results of cryopreserved allograft and xenograft valved ventricle to pulmonary artery conduits

J. K. Kirklin, J. W. Kirklin, A. D. Pacifico, E. H. Blackstone

University of Alabama Medical Center, Department of Surgery, University Station, Birmingham, U.S.A.

Introduction

The use of fresh aortic homograft valves in the reconstruction of ventricle to pulmonary artery connections in many forms of congenital heart disease was introduced by Ross and Somerville in 1966 (12). Subsequently, a large amount of experience has accumulated on the use of glutaraldehyde-preserved heterograft porcine valves mounted in a woven dacron tube (3, 9, 11). The intermediate-term results of heterograft valved conduits have been disappointing (2, 4, 10), and improved results have now been reported with the use of fresh, antibiotic sterilised homograft aortic valves in ventricle-pulmonary artery pathways (5, 6, 8). Little information is currently available on the use of cryopreserved aortic valve homografts in ventricular-pulmonary artery connections (9).

Experience at the University of Alabama at Birmingham (UAB)

Between 1968 and 1981, glutaraldehyde-preserved heterograft porcine valves (n = 64) and, prior to that, irradiated homograft aortic valves (n = 14), employing a dacron conduit were used in 78 patients undergoing repair of tetralogy with pulmonary atresia. These groups were analysed together, since these two conduits have been shown to behave similarly (1).
Between 1981 and 1986, cryopreserved (n = 131) or fresh (n = 19) homograft aortic valves and ascending aortas were inserted between a ventricle and the pulmonary arteries as part of the repair of various congenital cardiac anomalies in 149 patients. These two groups were analysed together, since no published information indicates differences in their behaviour. 94 of the homografts were inserted during the original cardiac repair and 56 were placed at re-operation (Table 1).

Technique of insertion

The technique of procurement, processing, and cryopreservation has been described elsewhere (7). At the time of operation, the largest homograft was selected which could be inserted without distortion. The graft was trimmed so as to leave about 5 mm of muscle, about 4 mm thick, and about 5 mm of anterior mitral leaflet beneath the nadir of the aortic cusps. The coronary arteries were securely ligated. The homo-

Table 1. Insertion and type of aortic valve homograft conduit and the relationship with obstruction (UAB, 1981—1986)

Category	n	Removal of conduit	n	PO cardiac catheterization		
		No.		Ventricle-PA gradient > 40 mmHg		
				No.	% of N	Cl
Primary insertion	94	2				
Extracardiac conduit	88	2	17	2	12	4—26%
Orthotopic conduit	6	—	—	—	—	—
Secondary insertion	56	2				
Extracardiac conduit	32	—	2	1	50	7—93%
Orthotopic conduit	24	2	5	2	40	14—71%
Total	150	4	24	5	21	12—33%

Abbreviations: PA, pulmonary artery; PO, postoperative.

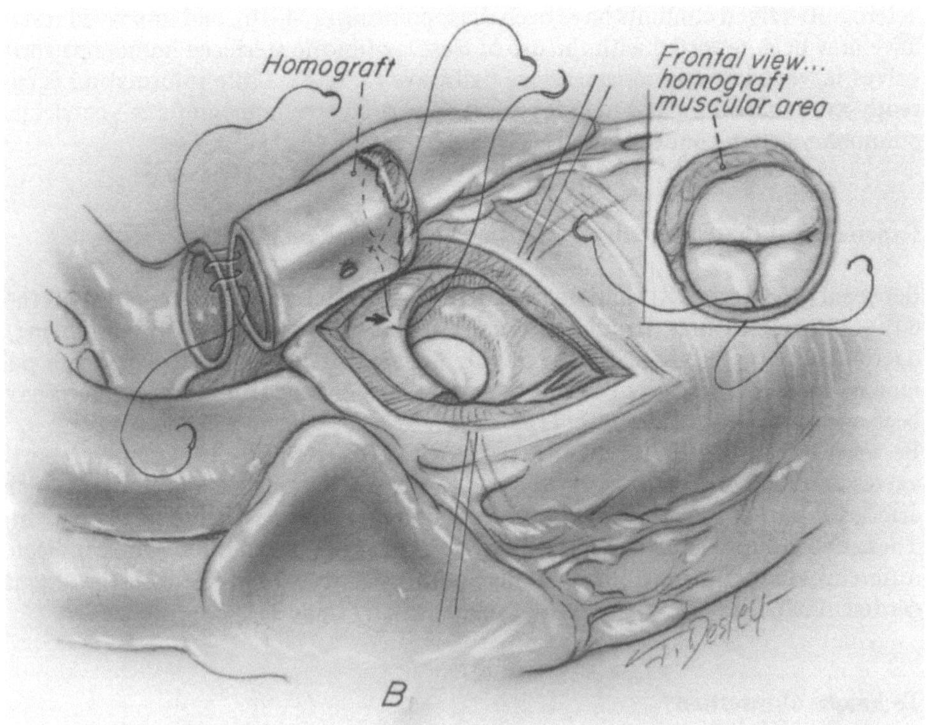

Fig. 1. The homograft of aortic valve and ascending aorta are placed as an orthotopic conduit, positioning it so that the convexity of the natural curve of the homograft is anterior. The proximal anastomosis is posterior to the infundibular septum, and when the ventriculotomy is shorter than shown, a supplementary patch is not needed anteriorly. Distally, the anastomosis between the homograft and pulmonary trunk is end-to-end.
(Reproduced with permission from ref. (8)).

graft was used in this condition as an orthotopic conduit. When used as an extra cardiac conduit, it was generally prolonged proximally by suturing it to a preclotted double-velour woven dacron tube, 2—4 m larger in diameter than the homograft valve. Less commonly, a portion of the transverse arch was used instead of a dacron tube graft.

When the homograft valve was inserted orthotopically, it was simply interposed between the right ventricle and the pulmonary artery (Fig. 1). When the homograft valve was placed as an extra cardiac conduit, the proximal end of the dacron extension was cut obliquely so that the actual circumferential portion of dacron was only 4 or 5 mm long (Fig. 2), and the more proximal portion was a hood over the ventriculotomy. In patients with atrial situs solitus and ventricular D-loop, the extra cardiac conduit was positioned in a somewhat reverse "C" configuration so that it lay to the left of the sternum and on the side opposite that of the ascending aorta. In patients with atrial situs olitus and ventricular L-loop, the conduit was similarly

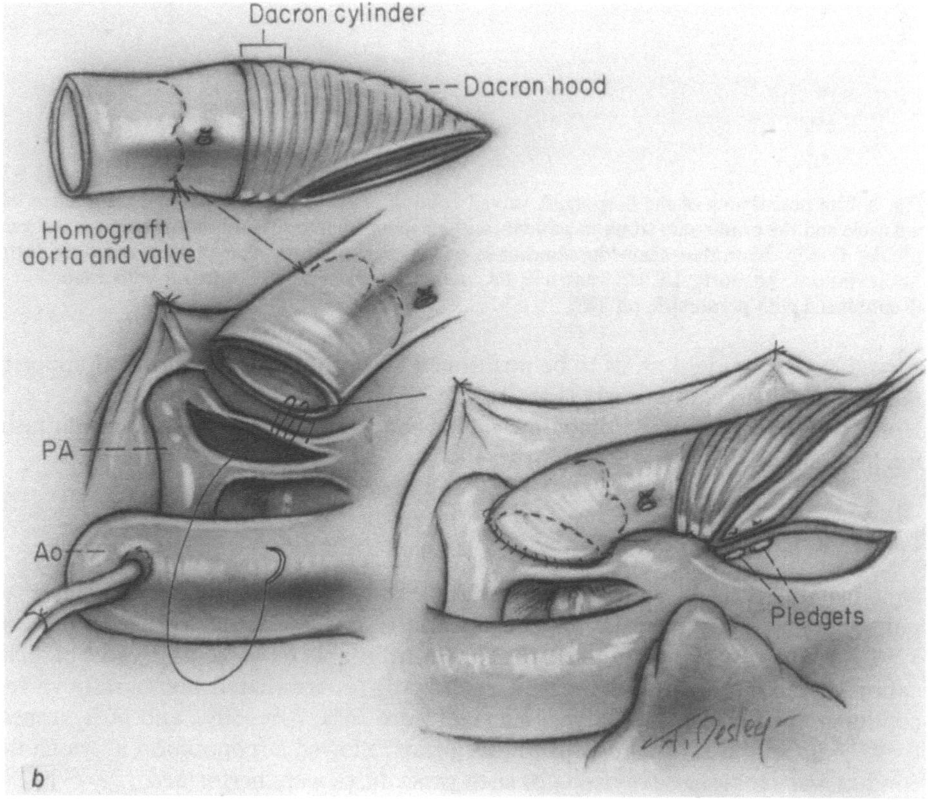

Fig. 2. The homograft has been prolonged proximally by anastomosing it to a preclotted segment of a double velour woven dacron tube. The tube is cut so that the tubular segment of dacron is only 4 to 5 mm long. Both proximal and distal anastomoses are end-to-side. The extracardiac conduit is positioned on the side opposite that of the ascending aorta. Abbreviations: Ao, aorta; PA, pulmonary artery.
(Reproduced with permission from ref. (8)).

293

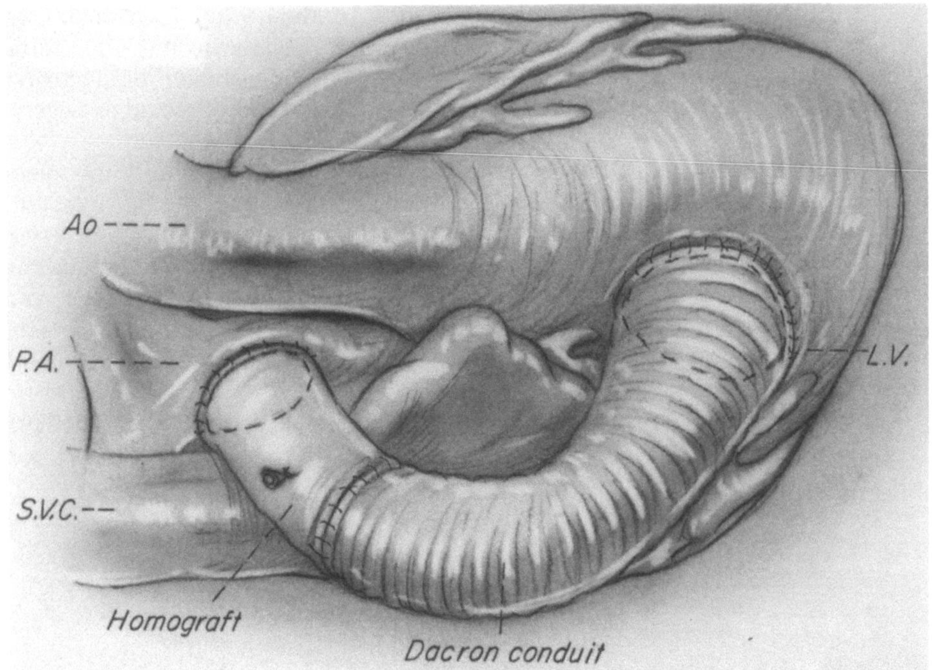

Fig. 3. The positioning of the homograft valved conduit between the anterior and right sided left ventricle and the pulmonary trunk in patients with atrioventricular discordant connection and ventricular L-loop. Note that again the conduit is on the side opposite that of the ascending aorta. Abbreviations: Ao, aorta; LV, left ventricle; PA, pulmonary artery; SVC, superior vena cava. (Reproduced with permission ref. (8)).

curved but to the right, so as to be positioned away from the sternum and opposite the side of the ascending aorta (Fig. 3).

Homograft and irradiated homograft valved conduits were placed in a similar fashion after about 1973.

Patient survival

Among patients receiving cryopreserved or fresh homograft valves in ventricular to pulmonary artery reconstruction, the actuarial 1 and 5 year survival was 76% and 72%, respectively. None of the deaths were attributable to homograft valve complications. Among patients receiving a heterograft (or irradiated homograft) valved conduits, the 1, 5, 10, and 15 year survival were 74%, 70%, 60%, and 60%, respectively. Four of the 28 total deaths in this group followed a reoperation in which the conduit was replaced or revised (20 such procedures were performed).

Early haemodynamic data

Unfortunately, early postoperative haemodynamic data regarding ventricular to pulmonary artery gradients were not systemically obtained in all patients. Among

294

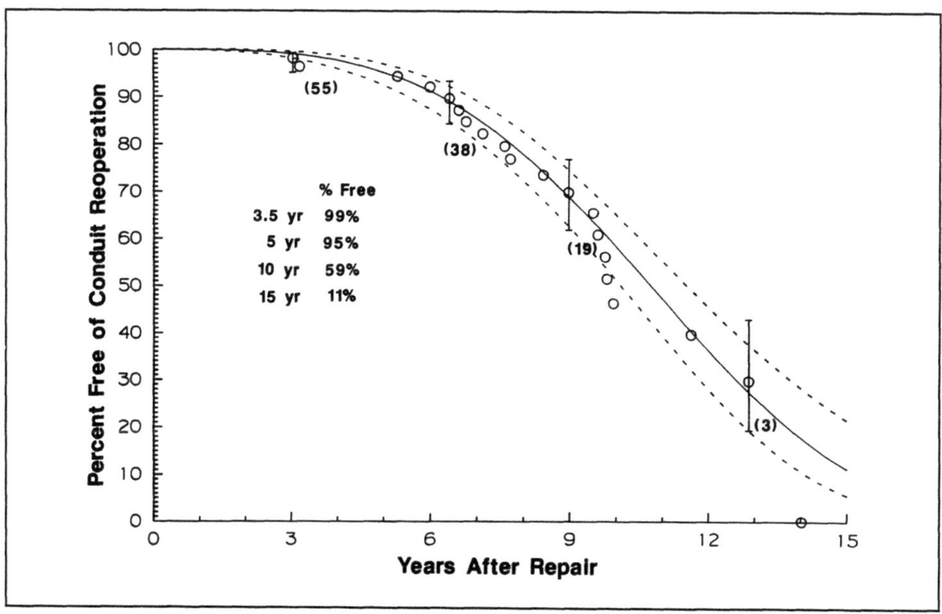

Fig. 4. Actuarial (○ and I) and parametric (——— and ------) depiction of percentage freedom from reoperation of heterograft (and irradiated homograft) valved conduits between right ventricle and pulmonary artery in patients with tetralogy of Fallot and pulmonary atresia (1967—1982: n = 78; events = 20). The lines (----) enclose the parametric 70% confidence limits.

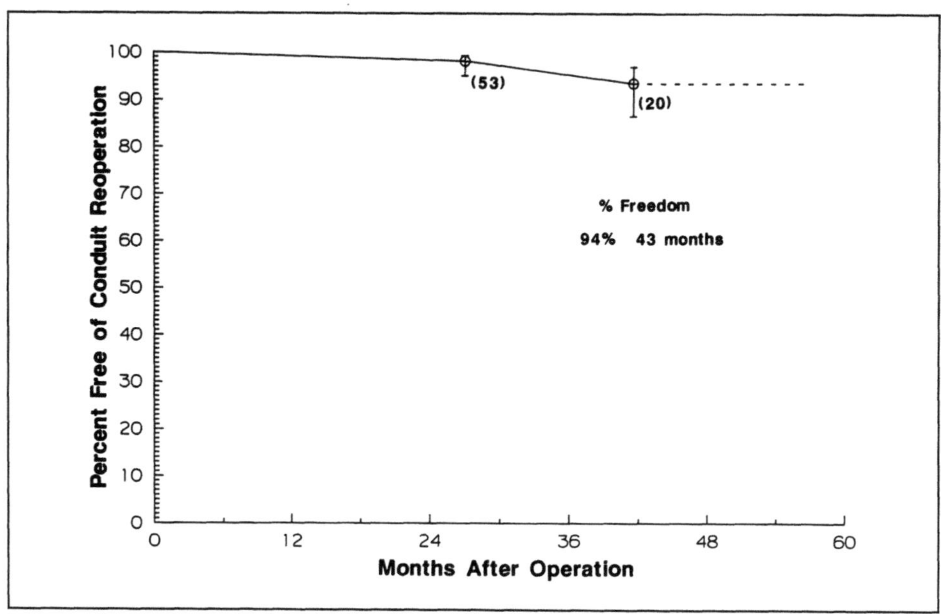

Fig. 5. Actuarial freedom from reoperation for replacement of cryopreserved (or fresh) homograft aortic valves used in ventricle-pulmonary artery reconstruction (1981—1986: n = 150; reoperation = 2). The verticle bars enclose the 70% confidence intervals (limits). The line (---) represents patients traced beyond the last event. The numbers in parentheses describe the number of patients traced beyond that point in time.

Reproduced with permission from ref. (9).

eight patients with cryopreserved (or fresh) homograft valved conduits, in whom withdrawal pressure tracings could be made on the first postoperative day, the ventricular to pulmonary artery systolic gradient was 0 in two patients, 12 mmHg in three, and 14, 18, and 20 mmHg in one patient each. The gradient was located at the distal anastomosis in three patients, at the proximal anastomosis in one patient, and at both anastomoses in one patient.

Conduit obstruction

Among the UAB patients with heterograft (or irradiated homograft) valve conduits, the percentage freedom from replacement of the xenograft (or irradiated allograft) valve conduit was 99% at 3.5 years, 95% at 5 years, 59% at 10 years and only 11% at 15 years (Fig. 4) (9). All reoperations were for obstruction. The hazard function (instantanous risk of replacement for 1 month) had a single decreasing phase and was 0.042 at 15 years.

At UAB, the follow-up for patients receiving cryopreserved (or fresh) valved conduits extends to only 5 years (Fig. 5) (9). At 4 years, however, the actuarial freedom from conduit reoperation is 94%. This is not significantly different from the freedom from conduit reoperation among patients with heterograft valve conduits over this same period. However, Ross, Somerville, and colleagues (6) have followed-up patients for up to 20 years with fresh homograft aortic valve conduits (Fig. 6). The

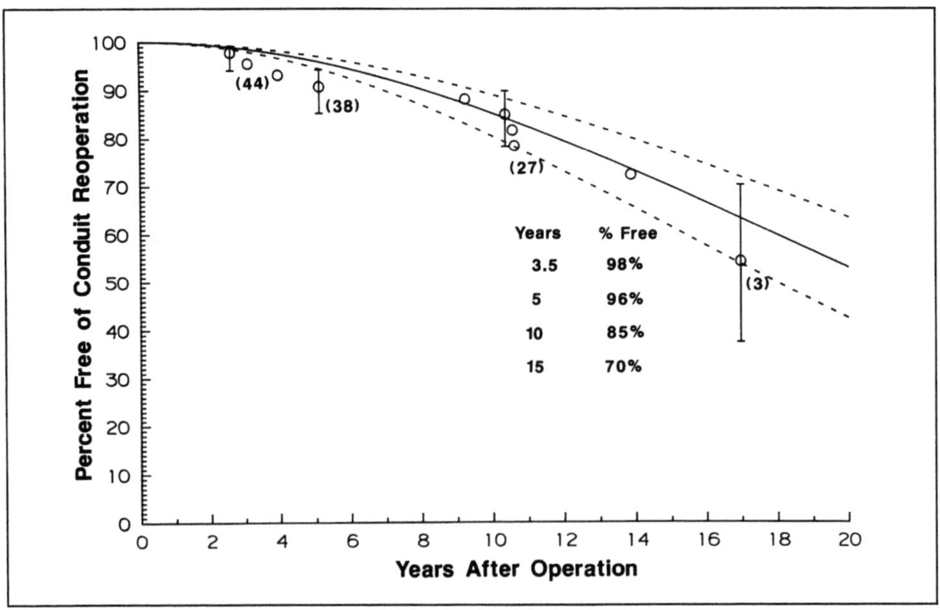

Fig. 6. Actuarial and parametric percentage freedom from reoperation on the conduit in patients with tetralogy of Fallot and pulmonary atresia in whom a fresh homograft aortic valve had been used in construction of a conduit between the right ventricle and the pulmonary artery (1966–1977: n = 49; events = 10). (Data supplied by J Somerville and DN Ross: personal communication).

296

actuarial freedom from conduit reoperation at 5 years was 96%, at 10 years 85 %, and at 15 years 70%. This is clearly different from the 11% freedom from reoperation at 15 years for heterograft conduits. Thus, the hazard function for conduit reoperation for homograft conduits is probably not different from that for heterograft conduits until after 5 years of follow-up, but is clearly different at 15 years. This underlines the importance of 5, 10, and 15 year follow-up before drawing firm inferences about other types of conduit valves such as pericardium or pulmonary valve allografts.

Valve sizes

The diameter of the cryopreserved (and fresh) homograft aortic valves that were inserted into the ventricular-pulmonary artery pathway was directly related to the size and age of the patient (with considerable variability (Fig. 7, 8) (9). A 20-mm homograft valve diameter was used in many patients aged 5 years and nearly all patients aged 10 years or more. Homograft valves with a diameter of 16 mm or more were nearly always used in patients over 2 years of age, or with a body surface area of 0.5 m² or more.

Although long-term preservation of ventricular function in many congenital heart conditions would favour an early complete repair, this must be weighed against the

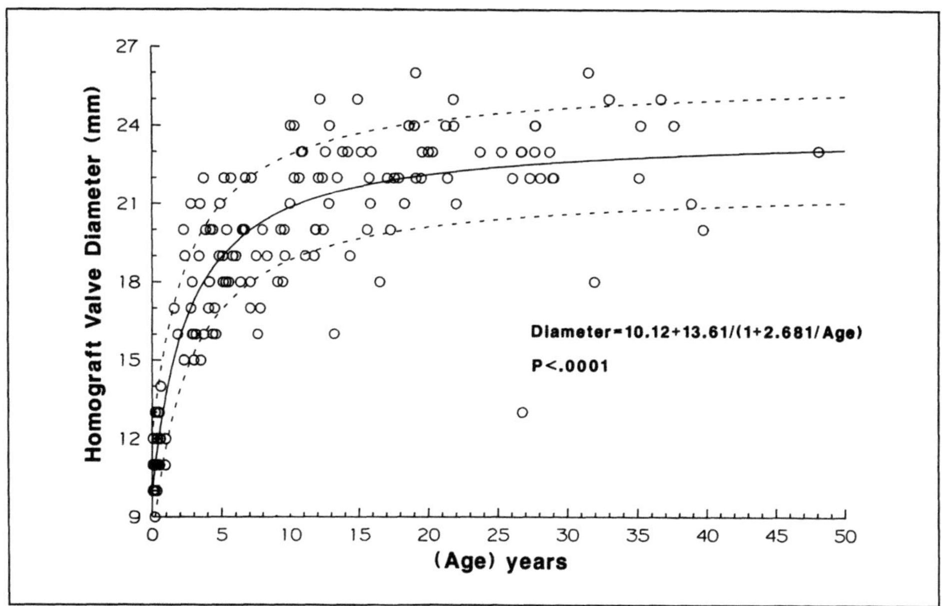

Fig. 7. The relation to patient's of the diameter of the cryopreserved (or fresh) homograft aortic valves used for ventricle-pulmonary artery reconstruction (1981—1986: n = 150). Each circle represents a patient, and (———) represents a solution of the regression equation. The lines (---) enclose the 70% confidence limits. Information is missing in one patient.
Reproduced with permission from ref. (9).

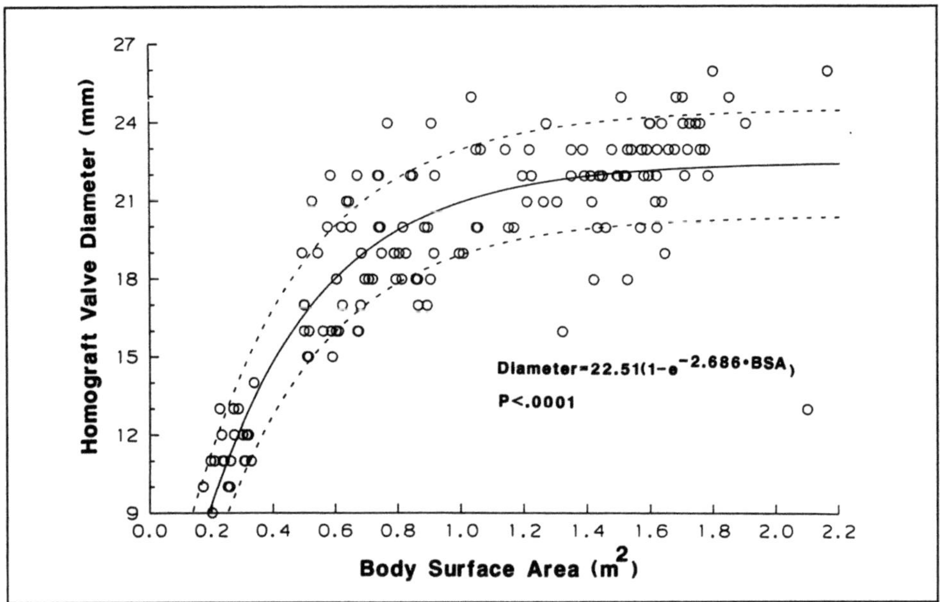

Fig. 8. The relation to the patient's body surface area of the diameter of the cryopreserved (or fresh) homograft aortic valves used for ventricle-pulmonary artery reconstruction (1981—1986: n = 150). Reproduced with permission from ref. (9).

nearly certain need for re-operation if a small valved conduit is inserted. Although the risk of reoperation for conduit replacement is low, it is currently not negligible, being perhaps 5%. Therefore, when placement of a valve conduit is known to be part of the repair of a congenital heart defect, it may be advisable, when safe, to delay total correction until age 3 to 5 years, at which time there is a reasonable chance that a conduit can be placed which is large enough (18 mm or greater) not to require replacement in adult life.

Inferences

Properly prepared and stored aortic valved homografts are the most durable proven devices for ventricular-pulmonary arterial reconstruction.
The past generation of heterograft valved conduits were distinctly less satisfactory, particularly after 5 years.

References

1. Bailey WW, Kirklin JW, Bargeron LM Jr, Pacifico AD, Kouchoukos NT (1977) Late results with synthetic valved external conduits from venous ventricle to pulmonary arteries. Circulation (Suppl II): 11—73

298

2. Bisset III GS, Schwartz DC, Benzing III G, Helmsworth J, Schreiber JT, Kaplan S (1981) Late results of reconstruction of the right ventricular outflow tract with porcine xenografts in children. Ann Thorac Surg 31: 437
3. Bowman FO, Hancock WD, Malm JR (1973) A valve-containing dacron prosthesis. Arch Surg 107: 724
4. Ciaravella JM Jr, Mcgoon DC, Danielson GK, Wallace RB, Mair DD (1979) Experience with the extracardiac conduit. J Thorac Cardiovasc Surg 78: 920
5. Fontan FM, Choussat A, Deville C, Doutremepuich CDC, Coupilland J, Vosa C (1984) Aortic valve homografts in the surgical treatment of complexcardiac malformations. J Thorac Cardiovasc Surg 87: 649
6. Kay PH, Ross DN (1985) Fifteen years' experience with the aortic homograft: The conduit of choice for right ventricular outflow tract reconstruction. Ann Thorac Surg 40: 360
7. Kirklin JK, Diethelm AG, Kirklin JW. Procurement, cryopreservation, and transplantation of aortic valve homografts, In: Fawcett K, Reynolds A (eds) Tissue Banking American Association of Blood Banks, Arlington, VA. In press
8. Kirklin JW, Barratt-Boyes BG (1986) Cardiac Surgery. John Wiley and Sons, New York, p 800, Tables 23—31
9. Kirklin JW, Blackstone EH, Maehara T, Pacifico AD, Kirklin JK, Pollock S, Stewart RW. Intermediate Term Fate of Cryopreserved Allograft and Xenograft Valved Conduits. Ann Thorac Surg, in press
10. Norwood WI, Freed MD, Rocchini AP, Bernhard WF, Castaneda AR (1977) Experience with valved conduits for congenital heart disease. Ann Thorac Surg 24: 223
11. Planche C, Binet J-P, Langlois J, Conso J-F (1972) Reconstruction de la voi d'ejection du ventricule droit a' l'aide de tubes valves. Nouv Presse Med 1: 541
12. Ross DN, Somerville J (1966) Correction of pulmonary atresia with a homograft aortic valve. Lancet 2: 1446

Authors' address:
James K. Kirklin, M.D.
UAB, Department of Surgery
University Station
739 Zeigler Bldg.,
Birmingham, AL 35294,
U.S.A.

Functional evaluation of allografts by non-invasive techniques

A. Wessel, P. E. Lange, J. H. Bürsch, H. H. Sievers[1], A. C. Yankah[1],
A. Bernhard[1], P. H. Heintzen

Department of Paediatric Cardiology and Biomedical Engineering and
Department of Cardiovascular Surgery[1], University of Kiel, F.R.G.

Introduction

Heart valve replacement aims to substitute malfunctioning valves by devices with
perfect haemodynamic profiles. Although there is some evidence that promising
results in this field may be achieved by allograft transplantation (1, 5) follow-up
remains mandatory to answer the question "What have you really done?" in the
individual patient.

Data for answering this question may be evaluated by invasive and non-invasive
techniques. Since, for children, non-invasive follow-up seems preferable, we tried
to evaluate the potential of non-invasive methods for quantitative assessment of
haemodynamics after allograft transplantation in the paediatric age group.

Patients and Methods

Our institutions transplanted 24 allografts (16/24 in pulmonary position, 8/24 in
aortic position) in children and adolescents, between 1983 and 1987. Patient data
are listed in Table 1. Indications for allograft transplantation were residual pulmonary stenosis or insufficiency after previous surgery for tetralogy of Fallot or valvular
pulmonary stenosis in 14/16 patients. In the remaining 2/16 cases with tetralogy of
Fallot, allografts were used primarily for reconstruction of the right ventricular outflow tract. Mean age was 12.8 ± 5.1 years (range: 4.8—19.2 years); mean body
weight, 37.4 ± 16.8 kg (15—65 kg). Indications for allograft transplantation in aortic
position was severe aortic incompetence in four out of eight, incompetence combined with stenosis in two out of eight, and stenosis in two out of eight patients.
Mean age in this group was 16.3 ± 2.3 years (range: 11.9—19 years) with a mean
body weight of 62.8 ± 15 kg (37.5—85 kg).

Transplantations either of fresh or preserved allografts were performed according to
blood groups (ABO system) of recipients and donors. Allograft were sterilised by
antibiotics and preserved in culture solution or cryopreserved (11). Donor's age
ranged from 11—41 years (mean, 24 years).

The only death among all 24 patients (1/24 = 4%) occurred on the first postoperative
day and was not related to the allograft, transplanted in the pulmonary position.

Post-transplantation heart catheterisations were performed a mean of 1.09 years
after allograft transplantation in the pulmonary position (9/16 patients) and a mean

of 0.55 years after transplantation in the aortic position (4/8 patients). Data revealed by these investigations are shown in Table 1. Allograft stenosis was measured in terms of peak systolic pressure gradients from pullback tracings. Valve incompetence was determined by videodensitometry as regurgitant fraction (RGF), which is defined as the ratio of regurgitant volume (RV) over total stroke volume (RGF = RV/TSV) (2). These data, obtained invasively, are compared with non-invasive findings in order to evaluate the reliability of non-invasive parameters for quantitation of allograft function.

Non-invasive follow-up investigations could be performed in 15/16 patients, who underwent allograft transplantation in pulmonic position between 0.1 and 4.3 years (mean follow-up time: 1.8 ± 1.1 years). The mean non-invasive follow-up time was the same in the eight patients with aortic allograft transplantation (range: 0.1—3.3 years). Investigations included chest X-rays to assess calcification, phonocardio-

Table 1. Data of patients who underwent allograft transplantation in pulmonary and aortic positions.

No./ Name	Sex	Diag- nosis	Age (years)	BW (kg)	pre-Tp dp (mmHg)	pre-Tp RGF (%)	post-Tp t (Y)	post-Tp dp (mmHg)	post-Tp RGF (%)
Pulmonary position									
1 SK	m	TOF/PS	8.6	21.4	56	0	0.1	2	0
2 AW	m	TOF/PI	18.9	55	7	47	1.1	25	65
3 GB	m	TOF/PI	16.1	65	5	50	0.05	3	10
4 JA	m	TOF/PI	6	18.8	4	78	1.08	40	23
5 GA	m	TOF/PI	19.2	62	25	50	0.9	2	10
6 BK	f	TOF/PS	17	48.6	60	15	3	40	15
7 SK	f	TOF/PS	18.7	45.8	65	0	0.01	6	0
8 FS	m	PS/PI	18	56	0	52	2.5	5	0
9 AZ	m	PS/PI	9.6	24	31	73	1.0	10	0
10 MM	f	TOF/PI	10	22.3	2	60			
11 SS	f	TOF/PI	9.1	29.9	4	50			
12 TS	m	TOF/PI	6.6	19.8	8	53			
13 MH	m	TOF/PI	16.5	46.4	9	55			
14 NH	m	TOF/PS	17	47					
15 LK	f	TOF	4.8	15	70				
16 JL	f	TOF	8.8	22	80		— died —		
Aortic position									
1 DH	m	AI	15	64	0	44	0.01	51	46
2 DK	m	AI	18.2	65	20	47	0.1	38	7
3 LN	m	AI	14	68	13	45	1.1	59	50
4 KP	f	AS/AI	18.1	56	10	39	1.0	10	37
5 OW	m	AI	11.9	37.5	22	65			
6 SF	m	AS	19	85	65				
7 JA	m	AS	16.2	82	65	12			
8 PK	f	AS/AI	17.7	45	30	44			

Abbreviations: BW, body weight; Tp, allograft transplantation; dp, pressure gradient; RGF, regurgitant fraction; t, time interval between transplantation and invasive investigation (years); AS, AI, PS, PI, aortic or pulmonary stenosis or insufficiency; TOF, tetralogy of Fallot. Indication for first operation on the left of "/"; indication for allograft transplantation on the right of "/".

graphy for documentation of murmurs, and echocardiography. M-mode techniques were performed to evaluate patterns of valve motion. 2D-echocardiographic studies were performed to determine valve size, before and after allograft transplantation, from long-axis views of the great arteries. Diameters were measured at cusp level using the leading edge method before, less than 1 month, 2—12 months, 1—3 years and more than 3 years after transplantation. Data are compared with normal ranges for valve diameters (mean $\pm$ relative error (s)), being derived from n healthy children with respect to body weight (BW) (7, 10):

Aortic valve diameter: $\quad$ AoD = 4.66 $\cdot$ BW$^{0.36}$ $\quad$ s = $\pm$ 12% $\quad$ n = 66
Pulmonary valve diameter: PuD = 5.45 $\cdot$ BW$^{0.36}$ $\quad$ s = $\pm$ 7% $\quad$ n = 83.

Results

Chest X-rays revealed calcification in 2/15 allografts in the pulmonary position (Fig. 1) and 1/8 in the aortic position. Calcification affected the walls of the allografts rather than their cusps. Thus, a calcification rate of 3 % results, for pulmonic as well as aortic position. With respect to the time course — the first hints for calcification became evident a mean of 1 year after transplantation — a calcification rate of 4 % per patient-year may be calculated. 2D-Echocardiograms were suggestive of calcification only in a patient with severe calcification of an allograft in the aortic po-

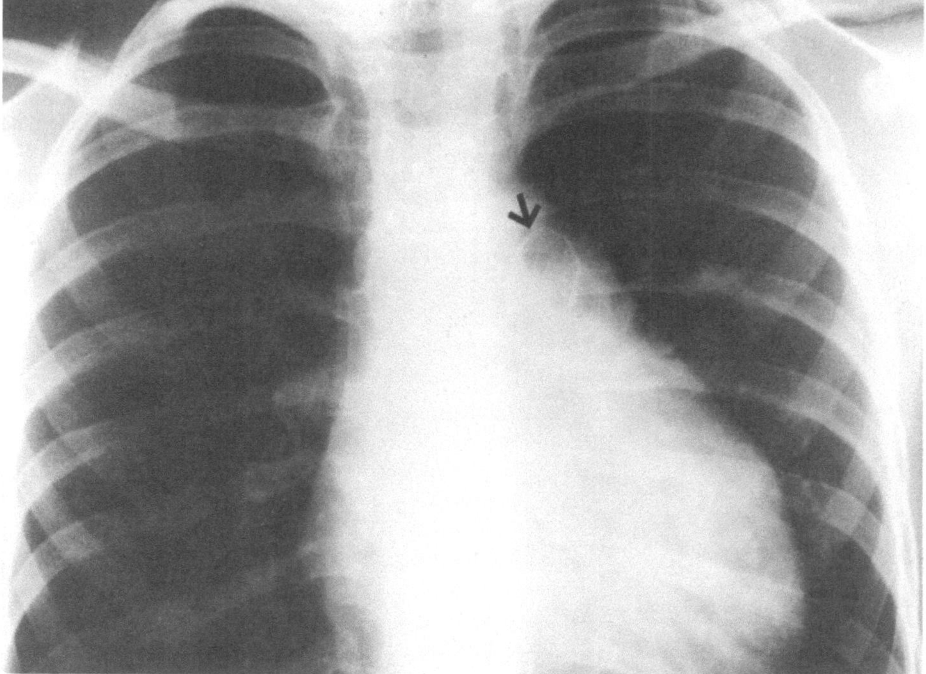

Fig. 1. Chest X-ray from an 8-year-old boy, 2.5 years after allograft transplantation in pulmonary position. The allograft walls are calcified showing the typical egg-shell fashion (arrow).

sition. In this case, increased echodensity suggested calcific degeneration of wall and cusps, which was proven by reoperation.

Systolic murmurs could be documented in all patients. They are related to allograft obstruction being responsible for pressure gradients detected by pullback tracings in all patients investigated invasively. Peak systolic pressure gradients ranged from 2—40 mm Hg (mean: 14.8 $\pm$ 15.0 mm Hg) in the pulmonary position and 10—59 mm Hg in the aortic position (mean: 39.5 $\pm$ 18.8 mm Hg). Decrescendo-shaped diastolic murmurs were found in 11/16 (69%) patients with allografts in pulmonic position and 6/8 (75%) patients who had allografts in aortic position. All diastolic murmurs appeared within the first week after surgery. Duration of these murmurs (calculated as percentage of total diastole) was not related to the degree of valve incompetence, measured in terms of regurgitant fraction by videodensitometry (Fig. 2). The amplitudes of diastolic decrescendo murmurs (relative to the initial component of the second heart sound) were also independent of the degree of regurgitation (Fig. 2).

M-mode echocardiography revealed normal pattern of pulmonary allograft valve motion in 8/15 patients (53%) and in 7/8 patients (88%) with allografts in the aortic position. In contrast to severe valvular stenosis, which be may be detected by echocardiography, a reliable quantitative evaluation of incompetent valves could not be established by ultrasonic techniques. Therefore, we tried to gain information about the degree of valvular insufficiency by comparison of echocardiographic patterns of valve motion and regurgitant fraction measured by videodensitometry. In this respect, there seems to be a difference between allografts in the aortic and pulmonary position (Fig. 3). In the aortic position, normal valve motion does not exclude a

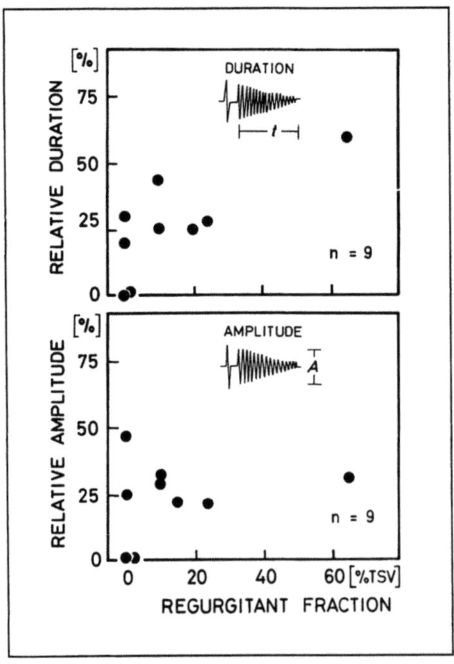

Fig. 2. Diastolic murmurs and valve incompetence after allograft transplantation in pulmonary position. Neither duration (% of total diastole, upper panel) nor maximal amplitude of the murmur (% of II_A, lower panel) correlate with the degree of pulmonary insufficiency in terms of regurgitant fraction.

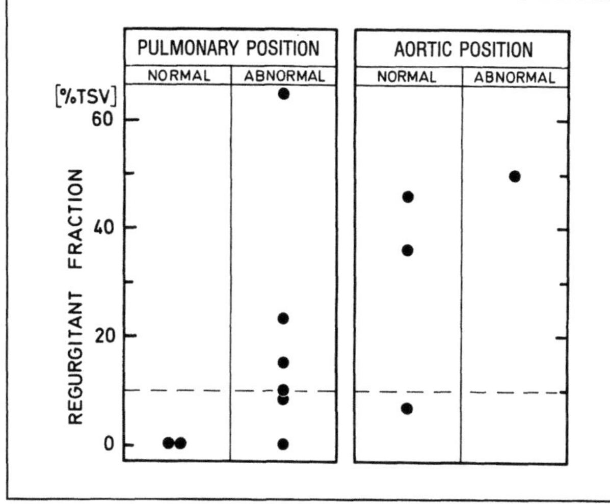

Fig. 3. Echocardiographic pattern of valve motion (M-mode) and degree of valvular insufficiency in terms of regurgitant fraction (RGF) evaluated at allografts in pulmonary and aortic position. Broken horizontal line indicates RFG = 10%, up to which valvular incompetence is regarded as trivial. Pattern of valve motion is not a reliable diagnostic criterion for the degree of allograft insufficiency.

significant valvular incompetence. But in the pulmonary position, normal valve motion only appeared in competent allografts. On the other hand, abnormal valve motion is not necessarily suggestive of significant insufficiency but may also be found in trivial regurgitation or even in valves with RGF = 0 (Fig. 3).

Due to the surgical technique used ("inlay technique", see contribution of Lange et al.) the original diameters of aortic and pulmonary valves may be altered by allografts. In cases of aortic insufficiency, valve diameters were increased preoperatively. After insertion of the allograft, these diameters were reduced to almost normal values (Fig. 4). Diameters of stenotic pulmonary valves were measured to be in the lower normal range or subnormal (Fig. 5). After transplantation, the diameters of all three stenotic valves increased and two of them were in the normal range

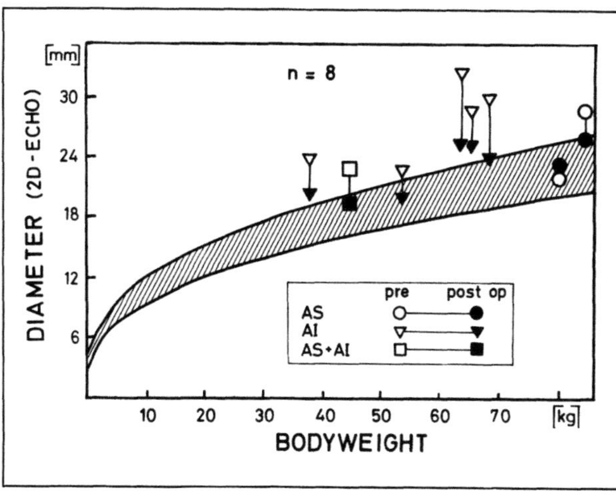

Fig. 4. Diameter of original preoperative valve and allograft valve after transplantation in aortic position, as measured by 2D-echocardiography. Eight patients had different valve diseases: AS, aortic stenosis; AI, aortic insufficiency; AS/AI, combined lesion. Normal range shaded.

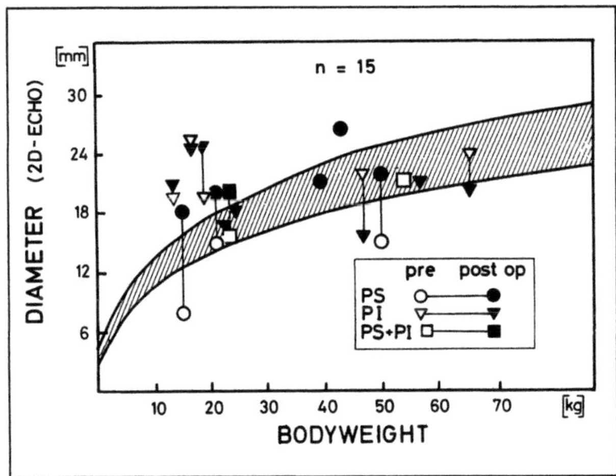

Fig. 5. Diameter of original pre-operative valve and allograft valve after transplantation in pulmonary position, as measured by 2D-echocardiography. 15 patients with different valve diseases: PS, pulmonary stenosis, PI, pulmonary insufficiency, PS/PI: combined lesion, Normal range shaded.

postoperatively. In children weighting less than 20 kg who received allografts because of pulmonary insufficiency, valve diameters were too large pre- as well as post-transplantation (Fig. 5). In contrast, post-transplantation diameters were usually normal in patients weighting more than 40 kg. This is true for the aortic and pulmonary position, irrespective of the indication for valve replacement (stenosis or incompetence) and is caused by the size of the allografts used. Their diameter averaged 21.4 ± 3.2 mm which equals the normal aortic valve diameter of a person weighing 65 kg. Moreover, there seems to be some evidence that the allograft valve function may depend on its proper size. Inappropriately large allografts, i.e. of diameter above the normal 2s-range seem to coincide with significant regurgitation (Fig. 6). If allograft diameters were within the mean range ± 2s, regurgitation did not exceed RGF = 15 % in six cases. Five out of six cases had only trivial or even no regurgitation with RGF < 10%.

As shown above, allograft transplantation leads to a change in valve diameter. Serial follow-up measurements of this parameter from 2D-echocardiograms revealed that the diameter achieved early after transplantation (i.e. less than 1 months) did not change significantly during the postoperative course, up to 4.3 years. This is true for allografts in the pulmonary (Fig. 7) and aortic position.

Discussion

Since allograft transplantation for heart valve replacement was introduced by Ross et al. in 1962 (8) this technique has become widely used for both aortic valve replacement and reconstruction of the right ventricular outflow tract in all age groups (1, 4, 5, 6, 10). Investigation of the haemodynamic profile of transplanted allografts is usually done by heart catheterization. Especially for follow-up in the paediatric age group, the reliability of non-invasive techniques for evaluation of allografts' haemodynamics seems worth knowing.

306

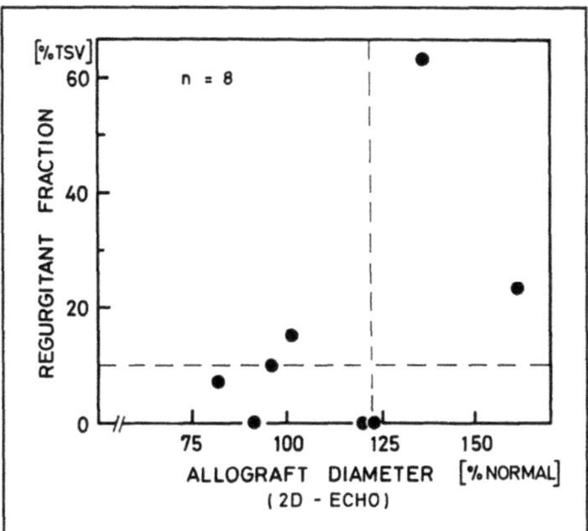

Fig. 6. Comparison of allograft diameter (% of normal) measured by 2D-echocardiography and regurgitant fraction (% TSV) as determined by videodensitometry in eight children who received allografts in the pulmonary position. Broken horizontal line indicates RGF = 10%; vertical broken line gives the values of mean + 2 s (i.e. 124% of normal). If allograft diameters exceed this value, significant insufficiency seems more likely than below this value.

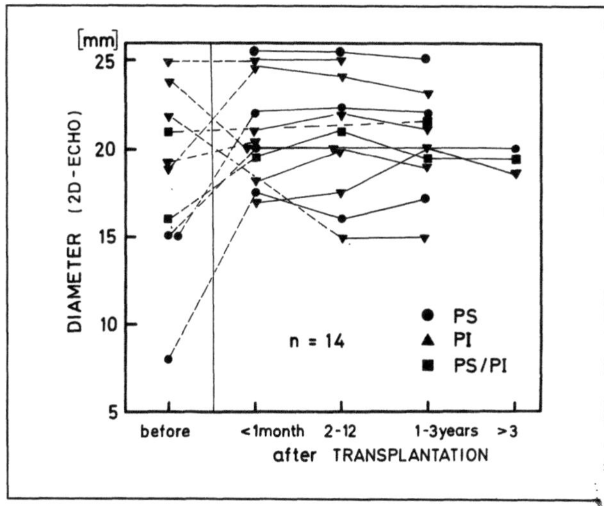

Fig. 7. Serial follow-up of valve diameters by 2D-echocardiography from 14 patients with allografts in pulmonary position. Preoperative data are to the left of the vertical line; (---) lines indicate the change achieved by transplantation. Symbols for valve lesions and abbreviations as in Fig. 5. Diameters achieved by transplantation show no significant change during this follow-up period.

From aortic valve replacement in adults, it is known that calcific degeneration of allografts may occur (1, 5). Usually, calcification of an allograft is limited to the remaining aortic wall, thus causing a typical egg-shell fashion in the chest X-ray, which was also found in two of our patients with allografts in the pulmonary position (Fig. 1). From our limited experience, it seems evident that in the pulmonary position, calcification of an allograft is better recognized by chest X-ray than by 2D-echocardiography. But for recognizing the severely calcified allograft in the aortic position, we found 2D-echocardiography more helpful than chest film. In this special case, the allograft was invisible within the silhouette of the heart. The finding that both wall and leaflets are calcified, thus causing severe valve dysfunction, is uncommon and may be related to antibiotic preservation of the allograft (1). In the large series by Barratt-Boyes et al. (1), allograft calcification is reported to be unusual in adults and in the series by Penta et al. (5) this occurred in 6/140 patients between

4 and 11 years after surgery. Unfortunately, larger series about allograft transplantation in children are not available for comparison.

The surgical "inlay technique" in allograft transplantation might cause a slight narrowing of the artery. Thus, it is not surprising that a — usually small — pressure gradient and systolic murmur result. This murmur may be regarded as a normal finding after allograft transplantation, irrespective of the position. On the other hand, diastolic murmurs should be absent if an aortic or pulmonary valve substitute is completely competent. But in the majority of our children, auscultation revealed diastolic murmurs (pulmonic position: 69%; aortic position: 75%), which all appeared early after surgery. Thus, the question arises of whether allografts are competent valve substitutes and to what extent a diastolic murmur is a reliable criterion for the degree of pulmonary insufficiency. In those cases in which pulmonary insufficiency was quantified by videodensitometry, it becomes possible to compare diastolic murmurs with the amount of allograft incompetence in terms of regurgitant fraction. But neither duration nor amplitude of these murmurs correlated with the degree of regurgitation. The fact that the degree of regurgitation in pulmonic insufficiency cannot be assessed from the diastolic murmur was also described by us after patch reconstruction of the right ventricular outflow tract in tetralogy of Fallot (3). That emphasizes the need for videodensitometric investigation in cases with pulmonary insufficiency. This is in contrast to aortic insufficiency where blood pressure and diastolic murmur may allow rough grading of the severity of aortic incompetence.

In transplanting allografts in children, problems may arise if the allograft size differs from that of the valve to be replaced. In this respect, two factors may be considered. The first concerns the normal difference in size of pulmonary and aortic valves. Our echocardiographic measurements from healthy children reveal that diameters of both valves grow identically with respect to body weight (power of the functions depicted above). But pulmonary valve diameters are about 17% larger than those of aortic valves, which is confirmed by necropsy measurements (9). Although this normal difference favours the "inlay technique" for allograft replacement of pulmonary valves, these differences seem to be of minor importance because of the fact that donors are usually adults (mean age: 24 years, in our group). This leads to the consequence that aortic allografts serving as pulmonary valve substitutes are often oversized with respect to the recipient's body weight. This becomes evident from Fig. 5, where one can see that in patients with a body weight above 40 kg, allograft diameters usually lie within, or close to, the normal range. But if the recipient's body weight is below 30 kg, only two out of eight diameters are normal. These diameters, achieved after transplantation, did not increase or shrink during the follow-up period (Fig. 7).

In this context, the question arises of whether appropriate allograft size contributes to proper valve function. Although our experience is limited, there seems to be evidence that allografts with diameters exceeding 124% normal (i.e. greater than mean + 2 s) carry an increased risk of significant regurgitation (Fig. 6). It might be speculated that in such cases, an oversized allograft is compressed within the thoracic cavity, thus disturbing the integrity of the valve geometry and causing incompetence. This is of major concern in children weighting less than 30 kg who have smaller thoracic cavities and whose normal valve diameter remains less than 20 mm, despite rapid growth. As the slope of the curves for normal valve diameters are flattened above 40 kg body weight, allografts from adults fit better in this group. This could mean, as a consequence, that for children up to 30 kg in weight (approximately 12 years of age) a smaller allograft than usual should be chosen, whereas for adolescents, normal adult allografts are suitable.

Conclusion

Non-invasive investigation alone does not allow reliable assessment of allograft function in children. Complementary invasive evaluation is necessary because diastolic murmurs and/or echocardiographic patterns of valve motion are of limited diagnostic value, especially with respect to pulmonary insufficiency.
However, one can state that significant pulmonary insufficiency seems to be unlikely if echocardiography reveals normal valve motion *and* normal diameter of the the allograft. Such findings may be due to an intact geometry of the valve and they emphasize the necessity of transplanting allografts of appropriate size in children.

References

1. Barratt-Boyes BG, Roche AHG, Subramanyan R, Pemberton JR, Whitlock RML (1986) Long-term follow-up of patients with the antibiotic-sterilized aortic homograft valve inserted freehand in the aortic position. Circulation 75: 768—777
2. Bürsch JH, Heintzen PH, Simon R (1974) Videodensitometric studies by a new method of quantitating the amount of contrast medium. Eur J Cardiol 1: 437—446
3. Bürsch JH, Lange P, Hüttig G, Johs R, Heintzen PH (1978) Videodensitometric quantitation of pulmonary insufficiency in operated Tetralogies of Fallot. In: Heintzen PH, Bürsch JH (eds) Roentgen-video-techniques for dynamic studies of structure and function of the heart and circulation. Thieme, Stuttgart, pp 74—79
4. Di Carlo D, Stark J, Revignas A, de Laval MR (1982) Conduits containing antibiotic preserved homograts in the treatment of complex congenital heart defects. In: Cohn LH, Gallucci V (eds) Cardiac bioprostheses. Yorke Medical Books, New York, pp 259—265
5. Penta A, Qureshi S, Radley-Smith R, Yacoub MH (1984) Patient status 10 or more years after "fresh" homograft replacement of the aortic valve. Circulation 70, Suppl I: I—182 — I-192
6. Radley-Smith R, Yacoub MH (1986) Aortic homograft replacement in children — a 15 year experience. In: Bodnar E, Yacoub MH (eds) Biological and bioprosthetic valves. Yorke Medical Books, New York, pp 299—304
7. Rimoldi HJA, Lev M (1963) A note on the concept of normality and abnormality in quantitation of pathologic findings in congenital heart disease. Pediatr Clin North Am 10: 589—591
8. Ross DN (1962) Homograft replacement of the aortic valve. Lancet 2: 487
9. Rowlatt UF, Rimoldi HJA, Lev M (1963) The quantitative anatomy of the normal child's heart. Pediatr Clin North Am 10: 499—588
10. Wessel A, Lange PE, Bürsch JH, Yankah AC, Sievers HH, Bernhard A, Heintzen PH (in press) Frühergebnisse nach Transplantation homologer Taschenklappen bei Kindern. In: Nars PW (ed) Pädiatrische Intensivmedizin IX. Thieme, Stuttgart
11. Yankah AC, Hetzer R (1987) Derzeitige und zukünftige Trends bei der Transplantation allogener Herzklappen. Z Herz-, Thorax-, Gefäßchir 1: 12—19

Authors' address:
Armin Wessel, M.D.
Department of Paediatric Cardiology
Schwanenweg 20
D-2300 Kiel 1
F.R.G.

Cryopreserved viable allograft aortic valves

M. F. O'Brien, E. G. Stafford, M. A. H. Gardner, P. Pohlner,
D. C. McGiffin, N. Johnston, P. Tesar, A. Brosnan, P. Duffy

The Prince Charles Hospital, Brisbane, Australia

Introduction

The clinical experience of allograft aortic valve replacement (AVR) began at the Prince Charles Hospital in 1969. From the commencement of this experience until May 1975, the method of valve sterilisation was antibiotic exposure, and the valves were stored in nutrient medium at 4 °C for periods up to several weeks before implantation. There is considerable evidence from this and other clinical experience (1, 6, 15, 16), as well as from experimental evidence (9, 10), that this process produces a non-viable valve, incapable of self-repair. Its clinical performance is characterised by an unacceptable incidence of late cusp rupture, reflecting leaflet degeneration (5). At the same time, experimental work was progressing at the Prince Charles Hospital (17), as well as at other centres (2, 8, 11, 12) in an endeavour to develop a method of storing valves indefinitely with maintenance of leaflet cell viability. This direction was taken as a result of work by Angell (3, 12) indicating the importance of leaflet viability as a determinant of long-term valve durability.
At the Prince Charles Hospital the use of antibiotic sterilised 4 °C refrigerated valves was discontinued in June 1975, and an era of cryopreservation of allograft aortic valves commenced. A description of the cryopreservation methods have been detailed elsewhere (14, 15), but in essence it involves "sterile" procurement, low-dose antibiotic exposure for 24 h and cryopreservation in the vapour phase of liquid nitrogen (approx. − 180 °C to − 190 °C) with the valve packaged and immersed in the cryoprotectant 10% dimethyl sulphoxide. At the time of thawing of the valve, viable leaflet cells can be demonstrated by resumption of metabolic processes and by tissue culture (15, 17). Van der Kamp (7) has confirmed the presence of post cryopreservation fibroblast viability and the absence of any damaging effect on the microscopic structure of the valve as well as the ultrastructural pattern of the collagen fibrils. In addition, he showed that the stress-strain characteristics and aortic wall elasticity remain unaffected by the cryopreservation.
A previous report (16) from this institution compared the long-term clinical results of an era of valve storage by refrigeration at 4 °C (1969—1975) and a more recent era of cryopreservation (1975—1987). Superior durability of the cryopreserved allograft aortic valve was demonstrated, reflecting the absence of leaflet degeneration necessitating reoperation.
The purpose of this paper is not only to update this experience, but also to present evidence that viability may not necessarily be perfectly maintained with cryopreservation and subsequent leaflet degeneration may occur.

311

Allograft valve failure

Allograft valve failure which requires reoperation may be due to leaflet degeneration, allograft valve endocarditis, paravalvar leak and technical malalignment of the valve pillars. It is the development of aortic incompetence due to leaflet degeneration which is of crucial additional importance to the analysis of the long-term performance of allograft aortic valves. Only by careful documentation of the evidence for leaflet degeneration, including examination of operative and autopsy allograft valve leaflet tissue, can inferences be made regarding leaflet viability and leaflet degeneration. Refinements can then be made to improve collection and storage techniques in order to enhance valve durability.

There are three ways in which leaflet degeneration may be noted:

a. Development of new aortic valve incompetence

In the absence of endocarditis, the development of this finding as a late event during the follow-up is highly likely to be the result of leaflet degeneration. The degree of aortic incompetence may not be of such severity to require reoperation at that time. On the other hand, allograft valve incompetence of more than a mild degree, present soon after the operation, usually progresses requiring reoperation in 1 to 2 years and is due to technical insertion problems.

b. Reoperation for leaflet perforation or rupture

In the absence of endocarditis or technical insertion problems, reoperation for aortic incompetence is invariably due to leaflet degeneration, seen macroscopically as either perforation or rupture. It is this event which is used to reflect allograft valve failure as a result of leaflet degeneration in virtually all analyses.

c. Histological assessment of leaflet tissue

In our experience, leaflet degeneration is regarded as being present if valve tissue at autopsy or at reoperation is very thinned with the likelihood of subsequent perforation, and if histological examination confirms acellularity and degenerative changes in the leaflet. Recognition of degeneration both macroscopically and histologically before a clinical event of valve failure has taken place assists both in the understanding and forecasting of structural changes that are likely to become clinically apparent.

Inclusion of all these three modes of valve failure in the analysis of long-term results of allograft aortic valves should attest to the veracity with which evidence of degeneration is being sought.

Comparison of 4 °C refrigerated valves and viable cryopreserved valves
Follow-up and survival

Between 16th December 1969 and 31st August 1987, 337 allograft aortic valve replacements were performed at the Prince Charles Hospital. There were 124 antibiotic 4 °C-refrigerated allografts inserted from December 1969 to May 1975 (Series I) and 213 viable cryopreserved valves from June 1975 to August 1987 (Series II). The follow-up data is complete and in this analysis the closing date for inclusion of events was the 31st August 1987.

The patient characteristics are outlined in Table I. Concomitant procedures were carried out in 36 (29%) of the 124 Series I patients and in 84 (39%) of the 213 Series II patients, coronary bypass grafting and mitral valve replacement being the commonest procedures in both groups (Table 2).

The Series I, median follow-up was 13.7 years (range 12.3—17.7 years). The Series II median follow-up was 4.3 years (range 4 days to 12.3 years).

The actuarial patient survival (Fig. 1) was similar for both groups, being 82%, 67% and 57% at 5, 10 and 15 years for Series I and 86% and 73% at 5 and 10 years for Series II.

Ten patients in Series I died in hospital or within 30 days, a mortality of 8.9% (C.L. 70%, 6.2%—12.3%), and in Series II, 9 patients died in hospital or within 30 days, a mortality of 4.2% (C.L. 70%, 2.8%—6.2%).

There was no difference in the incidence of late death in those patients having an isolated AVR and patients having AVR with an associated procedure. The commonest cause of death in both series was cardiac failure and cancer. Six of the 14

Table 1. Patient characteristics: Age at operation.

	Series I n = 124	Series II n = 213
Male	83 (67%)	108 (51%)
Female	41 (33%)	105 (49%)
Median age	50.5 years	58 years
Age range	13—72 years	3—80 years

Table 2. Concomitant procedures.

	Series I	Series II
CABG	2	35 (2)
MVR ± CABG ± TV surg	20 (1)	25 (1)
MV repair	6	6
Left ventricular myotomy	5	1 (1)
Ascending aortic root replacement	—	14
Miscellaneous	3	3 (1)
	36 (1)	84 (5)

CABG = Coronary artery bypass grafts; MVR = mitral valve replacement; MV = mitral valve; TV = tricuspid valve. Hospital deaths in parentheses.

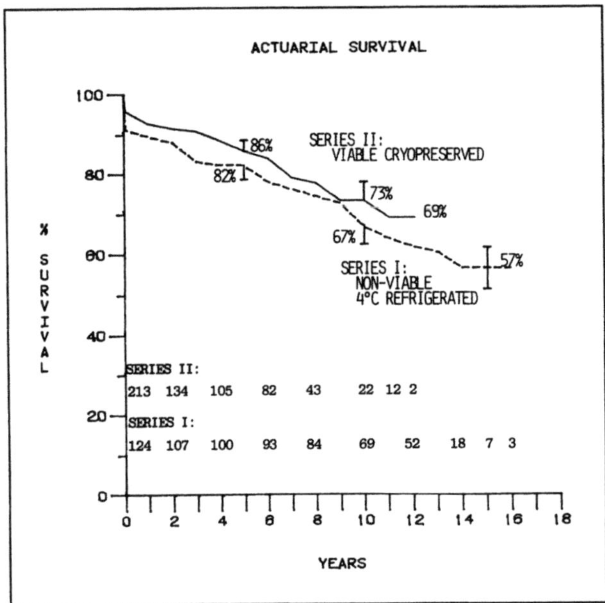

Fig. 1. Actuarial survival after allograft AVR for Series I (124 patients, 47 deaths) and Series II (213 patients, 34 deaths). The horizontal axis represents the years after operation and the vertical axis the percent survival. The numbers along the horizontal are the patients at risk at each interval. The standard error is recorded at the 5th, 10th and 15th year.

patients of Series I who died of cardiac failure had severe aortic incompetence and did not undergo reoperation for various reasons. No patient in Series II died late of any cause with moderate or severe aortic incompetence in the absence of endocarditis.

Endocarditis

Allograft valve endocarditis (AVE) occurred in 14 patients, nine in Series I and five in Series II, there being no difference in the occurrence of this event between the two series (p = 0.6). In a previous report (16) concerning these patients, the actuarial freedom from endocarditis (Series I and II combined was 92% at 10 years and 89% at 15 years.
Eight of the 14 patients had reoperation for AVR with one death from multi-organ failure. Six were treated non-surgically, of whom four patients died.

Thromboembolism

A previous report (16) of this series has shown thromboembolism to be a very uncommon event. The actuarial freedom from thromboembolism was 97% at 10 years and 96% at 15 years.

Moderate and severe incompetence

Excluding patients with allograft valve endocarditis there were 39 of the 124 patients in Series I and 12 of the 213 patients in Series II with moderate to severe allograft

314

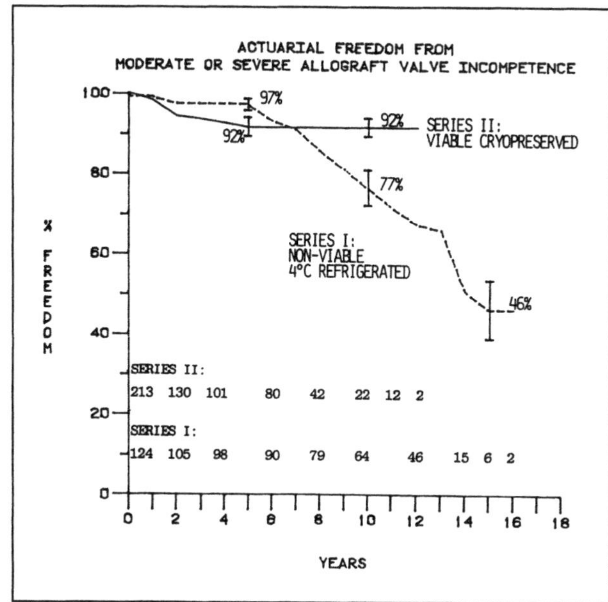

Fig. 2. Actuarial freedom from moderate or severe allograft valve incompetence in Series I (39 events) and II (13 events). (Depiction as in Fig. 1).

aortic valve incompetence. Reoperation was undertaken in 25 and five patients respectively in the two series. The actuarial freedom from moderate or severe allograft valve incompetence at 10 years was 92% (Series II) and 77% (Series I) (Fig. 2). In Series II seven patients had aortic valve incompetence that was present early after operation (within one month) and was presumed to be technical in origin. The degree of incompetence has been slowly increasing but reoperation has not yet been required.

The difference between the two curves continues to widen, and reflects firstly an increasing incidence of leaflet degeneration in the Series I patients, and secondly the fact that no patient in Series II developed moderate or severe allograft valve incompetence beyond 5 years.

Reoperation

Reoperation was performed for intrinsic leaflet degeneration, allograft valve endocarditis and valve incompetence due to technical factors, usually pillar malalignment at the time of surgical insertion. Allograft valve incompetence requiring reoperation is invariably due to technical factors when moderate incompetence appears early after operation and progresses in the absence of leaflet degeneration.

In Series I, 27 patients underwent reoperation for degeneration, four for endocarditis and two for technical factors. In Series II, the aortic allograft valve was replaced for degeneration in two patients, for endocarditis in four patients and for technical factors in six patients (Table 3). The two patients in Series II who underwent reoperation for degeneration, both had mitral valve bioprostheses inserted at the orig-

Table 3. Reoperation for allograft AVR removal.

Indication	Series I Antibiotic 4 °C Refrigerated			Series II Viable Cryopreserved		
	N	% of 124	70% C.L.	N	% of 213	70% C.L.
Degeneration	27	21.8%	17.8%—26.3%	2	0.9%	0.3%—2.2%
Endocarditis	4	3.0%	1.6%— 5.8%	4	1.8%	0.9%—3.4%
Technical	2	1.6%	0.5%— 3.8%	6	2.8%	1.7%—4.5%
	33			12		

inal operation. The indication for reoperation was bioprosthetic valve degeneration with severe mitral regurgitation, although one patient had mild and the other moderate allograft aortic valve incompetence. At reoperation, (one at 5 years, the other at 10.8 years) the allograft valve leaflets were excessively thinned in one patient and a small perforation was present in the other, and replacement of the valves was felt to be advisable.

The actuarial freedom from reoperation in Series I at 10 and 15 years was 83% and 55% respectively, while for Series II, at 10 years it was 88% (Fig. 3). Of critical importance to the analysis of the long-term performance of the allograft aortic valve is the incidence of reoperation for leaflet degeneration. The actuarial freedom from reoperation for degeneration at 10 years was 89% (Series I) and 99% (Series II). At 12 years, actuarial freedom from the event was 79% (Series I) and 93% (Series II),

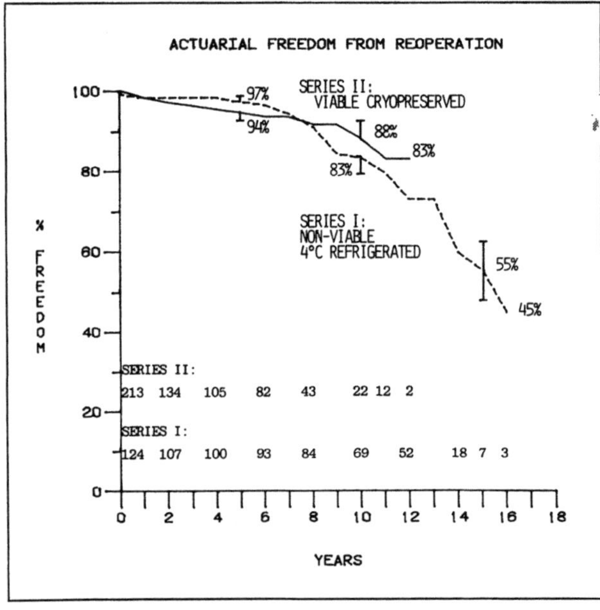

Fig. 3. Actuarial freedom from reoperation (due to leaflet degeneration, endocarditis and technical factors) in Series I (33 events) and Series II (12 events). (Depiction as in Fig. 1.)

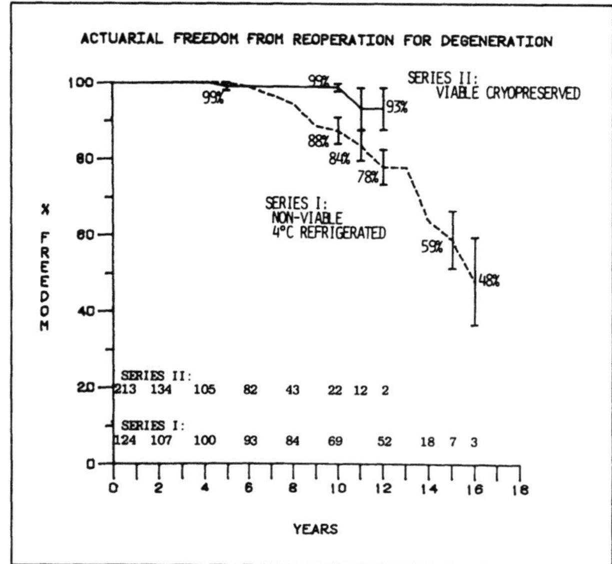

Fig. 4. Actuarial freedom from reoperation for intrinsic degeneration of the allograft valve in patients from Series I (26 events) and Series II (2 events). (Depiction as in Fig. 1.)

and at 15 years in Series I, 60% (Fig. 4). The two previously mentioned reoperations for mitral bioprosthetic degeneration at which time allograft aortic valves were replaced are included as events, although aortic incompetence was not the indication for reoperation. The reoperation at 10.8 years does make a significant impact on the actuarial curve because of the smaller numbers of patients at that point in time.

Histological studies

Examination of allograft valve leaflet tissue obtained at autopsy or reoperation is important to confirm viability and the integrity of the stroma, as well as to detect evidence of leaflet degeneration which may be neither clinically apparent nor clinically important.

Histological assessment of the histological fate of the allograft aortic valve at the Prince Charles Hospital has been reported elsewhere (15, 16) and shows the marked differences between the non-viable and viable preserved valves of Series I and II. The uniform picture of acellularity and loss of morphology of the matrix characterizes the Series I allograft valves. The preservation of cellular viability and of stroma (elastin and collagen fibrils) has been the pattern in leaflets obtained at 2 months, 10 months, 20 months, and 9.2 years following implantation in the Series II allograft valves (16). In the valve removed at 9.2 years chromosomal studies of the male donor and female host verified the presence of donor cells in the viable allograft.

Three allograft valves from the cryopreserved group have shown degeneration. The two previously mentioned patients who underwent reoperation for mitral bioprosthesis degeneration had replacement of the allograft aortic valve because of evidence

317

of degeneration. Histologically, the allograft aortic valve leaflet tissue was acellular, and cells could not be tissue cultured from the leaflets.

The third example was seen in a patient with a competent allograft aortic valve who died of carcinoma of the breast, 8.3 years after operation. This allograft was also non-viable on tissue culture studies and on histological examination (Fig. 5A). There was a marked difference between the appearance of this non-viable valve and the viability of the valve examined at 9.3 years (Fig. 5B).

Results of cryopreserved allograft valve replacement with patient follow-up of 10 years or more

Because the median follow-up time for the viable cryopreserved allograft group is only 4.3 years, examination of the fate of the 34 patients who had cryopreserved valves from June 1975 to August 1977 (minimum follow-up of 10 years) is of importance.

There were four early hospital deaths due to myocardial infarction (two patients), intra-operative haemorrhage from an associated left ventricular myotomy (one patient) and cerebral haemorrhage (one patient).

There were seven late deaths (mean survival 7.6 years) due to cardiac failure (three patients), malignancy (one patient) arrhythmia (one patient), endocarditis (one patient) and pulmonary infection and cardiac failure (one patient). Except for the patient with endocarditis, no patient had moderate or severe aortic valve incompetence at the time of death.

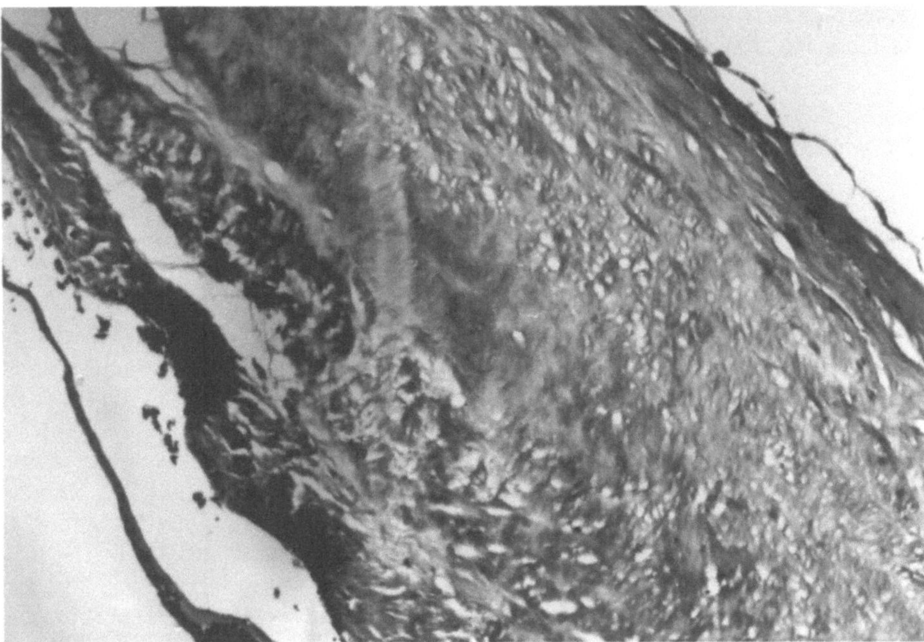

Fig. 5A.

318

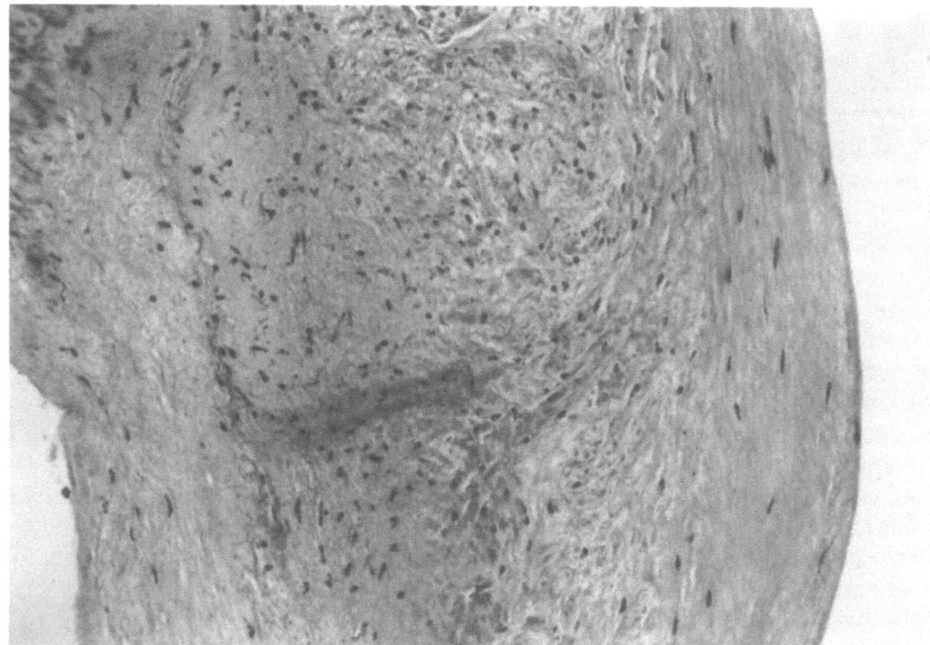

Fig. 5B.

Fig. 5A. Allograft, removed for progressive, incompetence 9.3 years after operation. The cusp shows persistent endothelium in most areas. The elastic layers are well preserved. The collagenous areas also are mostly well preserved, but, in the fibrosa, and, to some extent in the spongiosa, there are areas of immature collagenous tissue. Within the cusp, cells are mostly scattered uniformly. Some cells have round nuclei and lie in small clear spaces but show no evidence of phagocytic activity. Others have elongated nuclei and closely resemble fibroblasts or mature fibrocytes. There are also other plump cells associated with the immature collagenous tissue and strongly resemble active fibroblasts. There are relatively few obvious macrophages present. ($\times$ 100, H & E)
B. Allograft removed at autopsy (cancer death): operation 8 years previously. Endothelium is still present, but on both surfaces cells are lifting away. This shows particularly on the aortic aspect where there is evidence of haemorrhage and fibrin deposition. Elastic layers are present but are moderately disrupted. Mature collagen tissue is present but is disrupted and virtually acellular. The spongiosa shows an amorphous almost completely acellular appearance. Overall, there are only occasional cell nuclei visible, a few in the fibrosa and a few in the junctional area between elastic region and spongiosa. ($\times$ 100, H & E)

21 of the 34 patients are alive and have their original allograft valve as on 31st August 1987. No patient has moderate or severe incompetence. Two patients have undergone successful reoperation at 10 months because of technical malalignment of the valve, and at 10.8 years during mitral valve replacement of a second xenograft, as previously outlined.

Comments

This paper updates previous reports (15, 16) of the allograft valve experience at the Prince Charles Hospital, presents an argument for including other markers of leaflet degeneration (allograft valve incompetence and histology of leaflet tissue) and shows the performance of cryopreserved allograft valves with the follow-up greater than 10 years.

While the patient survival actuarially is similar in the two series and parallels an age and sex-matched normal population (15), there is an obvious difference in durability between the antibiotic sterilised 4 °C-refrigerated aortic allograft valve and the viable cryopreserved aortic allograft valve. This difference is apparent whenever the incidence of intrinsic valve leaflet degeneration is analysed. The superior durability of the cryopreserved allograft aortic valve is highlighted by comparisons between Series I and II patients for incidence of allograft valve incompetence, reoperation for degeneration, and histological evidence of loss of viability and degeneration. Analysis of Series II patients with 10 or more years of follow-up supports this contention of superior durability.

The potential reoperation rate of the Series I non-viable allografts is underestimated because several late deaths were due to severe allograft valve incompetence in patients who did not undergo reoperation. This difference would be greater if the two "non-clinical" degeneration events in Series II had not been included.

Nevertheless, there is some evidence of tissue degeneration verified by histological examination of the viable cryopreserved allografts. The protocol of collection, sterilisation, cryopreservation and thawing has not been changed since its inception 12 years ago. However, despite this, leaflet viability can vary considerably. The allograft aortic valve from an organ donor has superior metabolic glucose utilisation and tissue culture results compared to the autopsy-derived allograft retrieved within 24 h of donor death. To improve viability, refinements of the protocol may need to include firstly, changes in collection (obtaining more valves from organ donors, or harvesting sooner, i.e. within 12 h after death, from the autopsied donor), secondly, reducing the exposure time to antibiotics and varying the antibiotic concentration and constituents according to the "sterile" or "clean" harvesting and thirdly, cryopreserving within 12—18 h after donor death. Use of potentially less viable valves for older recipients, and very viable valves for younger patients may be preferable. This clinical experience has demonstrated that patients receiving viable cryopreserved allografts can expect, in most instances satisfactory valve performance well into the second decade of follow-up. The understanding of the need for viability to confer durability has been an important milestone and further work to enhance viability appears to be an important direction.

References

1. Al-Janabi N, Gonzalez-Lavin L, Neirotti R, Ross DN (1972) Viability of fresh aortic valve homografts: A quantitative assessment. Thorax 27: 83—86
2. Angell JD, Christopher Bs, Hawtrey O, Angell WM (1976) A fresh viable human heart valve bank: Sterilization, sterility testing and cryogenic preservation. Transplant Proc 8 (2 Suppl I): 139—147
3. Angell WW (1969) Personal communication
4. Angell WW, Angell JD, Oury JH, Lamberti JJ, Grehl TD (1987) Long-term follow-up of viable frozen aortic homografts. A viable homograft valve bank. J Thorac Cardiovasc Surg 93 (6): 815—822

5. Barratt-Boyes BG, Roche AH, Subramanyan R, Pemberton JR, Whitlock RM (1987) Long-term follow-up of patients with the antibiotic-sterilized aortic homograft valve inserted freehand in the aortic position. Circulation 75 (4): 768—777
6. Bodnar E, Wain WH, Martelli V, Ross DN (1979) Long-term performance of 580 homograft and autograft valves used for aortic replacement. Thorac Cardiovasc Surg 27 (1): 31—38
7. Kamp van der AW, Visser WJ, Dongen van JM, Nauta J, Galjaard H (1981) Preservation of aortic heart valves with maintenance of cell viability. J Surg Res 30 (1): 47—56
8. Kamp van der AW, Nauta J (1979) Fibroblast function and the maintenance of the aortic valve matrix: Cardiovasc Res 13 (3): 167—172
9. Kosek JC, Iben AB, Shumway NE, Angell WW (1969) Morphology of fresh heart valve allografts. Surgery 66 (1): 269—274
10. McGregor CG, Bradley JF, McGee JO and Wheatley DJ (1976) Tissue culture, protein and collagen synthesis in antibiotic sterilized canine heart valves. Cardiovasc Res 10: 389—393
11. Mermet B, Angell WW, Dor V (1971) Viabiliti des homogriffes fraiches sterilisies par les antibiotiques et conservies au grant froid (— 196 °C). Ann Chir Thorac Cardio-Vasc 10: 463—469
12. Mermet B, Buch WS, Angell WW (1970) Viable heart graft: Preservation in the frozen state. Surg Forum 21: 157
13. Mochtar B, Kamp van der AW, Roza-de Jongh EJ, Nauta J (1984) Cell survival in canine aortic valves stored in nutrient medium. Cardiovasc Res 18 (8): 497—501
14. O'Brien MF, McGiffin DC. Aortic and pulmonary allografts in contemporary cardiac surgery. In: Karp R (ed) Advances in Cardiovascular Surgery (in press)
15. O'Brien MF, Stafford G, Gardner M, Pohlner P, McGiffin D, Johnston N, Brosnan A, Duffy P (1987) The viable cryopreserved allograft aortic valve. J Cardiac Surg I (3: Suppl): 153—167
16. O'Brien MF, Stafford EG, Gardner MA, Pohlner PG, McGiffin DC (1987) A comparison of aortic valve replacement with viable cryopreserved and fresh allograft valves with a note on chromosomal studies. J Thorac Cardiovasc Surg 94: 812—823
17. Watts LK, Duffy P, Field RB, Stafford EG, O'Brien MF (1976) Establishment of a viable homograft cardiac valve bank: A rapid method of determining homograft viability. Ann Thorac Surg 21 (3): 230—236

Authors' address:
Mark O'Brien
Cardiac Surgeon-in-Charge
The Prince Charles Hospital
Rode Road
Chermside
Brisbane 4032
Australia

Short-term follow-up of cryopreserved allograft valves and valved conduits from the CryoLife clinical registry

R. T. McNally, A. E. Heacox, and K. G. M. Brockbank

CryoLife Inc., Marietta, Georgia, U.S.A.

Introduction

CryoLife, a laboratory which specializes in the cryopreservation of human tissues for transplant, first started preserving valves in Autumn 1984. The hearts which arrive at CryoLife are currently procured by 144 independent organ and tissue procurement agencies in the United States, Canada and West Germany. This procured tissue is preserved by CryoLife as a service to those agencies or doctors to whom the tissue has been assigned. In order to assure consistent quality control, all agencies follow the guidelines printed in the CryoLife (3) heart valve procurement protocol. The protocol provides information for screening for infectious diseases and diseases of the heart which would render the tissue less than ideal. For instance, when the required serum sample is returned by the procuring group, tests are performed for HIV (AIDS), hepatitis, syphilis and CMV (cytomegalovirus). These internal tests are compared with pretest data which accompanies the organ and are used as a double check to confirm that the possibility of transmission of these diseases is eliminated. The donor form also contains a detailed medical history of the donor, which helps eliminate donors of questionable standards or with a history of cardiac complications. The protocol also contains the precise details for the surgical extraction of the heart so that uniformity amongst participating centres is maintained. Since the donors are uniformly screened and the heart procured in the same manner, it is possible for participating implanting surgeons to exchange or transfer tissue; thus, paediatric centres which desire smaller valved conduit sizes may obtain tissue from centres who specialize in adult surgery and require larger sizes.

During the year 1984, 32 hearts were procured, followed by 383 in 1985, 895 in 1986 and an estimated 1235 for 1987. By September 1987, 2135 hearts had been procured by 144 procurement centres. Figure 1 describes the donor and recipient age distribution: 54% (mean 17 years) were male; 46% (mean 14.8 years) were female. Note that there are considerably more recipients in the under-20-year-olds age group than donors. Although this would lead one to believe that there would be fewer tissues available for this age group, this is not the case in children over the age of 10, since it appears that right ventricular outflow tract reconstructions may be performed utilizing larger sized valves. Donors are rarely accepted past the age of 50 and valves are carefully screened after dissection for evidence of plaque. Any plaque on the leaflets would be reason for discarding tissue. Donors in the 15—25 age group are usually from traumatic accidents resulting in closed head injuries which require that the donor remain on life support systems for a mean of 2.5 days (range 0—18 days), thereby giving adequate time for a thorough screening. Figure 2 summarizes the cause of death from 90 consecutive donor hearts received during the month of February 1987. Note that 34% were closed head injuries (CHI) and

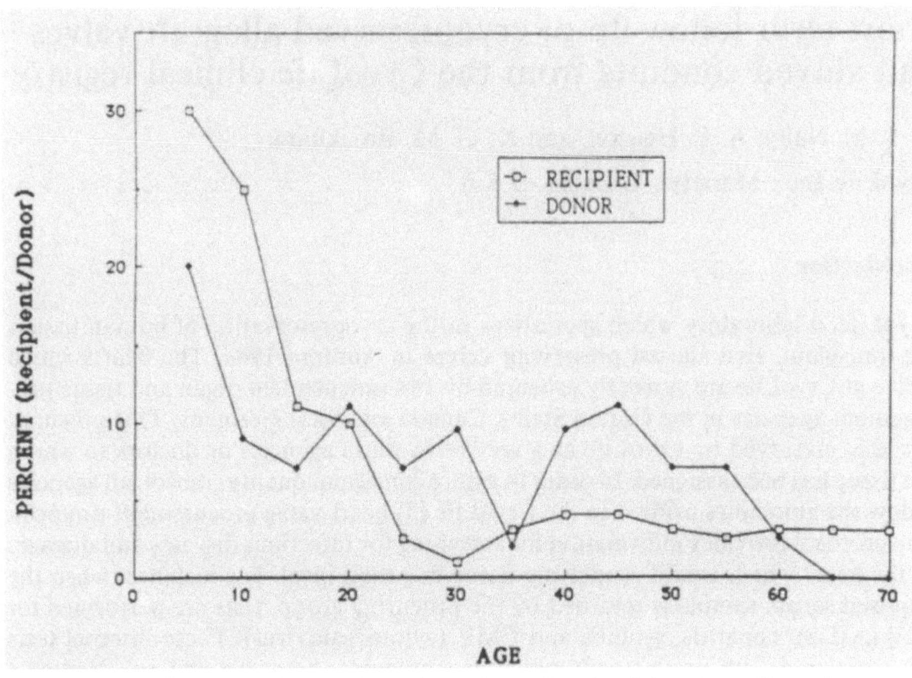

Fig. 1. Percent distribution of valve donor (————◆————) and recipient (————□————) versus age distributions.

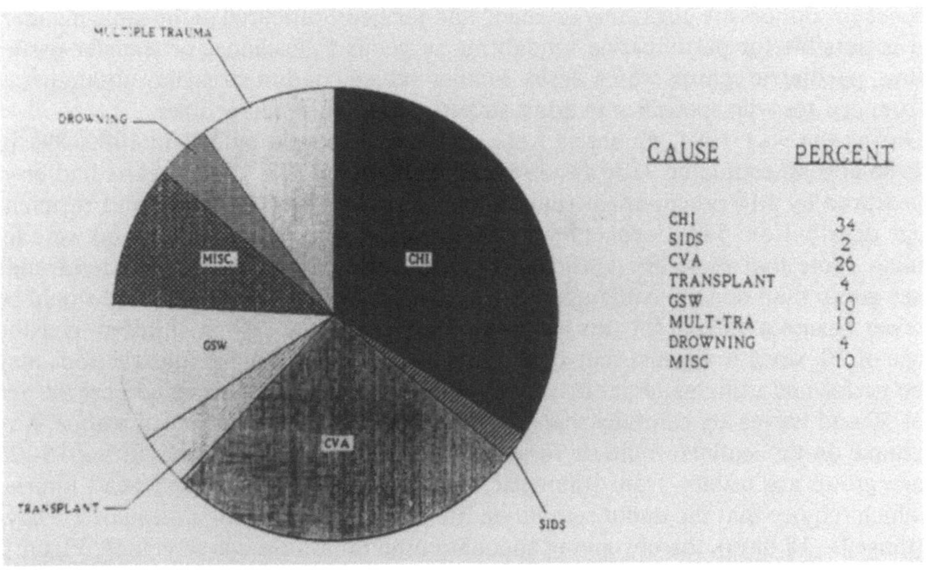

Fig. 2. Cause of death of valve donors: CHI (closed head injury), SIDS (sudden infant death syndrome), CVA (cerebral vascular accident). GSW (gun-shot wound).

324

26% cerebral vascular accidents (CVA). Few, of any, if the donors had trauma which would have allowed systemic infection, and less than 2% of the donor pool are pathology referrals. Pathology referrals may not allow for the appropriate quality control and donor screening, and may result in time delays. Acceptable limits are 8 h warm ischaemia with an upper maximum of 24 h combined warm and cold ischaemia from the time of cessation of heartbeat. Normally, tissue arrives at the preservation laboratory after a mean ischaemia time of 16 h (range 6—24 h). Nearly all the donors are multiple organ donors and 86% were primary kidney donors. Table 1 summarizes the frequency that other organs are procured at the same time as the heart. It should be noted that the heart is not procured for valves unless it cannot be utilised as a whole organ transplant.

Processing and preservation

Upon arrival at CryoLife, the package containing the hearts is inspected in an effort to identify any shipping damage or obvious deviations from the protocol. The container in which the heart is packed is then removed from the shipping box, labelled and numbered for identification and brought into the clean-room environment where it is unpacked. The hearts are dissected under class 100 biological safety cabinets in such a manner which should yield both an aortic and pulmonary valved conduit. In approximately 70% of the cases, it is possible to harvest both valves. Following dissection, the resulting valves and conduits are placed in a nutrient media containing the antibiotics: amphotericin B, lyncomycin, cefoxitin, polymixin and vancomycin, and incubated at 4 °C for 8 to 24 h. It should be noted that incubation periods in excess of 24 h reduce the number of viable fibroblasts (9). This decrease is in the range of 15% for each 24 h period that the tissue remains in antibiotics. For this reason, CryoLife is investigating alternative antibiotic sterilisation techniques which will allow for survival of the endothelial cells and improved maintenance of fibroblast cell viability. Following the antibiotic incubation, the tissue is placed into a tissue culture media and 10% DMSO (dimethyl sulphoxide) solution and frozen at a regulated rate in a microprocessor controlled liquid nitrogen freezer. Although a variety of freezing profiles have been used by others (6), CryoLife has found that the best profile is one that allows for an initial equilibration of tem-

Table 1. Frequency of procurement of other organs from donors of heart valves.

Organ	Frequency (%)
Kidney	86
Liver	31
Eye	14
Pancreas	13
Bone	13
Lung	3
Skin	1

perature at 4 °C, followed by a precise sequence at the heat of fusion point, again followed by an equilibration plateau, and finally a gradual freeze to the point where the tissue is removed and placed into liquid nitrogen for storage.

At several places during the laboratory processing, tissue and fluid samples are taken and evaluated for anaerobic and aerobic bacteria, and fungi. Tissue samples are sent for histological examination and the tissue remains in quarantine and is released for implant only after all results from these tests are satisfactory.

The typical valve sizes dissected from this same data set of 90 consecutive donors are shown in Fig. 3 and 4. The most frequently dissected aortic valve is 22 mm (average 19 mm, range 8—28 mm) whereas the corresponding pulmonary valve size is 26 mm (average 21 mm, range 6—30 mm). The size distribution is consistent with the age of the donors, as depicted in Fig. 1.

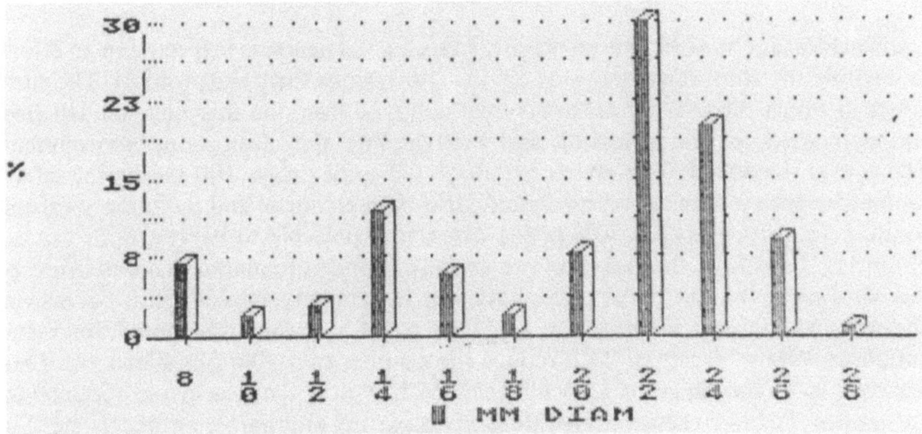

Fig. 3. Aortic valve size distribution (n = 90, average diameter 19 mm).

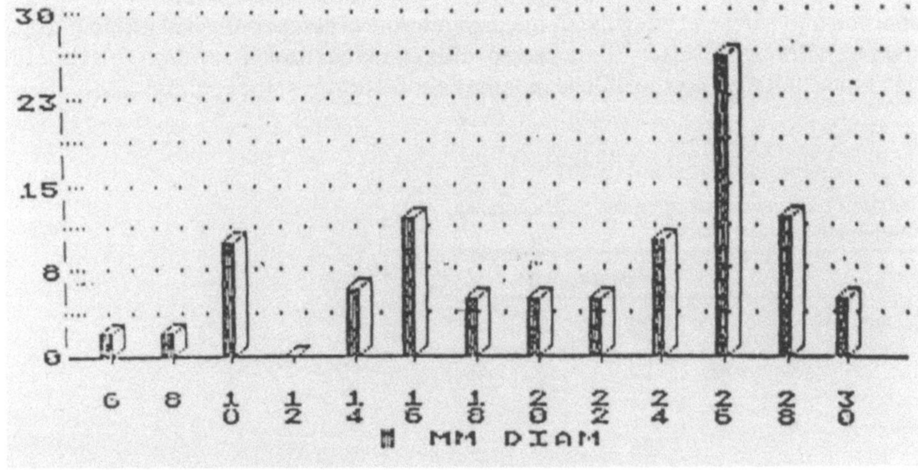

Fig. 4. Pulmonary valve size distribution (n = 90, average diameter 21 mm).

326

Cell viability

The processing technique just described has evolved due to the necessity of maintaining cell viability in order to maximize function and longevity and durability. The majority of studies on heart valve viability have concentrated on fibroblasts, because these cells are responsible for maintenance of the valve matrix (8) and are considered to be a prerequisite for long-term function of transplanted valves (1, 5). A variety of valve fibroblast assays have been utilised in the literature, as indicated in Table 2. We assess valve fibroblast function in specimens of valve tissue by analysis of collagen synthesis, as described by van der Kamp et al. (8, 9). The most effective way to study protein synthesis in tissues is to use isotopic uptake analysis by scintillation counting coupled with autoradiography. This combination of methods permits the determination of whether significant changes are due to changes in protein synthesis per cell or due to cell death. Using this approach, we have found that valves cryopreserved by this laboratory and subsequently thawed are essentially identical to fresh valves in their ability to synthesize collagen. Autoradiography results comparing cryopreserved and fresh valves are shown in Fig. 5. We have been

Table 2. Cell viability assays.

Component tested	Analytical method	Selected references
Fibroblasts	glucose utilization	10
	proliferation in vitro	10
	protein synthesis	8,9
	collagen synthesis	8
Endothelial cells	viability dye test	11
	protein synthesis	9

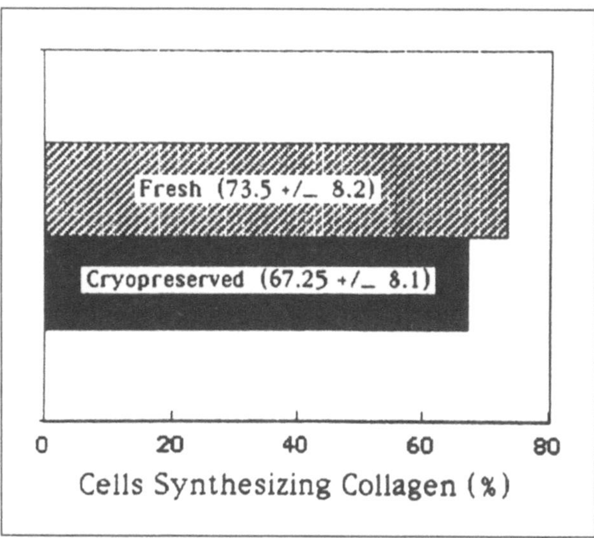

Fig. 5. Comparison of collagen synthesis by cryopreserved fresh valves. The data is presented as the mean ± 1 standard error in percent of total cells counted (n = 4). Pieces of valve were incubated in 3H-Proline for 6 h in 5 ml of F-10 medium containing 10% fetal calf serum. The valves were incubated with cold Proline and fixed in formaldehyde. Paraffin sections (5 μm) were processed for autoradiography using a Kodak emulsion. After 2 weeks of exposure the film was fixed and the sections stained with haematoxylin and eosin.

unable to demonstrate any significant differences in the percentage of cells synthesizing collagen in these two types of valves.

There have been few studies conducted regarding the viability of endothelial cells in cryopreserved heart valves. An independent study by van der Kamp of canine valves demonstrated 40% viable endothelial cells by autoradiographic means, while a study on rats (11) demonstrated approximately 94% viable endothelial cells by an alcian blue dye exclusion method. Our experience has generally corresponded to that of van der Kamp (9).

Occasionally we observe morphologically intact endothelium in cryopreserved heart valves. Indeed, most of the damage is done prior to the preservation process. We are currently developing a technique for the experimental preservation of endothelial cells in addition to the fibroblast component of heart valves. Animal transplantation studies will be required to determine whether the presence of endothelial cells is advantageous for cryopreserved valves, because even though endothelial cells may play a role in fibroblast nutrition, in the prevention of thrombus formation, and in the prevention of calcification, it is possible that the presence of these cells may induce immunological rejection phenomena (2).

Tissue use etiology

In the right heart, the etiology was exclusively congenital. Figure 6 summarizes the five largest classes of congenital abnormalities which were reported. Of particular note, of the right heart reconstructions, 17% were for the replacement of a previous artificial conduit obstruction and 2% were for an obstructed artificial pulmonary valve. As one can see in Fig. 6, 24% were for pulmonary atresia with the next largest category being tetralogy of Fallot. Almost evenly divided are truncus arteriosus

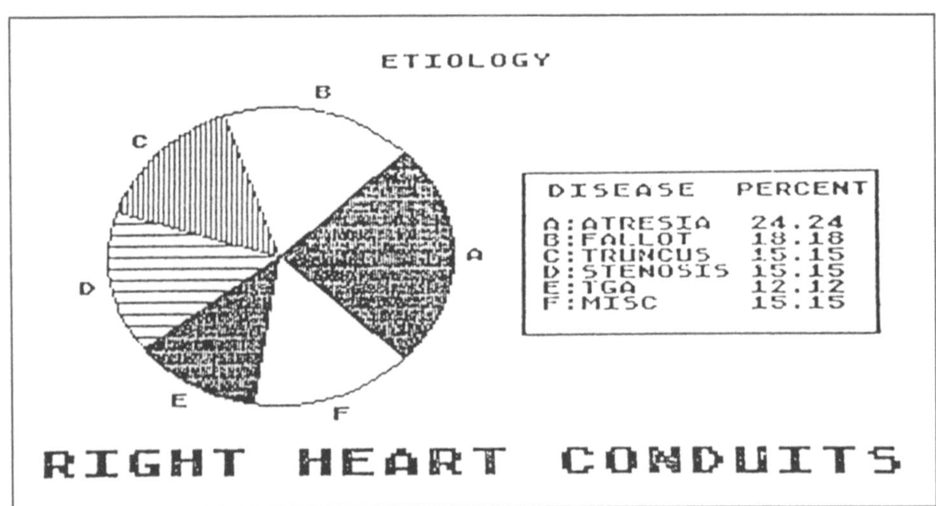

Fig. 6. This figure summarizes the etiologies of diseases affecting the right side of the heart from 114 consecutive clinical implant returns.

(15%), pulmonary stenosis (15%) and transposition of the great arteries (12%). All left heart procedures consisted of diseases of the aortic valve: rheumatic complications which resulted in aortic valve incompetance (19%) combined with degeneration (62%) which gave both calcific aortic stenosis and aortic insufficiency, and endocarditis (19%).

Tissue utilisation

Right heart reconstructions consisted of a variety of procedures which are summarized in Fig. 7. The most common application (76%) was for a valved conduit to be implanted between the right ventricle and the pulmonary artery. Concomitant surgical procedures consisted of closure of VSD, ASD, tricuspid annuloplasty, takedown of the Blalock Taussig shunt and intra-aortic balloon pump.
Left heart utilisation was exclusively for aortic valve and root replacement. Data is not available as yet to report the percentages of the different procedures.
Calculated ratio of cardiac output and gradient (AVA) which equals CO/(square root of gradient) were found to be preoperatively 0.70 and 1.53 for the replacement postoperative homograft. Regurgitation on a scale of 0 to 4 was a mean of 2.25 preoperatively and 0.04 postoperatively. The New York Health Association classification for patients improved from a value of 2.45 preoperatively to 1.15 postoperatively.

Implants

Figure 8 summarizes the homograft valves shipped and implanted from 1984 to 1987. The dramatic growth in implants is related to the acceptance on the part of the medical community to the results obtained by Ross (7), Barratt-Boyes (4), O'Brien (6) and others. As of early September 1987, 3296 aortic and pulmonary valved conduits have been processed from 2135 hearts. Out of this total, 2411 have been returned to the hospitals requesting the preservation service and approximately 2000 have been implanted.

Results

Table 3 summarizes all the incidents of valve related removals during the 3.5 years that cryopreserved homografts have been implanted by this laboratory. A total of nine (9) homografts have been removed, resulting in an overall rate of removal for this period to be 0.0045.
Several inferences may be deduced from this information which will lead to further refinements of the technology and/or surgical procedure:
1. Calcification was present in two cases and was always associated with a young recipient (10 days and 1 month respectively). Considering the overall numbers of implants being done in children under the age of 15 (approx. 60%), this is a very

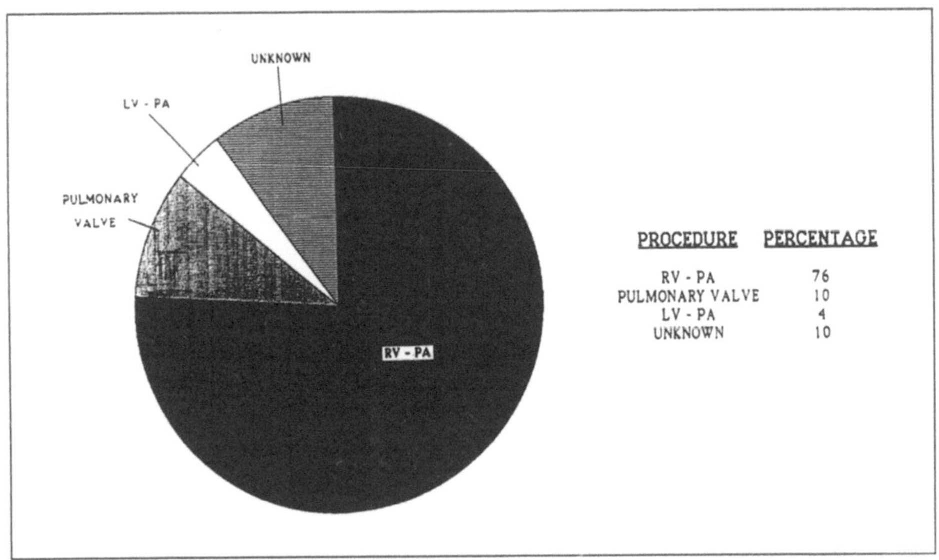

Fig. 7. The right heart operative procedures are summarized for 114 consecutive allograft clinical implant returns. RV-PA (right ventricle to pulmonary artery conduit), LV-PA (left ventricle to pulmonary artery conduit).

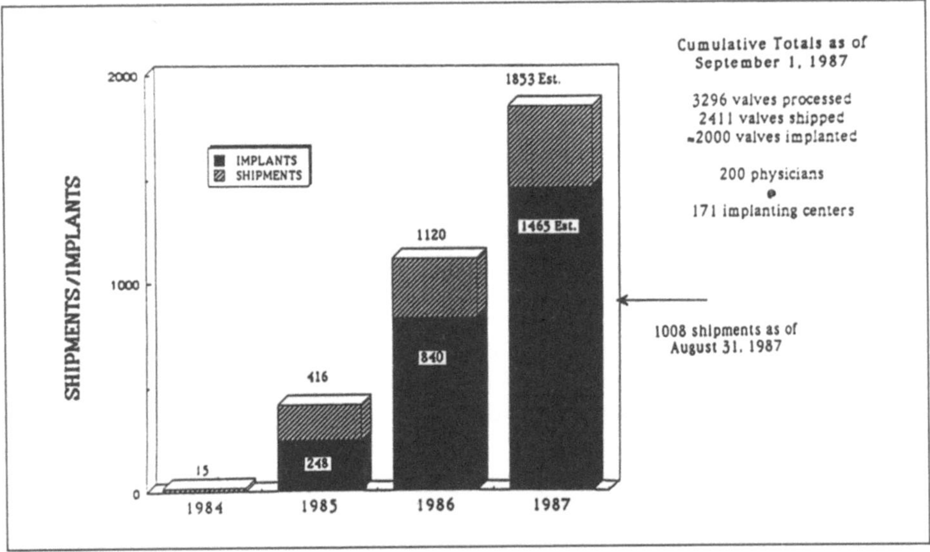

Fig. 8. This figure depicts the disposition of the valves and valved conduits obtained from 2135 hearts received by the laboratory during the period August 1984 to September 1987.

330

Table 3. Valve-related complications.

Complication	Cause	Procedure	Patient age	Time implanted
Calcification		Truncus	10 days	13 months
Calcification		RV-PA	1 month	9 months
Conduit rupture	Pro. Time	AV-root	62 years	1 day
Cusp degeneration	Pro. Time/IMM	AV	61 years	6 months
Cusp degeneration		AV	63 years	1 month
Cusp degeneration	Pro. Time/IMM	Truncus	1 month	6 months
Dehiscence		AV-MVR	27 years	3 weeks
Insufficiency		AV	28 years	5 months
Regurgitation		AV	39 years	10 months

small complication rate. It has been reported by a number of clinicians that homograft calcification is not uncommon in children but that it occurs less frequently in the homograft as opposed to other biological prosthetic valves. One investigator has an ongoing program to treat homografts in order to retard even this small amount of leaflet calcification with chemical pretreatment. Concurrent with this study will be another study to retard or eliminate conduit wall calcification which is very common in homograft conduit use.

2. One case of conduit rupture occurred when a patient was placed on post-operative balloon pumping. It is surmised from discussions with a group of clinicians that immediate post-operative balloon pumping might be contraindicated. This particular case had another contributory factor in that the procurement time (time from cessation of heartbeat to receipt in the laboratory) exceeded 24 h. This extended time has also been reported to be a contributory factor for cusp degeneration as well.

3. Three cases of cusps degeneration were reported. All occurred in 6 months or less. Two were aortic valve replacements and one was for a truncus repair. In two cases, AV and truncus, extended procurement time may have been a contributory cause. In one of these cases, lymphocitic infiltration was associated with the demise of the leaflet and in both of these there was donor: recipient blood group incompatibility.

Several investigators, but in particular Yankah (12), are currently attempting to ascertain the overall influence of ABO blood group compatibility for homografts by studies in the rat. Intuition would indicate that this might be a significant factor in any immunological degradation of the tissue. However, it will not be confirmed until implanting surgeons report a significant difference in the two groups.

4. Dehiscence was reported in one case at 3 weeks post implantation. Related to this, there have been several reports of suture pull-through, which are usually associated with inappropriate choice of suture material. Generally the use of 5—0 prolene has resulted in problems.

5. Valvular insufficiency occurred in one AV replacement at 5 months. No particular cause is associated with this data.

6. Regurgitation was reported in one AV patient at 10 months. This tissue is currently being evaluated to ascertain the genetic make-up of the tissue and the viability of the donor tissue in the recipient.

There have been no reported incidences of thromboembolism, endocarditis or patient death due to the use of the homografts.

Conclusion

The data reported here agrees favourably with the results achieved by O'Brien (6), in that cryopreserved viable tissue results in superior performance over both mechanical or other non-viable bioprostheses.

Although the homograft has been used clinically for 25 years, it perhaps has not received the scrutiny and evaluation which has been performed on bioprosthetic and mechanical valves. Obvious needs still exist to improve and refine preservation techniques, achieve better screening of the donor and perhaps increase longevity through improved implantation and donor: recipient matching.

References

1. Angell WW, De Lanerole P, Shumway NE (1973) Valve replacement: Present status of homograft valves. Prog Cardiovasc Dis 15: 589
2. Brockbank KGM, Bank HL (1987) Measurement of post cryopreservation viability. J Cardiac Surg Suppl II: 145
3. CryoLife Inc. Clinical Program 101 allograft heart valves (1987) CryoLife Inc., Marietta, Georgia, U.S.A.
4. Kirklin JW, Barratt-Boyes BG (1986) Cardiac surgery. John Wiley, New York. Chapter 12: Aortic valve disease, p 373—429
5. Lockey E, Al-Jenabi N, Gonzales-Lavin L, Ross DN (1972) A method of sterilizing and preserving fresh allograft heart valves. Thorax 27: 398
6. O'Brien MF, Stafford G, Gardner M, Phlner P, McGiffin D, Johnston N, Brosnan A, Duffy P (1987) The viable cryopreserved allograft aortic valve. J Cardiac Surg Suppl 2: 153—157
7. Ross D, Martelli M (1979) Allograft and autograft valves used for aortic valve replacement, In: Ionescu M (ed) Tissue heart valves. Butterworth, London, pp 127—172
8. van der Kamp AWM, Nuata J (1979) Fibroblast function and the maintenance of aortic valve matrix. Cardiovasc Res 13: 167
9. van der Kamp AWM, Visser WJ, van Dongen JM, et al (1981) Preservation of aortic heart valves with maintenance of cell viability. J Surg Res 30: 47
10. Watts LK, Duffy P, Field RB, Stafford EG, O'Brien MF (1976) Establishment of a viable homograft cardiac valve bank: A rapid method of determining homograft viability. Ann Thorac Surg 21: 230
11. Yankah AC, Randzio G, Wottge HU, Bernard A (1985) Factors influencing endothelial cell viability during procurement and preservation of valve allografts. In: Theide A, Deltz E, Engemann R, Hamelmann H (eds) Microsurgical models in rats for transplantation research. Springer-Verlag, Berlin, p 107
12. Yankah AC, Wottge HU, Muller-Hermelink HK, Feller AC, Large P, Wessel U, Dreyer H, Bernhard A, Muller-Ruchholtz W (1987) Transplantation of aortic and pulmonary allografts, enhanced viability of endothelial cells by cryopreservation, importance of histocompatibility. J Cardiac Surg Suppl 2: 209—220

Authors' address:
Robert T. McNally, Ph.D.
CryoLife, Inc., Suite 142
2211 New Market Parkway
Marietta, GA 30067
U.S.A.

Discussion

Part 1 chaired by: F. Fontan, France; H. Meisner, F.R.G.

FONTAN:

You mentioned in your tricuspid atresia patient that the imperforated valve is very rare. I agree with you that in our experience, we have only one or two that could be called imperforated valve. You said in your presentation that these patients have all the normal components of the right ventricle.

ALLWORK:

They are often underdeveloped but they are present. In most tricuspid atresia the inlet portion is never absent. Yes, it's underdeveloped.

ING-SH CHIU, TAIWAN:

I would like to ask: How do you know that the pulmonary artery inside the pericardium of truncus arteriosus is not derived from the sixth arch?

ALLWORK:

Because there's no sixth arch in a truncus, there's no conal truncal development; there's no need for there to be.

FONTAN:

Concerning timing following previous repair: What is your timing exactly, what is your decision-making parameter? Is it right ventricular ejection fraction, or exercise intolerance or cardiac enlargement?

LANGE:

We routinely tried to restudy those patients who, as a rule, are asymptomatic. 1 year or later after the previous, original repair and if the ejection fraction is then less than 85% of normal, and a volume load which is equivalent to QP:QS of more than 1.6—1.0, then we consider insertion of an allograft. But most of these patients were studied up to 11 years post previous repair, and it is very difficult to get the patients restudied 7 years after the original repair.

MEISNER:

This is quite early, isn't it?

LANGE:

Yes, it is early, but most of these patients were studied up to 11 years post previous repair. And it is very difficult to get the patients restudied 1 year after the original repair.

FONTAN:

Are there surgeons here sharing this concept who have already implanted allograft valves after previous repair in tetralogy of Fallot for the reasons indicated by Dr. Lange?

BARRATT-BOYES:

I think we've done it in two patients with 20 years follow-up, because they were clinically symptomatic.

KIRKLIN:

In Birmingham it was basically the same: we have used this in a situation with previous transannular patch, in patients in whom after 18—20 years there is progressive increase of right ventricular enlargement, not always with clinical signs of heart failure but certainly with important progression of right ventricular size. In that situation we have frequently put allografts in the orthotopic position under the patch.

MEISNER:

What happened to the right ventricular function afterwards?

KIRKLIN:

We don't have good follow-up but we suspect it doesn't change greatly; we hope that it doesn't worsen. You may have read a paper from Chicago where they said, if they repaired before 2 years postprevious repair the ejection fraction increases, and in all the other ones post 2 years it stays the same or decreases.

FONTAN:

Well, I think that's the source of the controversy.

ZIEMER, Hannover, West Germany:

First I want to congratulate Dr. Clarke on his experience with pulmonary homografts, especially in the tetralogy of Fallot. He has a good reason to use this: firstly, he lives at 5,000 feet altitude (most of the patients in the world live below 5,000 feet altitude), but I agree that pulmonary homografts have to be used in those patients with tetralogy of Fallot where we have a hypoplastic pulmonary artery system where you feel that you might get systemic or even suprasystemic pressure. This relates to my first question about patients with a systemic pressure or near systemic pressure on the right side. Are you not frightened by this bouncing up and down of the pulmonary homograft which has a very different consistency than the aortic homograft? My second question is, Dr. Pacifico shows that a 20-mm diameter valve is good for an adult. By squeezing a 20-mm valve into an 8-kg infant, you will end up with a 20-mm distal anastomosis. How do you view this allograft/patient size relationship?

CLARKE:

To answer your first question first, we too acknowledge that there was quite a lot of elasticity in the pulmonary allografts; this worried us, particularly because of the very frequent incidence of at least mild pulmonary regurgitation following placement of the pulmonary allograft. We have subsequently modified our method of preparing the pulmonary allograft in that we advent tissue in epicardium and the pulmonary allograft is left on, which I think adds to the integrity of the pulmonary valve ring and, to some extent, diminishes the elasticity of the graft.

In response to your second question, regarding the size of the allograft, I would say that almost always in these patients, the distal anastomosis is at least 20 mm, since the main pulmonary artery is opened and very frequently extended to the right or to the left or both, so that a large anastomosis can be achieved. So very frequently, the distal anastomosis is at least as big as the internal diameter of the conduit.

FONTAN:

I think you make an important contribution with this pulmonary allograft and I agree that the size could be convenient for an adult, but the point is that the patient is going to grow up and possibly in the future, as we have observed in aortic valve allograft, the conduit is going to be stressed. Sir Brian, would you like to make a comment?

BARRATT-BOYES:

I would just like to make a few comments about the question of the conduit. Follow-up of the homografts in the pulmonary position from Green Lane, compares the data with Donald Rosses National Heart Hospital experience, which was kindly given to John Coconun and myself for publication in our textbook, is an analysis of data in those 49 patients, provided by Mr. Donald Ross and Dr. Jane Somerville. The point I'd like to make is that both curves of course are virtually identical in the first instant, which is interesting, but if we look at them carefully, at 10 years, the reoperation rate for conduits is actually 20%, there's a 80% reoperation free incidence. Now that's very significant. A lot of people have said, well, it's small, but it isn't small. It's really very significant and if you go out longer than that, of course, the reoperation rate is higher. Now the reoperation rate, of course, is an underestimate of failure rate of the conduit. If you looked at the additional patients you'd have a significant gradient who haven't been reoperated, the curve is lower, so the incidence freedom from complications is at 10 years nearer to 65%. Now in fact these figures are almost identical to the incidence rate in the aortic position (the aortic position in our data we're using) and this is a antibiotic treated valve, it's not a viable valve. At 10 years the incidence of freedom from significant incompetence in the aortic position is 80%, and in the pulmonary position it's identical. So the statement, that they're different, is, I believe, not really correct. Now the other thing that we've got to remember is that when we reoperated on these conduits — and I reoperate on virtually all our own patients in this group — all the valves were incompetent, all the conduits were very stenotic with heavy calcification in the aortic wall, and there was also obstruction usually at valve level. None of the valves was normal. Now I think we've got to be very careful if we're going to advocate using this sort of conduit in infants, as a routine in tetralogy for example. I think that would be disastrous, because we know at 10 years, the reoperation rate for tetralogy is virtually zero for pulmonary obstruction, if the operation is done correctly, using pericardium or some other substance without a valve. And the message that I'm trying to put across is that I think that we are overstating the good function of this conduit on the right side of the heart; it's the best we've got, but it's not good enough to move to using it in a routine sort of way. And whether or not the viable ones are doing any better is a moot point. These are not viable conduits, they're antibiotic-treated, so maybe we've got to wait and see whether the pulmonary conduit is any better in a viable way or not. I doubt that it's going to be different.

MILLER:

I'm curious if Mr. Ross or Dr. Clark would care to comment on what they're doing with hoods. What material do you use; PTFE most of the time. I think we could be asking for trouble with our hoods, no matter what material we use.

Secondly, and this gets back to Dr. Angell's question earlier, about the paper from Chicago. I think it's a self-fulfilling prophecy that the postoperated patients who get a valve early do better than those who get it late, just by virtue of how they selected their patients and I would urge, as Sir Brian has just said, to be very cautious if we apply these valves.

ANGELL:

We've done 13 pulmonary conduits and they're all leaking, there's not one that has not some degree of pulmonary insufficiency. We do feel technically that pulmonary annulus need some sort of support other than being left free.
Secondly, we used the pulmonary patch either with a single or double cusp, 16 years or so ago with the fresh homograft. Most of those patients have serious pulmonary insufficiency but none of them has been reoperated for stenosis of the cusp.

TURLEY:

I think Mr. Ross uses autologous pericardium to extend, and to make a hood, that's not necessary in all cases. I think in a large number there's enough right ventricular outflow tract to simply use the conduit by itself.

ROSS:

Almost invariably we do need some sort of patching material. I have no anxieties about the ability of the pulmonary valves to withstand systemic or near systemic pressures, as someone expressed the anxiety, and I think the potential for the pulmonary as an aortic allograft is great because there's less calcium content, as one of my research people has shown. We think that it's going to reduce the incidence of calcification in the conduit at least. Whether it's going to last longer I don't know.
Can I just make a surgical point which Dr. Meisner really emphasized, and that is the importance of laying your conduit within the outflow tract if possible, or laying it in the alignment of the outflow tract. I think a lot of the bad results of conduits have been from redundant conduits looping out, from the right ventrical to the pulmonary artery rather than laying in it.
The other problem that I have had accounts for some of the reoperative problems that Dr. Somerville has mentioned has been distal sutureline stenosis where the conduit is attached to the distal pulmonary artery. It is very easy, for me at least, to create a purse ring effect there in using a running 4-0 proline suture and we found quite a number of stenoses of the distal suture line which we had thought had been in the homograft. We now not only interrupt that distal sutureline but lock the sutures entirely.
Thirdly, we used, in our learning stages a lot of different reconstructive patches, the most disastrous of which was the extension of dacron to the lower and of the homograft which ended up, as they usually do, with peel, so that we use only autologous pericardium in that position now.

RADLEY-SMITH:

I am a little bit concerned about the use of the pulmonary allograft in the right ventricular outflow tract in some of these complex cases, where the right ventricular pressure is raised, because I think — Dr. Somerville will correct me if I'm wrong — the architecture of the pulmonary artery is different from the architecture of the aorta and I am somewhat worried that this will be able to stand up to long-term high pressure particularly as we have been talking about viability of cells. I can't see that the pulmonary arterial wall is going to be able to stand up to high pressure for 20—30 years in some of these complex, particularly pulmonary arteries. Any comment?

336

MEISNER:

We don't know about that exactly.

RADLEY-SMITH:

I could foresee perhaps a rupturing late because of thinning of the wall.

ROSS:

I think there is no reason why it should rupture any more than any other allograft tissue that your're putting in.

RADLEY-SMITH:

But it is different, histologically, from the aortic wall.

ROSS:

Only a little thinner.

RADLEY-SMITH:

The linament is different.

MEISNER:

It is very close to the saphanous vein and there we don't see any ruptures.

FONTAN:

In the case of rupture, it should already have occurred, and we would know already.

JONAS:

There is a history of aortic homograft ruptures. I don't think we know the answer to Dr. Radley-Smith's question. We have cryopreservation and we have pulmonary tissue: it is a potential risk. As I said, if you go back to the vascular surgeons of the 1950s, there are certainly reports of homograft ruptures, there are two or three large series: I think Dr. Sikarskie reported about a 4% incidence of aortic abdominal homograft rupture. If you look at femoral artery homografts, about 40% of those became aneurysmal and, of course, they stopped using them.

FONTAN:

You have shown yourself that it can happen with pericardium.

JONAS:
We are going to continue to use them but we just don't know.

FONTAN:

Are there clinical situations in which the authors think that use of aortic valve or a pulmonary homograft is not required? Dr. Jonas, do you have a clear definition of when or when not to use a valve?

JONAS:

If I am going to do a conduit reconstruction, my conduit of first choice is a homograft; unfortunately it's not always available.

MEISNER:

Are we to understand that you changed your policy also in the tetralogy of Fallot cases, where you really were using a transannular patch freely? Do you do the same thing or do you implant an aortic allograft at the first operation now?

JONAS:

No, we would never electively place a valve at primary operation, but we do operate on very young tetralogies now and we do frequently place transannular patches. I think it's important that the patch is not too wide: that can result in late problems with the right ventricle because of excessive pulmonary insufficiency.

DAENEN:

I'm just wondering whether it is really necessary to put in a conduit in anomalous left coronary artery origin in tetralogy of Fallot.

BARRATT-BOYES:

We've had 18 cases of anomalous anterior descending coronary rising from the right, and in no patient have ι put in a conduit. They have all been reconstructable from within or in combination with elevation of the artery and a patch underneath the artery, and this includes very young children. This is not a contraindication in our hands to early primary repair, as it has been, but we have restudied all these patients: They're all alive and there are very few problems with them, very few gradients, so we do not think there is a primary indication for a homograft.
One other point I'd like to add to Dr. Somerville's presentation, and that is the question of age and the obstruction. Almost half our patients are under 2 years, they range from 13 or 15 days up to 2 years and the other half are over 2 years. The actual curve of the incidence of reoperation for obstruction, is identical in the two groups, the lines overlap. However, we are using a big sized conduit and by the time you get to 10, 15 years, the child has outgrown the conduit, but it needs replacement anyway. I think that's the point: if the patient is older, by 10—15 years, he's going to have the same sort of problems, so that actually the curves are identical.

ELLIOTT:

With regard to the anomalous coronary artery in tetralogy of Fallot, five patients had an anomalous coronary artery diagnosed who did not have a conduit. So it has not been an "every time" indication. Of those five patients, three were managed with elevation of the artery and a patch underneath, one

338

had to be reoperated in the immediate postoperative period because of ischaemic changes and another one subsequently developed ischaemic changes quite suddenly a little later, we think because the patch became aneurysmal, and the remaining two were managed by endocardial resection either through the valve or through the atrium and the Fallot repair in that way. Those are doing well. I think that one should not assume that it is an indication for a conduit replacement but it's something that one should bear in mind when an artery is present.

ZIEMER:

There are other techniques, which avoid the use of aortic homografts. Although I am basically fond of aortic homografts, they are not always available, and regarding the absent pulmonary valve syndrome, the plication and resection of the pulmonary arteries gives as good a result as a normal Fallot repair.
The second is, in the truncus repair where you usually deal with babies of about 2—4 kg in weight, you will not always have a small conduit available. Although I have heard of people putting in 17-mm valves in 3 kg babies, I still cannot imagine it, but I have to visit these centres to see for myself. Since we do not have a supply of small aortic homografts, we have been using for 5 years now in truncus arteriosus, a nonvalved conduit. Of those eight patients we have operated on in the first 4 months, two died. One patient certainly died because of a wrong indication, he had a stenosis and would have needed a valve. That makes just one death out of seven patients, which is a mortality of around 15% and this is a mortality rate which everybody has been experiencing with these valves. I just want to make the point that if there is no homograft valve available, one can still repair truncus.

TURLEY:

We have always felt that the use of a valve in infant truncus repair was very beneficial. All the measurements we have made of sudden acute pulmonary hypertensive episodes have been helped by the presence of a valve within the truncus, and when using a non-valve conduit we think your chance of an acute ventricular distension is much higher. I reported the results in that series of patients with non-valve conduit, but I think if you get a larger series, you'll find a significant number of patients who have acute right ventricular distension and early death.

MEISNER:

Yes, I have to ._ree completely with that.

BARRATT-BOYES:

I just wanted to make one brief comment to Dr. Turley about the technique of putting these in, because I've now altered our technique: now we no longer put the muscle at the back because, particularly in a small heart, it produces quite a bulge and I don't personally think the anterior mitral leaflet is much good. I don't agree either with Dr. Jonas about the having to turn it on the side like that. Maybe it does lie a little bit better that way, but we put the anterior mitral leaflet at the back and the muscle at the front, and extent it with pericardium. I think you get less obstruction than in these areas where every centimeter is important. Have you got any comment about that?

TURLEY:

I expected comment on that. I think the technique we use is to drop that muscle shelf down into the ventricle and then the suture line comes up out of the ventricle. The stitch begins outside the heart, goes through the patch (the teflon-felt patch inside ventricle which is brought right up to the ventricular edge) and then through the muscle band and tied inside the muscle band, bringing the conduit down. Any obstruction I think would be from bending back and that's what we're most concerned about. The significant thing about truncus repair is just an extremely short allograft and it is placed far out, next to the aorta, so that the distance is short and the chance of an acute bend in the conduit is lessened.

ELLIOTT:

With the absent pulmonary valve syndrome, there is such a recorded high incidence of arborization anomalies that I'd be quite worried about putting in a non-valved conduit. I would not put it in, I would just do a plication. You know that the palliative operations have not proved to be wonderfully successful in the published literature and I would choose, I think, to use a valved homograft.

SOMERVILLE:

I want to support Dr. Fontan. It may have shocked some of you, about the use of valves, but in our series, long-term results of the direct anastomosis are very much better, but there are some patients in whom you need something to bridge the gap and in those I'm sure the homograft is better. I'd also like to say we have quite a series of caval valves, and I regard them as completely useless.

FONTAN:

Well, I think that if there is a gap between the two parts of the anastomosis you may usually construct posteriorly wherever it is, the right ventricle or the peak of the septum distally, by placing anteriorly a hood of the material you prefer.

ROSS:

Although we've all used homografts in the Fontan-connection and in palliation of single ventricle, it doesn't really make any sense to do so, because, as Lamm pointed out way back in 1952, if you don't have a pulsatile flow, the homograft, of course, won't function. So putting them in the inferior vena cava and in the right atrial pulmonary artery connections, where you have a continuous flow, they're pushed aside. They won't function and it is not surprising. Perhaps we should give it up.

Part 2 chaired by: R. Radley-Smith, UK; E. Fleck, Germany

HETZER:

In the list of the donors, Dr. McNally, you show that 31% of donors were also liver donors. I would like to know whether those were not suitable as heart donors or if they were primarily considered as donor hearts for valves.

McNALLY:

The question is difficult to answer since we weren't actually doing the procurement. But generally speaking, if 86% of all the donors were kidney donors, then at least they would have been suitable for that. The liver would have been the third organ that generally would have been taken. We do histological analysis on every piece of tissue as well as the routine microbiological and fungal analysis.

HETZER:

You don't really understand what I mean. I would consider it as ethically questionable if you took viable hearts that may be suitable as transplants primarily only for the use of valves.

McNALLY:

Yes, that is an entirely different question. These hearts are procured by independent groups. We have no control over that and, of course, it is our opinion and the opinion of those who are doing the procurement that a whole organ transplant would be the first use of this kind of tissue. It would only be after there was no suitable donor or recipient that the tissue would come for processing.

SOMERVILLE:

Dr. Angell, how can you say anything has statistical significance when you have lost between 13 and 21% of it?

ANGELL:

That's a good question and I asked the statistician that question too. Fortunately, we only lost 3% of the frozen group and that is the small group. The patient loss was in follow-up in the larger groups. It is almost a philosophical question, because you have to assume that either those patients lost in follow-up have an impact on the valve failure rate or they don't, and how significant is that when they are 10 to 15% of the patients lost? In order for that lost patient group to have a significant impact on what we quoted as statistically significant, they would all have to be valve failures or all not valve failures. When you take all the patients we have lost and count them as valve failures, it does not change the statistical significance of the analysis.

BODNAR:

I would like to congratulate Dr. O'Brien for his 100% results because I think it is absolutely unique that someone has 100% follow-up of patients over a 17-year period and a 100% exclusion from valve degeneration. I have two questions:
(1) Are you therefore saying that the viable homograft which is to be considered as a living donor organ provokes no immunological reaction and that there is a zero-rate of rejection in these homografts? You reported to have experienced no degeneration.
(2) In the CryoLife-series I believe I recognized 16 early valve failures from which they experience calcification and degeneration following exactly your method. I believe the selection of the valves was even more meticulous than in your practice. How would you explain other people's experience? Am I right that a vast majority of the CryoLife valves went into the right-side position where as you were talking about free-hand grafting? The much better chance for the CryoLife valve provoked a considerable amount of numbers of early valve failures. Why do you think you did not experience those?

O'BRIEN:

I presented the facts exactly as I see them and compared them to another series at the same institution, and the difference is striking. There is no evidence of degeneration in that group followed up to the end of last year.
There are deaths that occurred and but without autopsy examination. The clinical assessment of the valve close to that patient's death has not suggested that the valve is falling to bits. I think that our curve is going to be superior to any other curves but is going to drop for certain. I am not sure whether the down curve will be at 13, 14 or 15 years. I have no doubt that there is going to be degeneration. I did quite clearly state the degeneration that we have seen this year and the patients we have reoperated on. I showed histologically the evidence at 7 years of a patient in this cryopreserved viable series, in whom we thought the valve was completely dead and histologically it was. We have degeneration that is appearing not leading to reoperation. I think it is there, histologically in the 7-year patient dying of cancer whose valve, although competent, was certainly completely acellular and so thin that it would have perforated at some time. I would think our protocol is much tighter than CryoLife because they've got an unknown variable of institutions delivering valves to them. But given that we have valves that are of variable viability, some of these will be quite viable and others, extended to near the 24-h donor death, will show a little less viability. But you have to look at it as a series where the valves are being taken at a mean of 15 h and cryopreserved within a mean of 39 h. The difference is that many of our valves will be, as Dr. Angell has said, thicker and less likely to perforate.

McNALLY:

I will answer that in two steps: (1) procurement and processing in the meantime is 15 h and (2) the actual freezing would occur at about 36 h, something in that range.

GONZALEZ-LAVIN:

Do you assess viability at the time of delivery of the valve, not at the time of processing?

McNALLY:

We do a different type of assessment, and that is, as we research a particular process, we send whole valve leaflets to Rotterdam in the Netherlands for Prolin uptake study. So, we do it on a batch sampling basis.

342

ROSS:

Dr. O'Brien, you are dealing in your series with two time frames: the first time frame being with fresh valves, and the second time frame where you require surgery. Do you think that this has a bearing on the results?

O'BRIEN:

We did not think so and we went to show how to analyse that. We looked at the patients just prior to and after the change and we could really not see any difference. One additional thing would be that five surgeons put the valve in, although now primarily four, whereas in the 1975 we used to have two surgeons. I probably would have put in the valves anyway.

Contribution for discussion:
A mathematical model of aortic valve vibration

D. L. Sikarskie, P. D. Stein, M. Vable

Michigan Technological University, Houghton, Michigan, U.S.A.

Introduction

A considerable amount of data has now been accumulated which clearly shows that the second heart sound is produced by diastolic vibration of the closed aortic and pulmonary valves (5, 6, 8). An understanding of the physical and physiological basis of production of the second heart sound has led to a better understanding of several auscultatory observations (8, 9), thereby permitting a more refined interpretation of some aspects of cardiac auscultation. Identification of the precise mechanism of production of the second heart sound has led to the prospective development of diagnostic techniques based upon the predicted behaviour of the heart sounds under various pathophysiological conditions. In particular, knowing that the stiffening of a structure raises its natural frequency enabled the prediction that the frequency of the second sound would increase as the valve stiffened due to disease. Analysis of the frequency content of the heart sound has confirmed this prediction (8, 10, 11) and has led to a diagnostic indicator of pathological stiffening of porcine bioprosthetic valves. This may serve as an early indicator of bioprosthetic valve degeneration.

Literature review

In light of the potential importance of these observations, quantitative modelling is an important step in helping to evaluate the effects of pathophysiological factors. Blick et al. (1) previously modelled valve vibration as a spring, mass, damper system with the parameters adjusted to match the experimental output. This model identified several constitutive properties of the valve which affect the amplitude and frequency of the second heart sound. The validity of the factors was subsequently shown in patients (9). Little other work has appeared related to modelling of the aortic valve response. In two papers, Mazumdar and Hearn (2, 4) modelled the free and forced vibration of a single valve leaflet. They did not, however, treat the problem as a coupled fluid/solid problem. Lim et al. (3) also developed a valve membrane vibration model. This model included only a linear material response and it did not have the proper forcing term.

Discussion of model

In an effort to evaluate in further detail the physiological factors that affect the second heart sound, a mathematical model for aortic valve vibration has been developed from first principles. The model assumes a one dimensional, but non-linear, fluid behaviour. The problem is coupled through a non-linear, planar valve. A solution is obtained using the method of characteristics developed in finite difference form. The resulting valve frequency and amplitude are in good agreement with patient data. The model predicts a strong dependency of response on the valve forcing function and valve stiffness; and a weaker dependency of response on valve mass. More importantly, perhaps, additional factors which affect sound frequency and amplitude are identified by a parametric examination of the model. Details of the model are thoroughly discussed in the cited reference (7).

References

1. Blick EF, Sabbah HN, Stein PD (1979) One dimensional model of diastolic semilunar valve vibrations productive of heart sounds. J Biomech 12: 223—227
2. Hearn TC, Mazumdar J (1981) A study of the dynamic response of atrio-ventricular valves using a membrane model. Math Model 2: 97—107
3. Lim KO, Liev YC, Oh CH (1980) Analysis of mitral and aortic valve vibrations and their role in the production of the first and second heart sounds. Phys Med Biol 25: 727—733
4. Mazumdar J, Hearn TC (1978) Mathematical analysis of mitral valve leaflets. J Biomech 11: 291—296
5. Sabbah HN, Stein PD (1976) Investigation of the theory and mechanism of the origin of the second heartsound. Circ Res 39: 874—882
6. Sabbah HN, Stein PD (1978) Relation of the second sound to diastolic vibration of the closed aortic valve. Am J Physiol (Heart Circ Physiol) 3: H696—H700
7. Sikarskie DL, Stein PD, Vable M (1984) A mathematical model of aortic valve vibration. J Biochem 17: 831—837
8. Stein PD (1981) A Physical Basis for the Interpretation of Cardiac Auscultation: Evaluations Based Primarily on the Second Sound and Ejection Murmurs. Futura, Mt Kisco, New York
9. Stein PD, Sabbah HN (1978) Origin of the second heart sound: clinical relevance of new observations. Am J Cardiol 41: 108—110
10. Stein PD, Sabbah HN, Lakier JB, Goldstein S (1980) Frequency spectrum of the aortic component of the second sound in patients with normal valves, aortic stenosis and aortic porcine xenografts: potential for detection of porcine xenograft degeneration. Am J Cardiol 46: 48—52
11. Stein PD, Sabbah HN, Lakier JB, Magilligan DJ, Jr, Goldstein S (1981) Frequency of the first heart sou   in the assessment of stiffening of mitral bioprosthetic valves. Circ 63: 200—203

Authors' address:
David L. Sikarskie
Dean of Engineering
Michigan Technological University
Houghton, Michigan
U.S.A.

25 Years' clinical experience of allograft surgery — A time for reflection

B. Barratt-Boyes

Cardiothoracic Surgical Unit, Green Lane Hospital, Auckland, New Zealand

The Green Lane Hospital (GLH) experience of freehand aortic allograft valve replacement extends back to August 1962, when the first such valve was inserted using a double suture line technique. In 1966, the aortic allograft was used as a conduit to reconstitute the right ventricular outflow tract and subsequent to that, stented aortic allografts have been used in both the mitral and tricuspid positions. Because of time constraints, I will confine my remarks to freehand aortic allograft valve replacement.

As can be seen from Table 1, our enthusiasm for its use in the aortic position has persisted over the 25 years despite various setbacks. Our first 16 valves were untreated (that is, they received neither chemical nor antibiotic treatment as they were collected sterilely and placed in Hanks' solution only, in which they were stored for varying periods of time extending from 2 days to about 31 days). Some of these valves contained viable fibroblasts at the time of insertion. In the next group of patients, up until August 1968, the valves were collected unsterilely and sterilised with betapropiolactone or ethylene oxide (chemical sterilisation). Some of these were freeze dried (lyophilised) and the others were stored wet at 4 °C in Hanks' solution. The next group of patients from 1968 to 1983 received valves sterilised with an antibiotic solution ("PSKA"). This was a relatively strong solution in which the valve was inserted for 8 days at 4 °C and subsequently stored wet in Hanks' solution or nutrient medium at 4 °C. In 1983, the antibiotic solution was changed to "CLPVA" which was a much less concentrated solution in which the valve was inserted for only 48 h. The details of these antibiotic solutions are presented later.

Hospital (30 day) mortality

Table 1 contains our entire experience with freehand aortic allograft valve replacement. It includes both isolated aortic valve replacement and aortic allograft valve replacement combined with replacement of the mitral valve with some other device, with or without tricuspid surgery. It includes first operations and reoperations (one or more) and patients who had additional non-valve surgery (mainly coronary artery bypass grafting). There has been a progressive reduction in 30-day mortality so that in the current cardioplegic era (1980 up to and including 1985) the mortality has been reduced to 2.3%. The mortality for isolated aortic valve replacement is noted in parenthesis. In the current era it has been 2.2% (n = 492) compared with 2.6% in multivalve replacement patients (n = 78). There is thus no significant difference in these two subsets. It is to be noted that during this current era, 327 prosthetic or bioprosthetic valves have also been inserted in the aortic position in other patients. The allograft is thus our valve of choice but it is not used in all patients.

Table 1. Aortic allografts: isolated + multivalve surgery. First and reoperation ± additional non-valve surgery.

Year of operation	n	Hospital deaths	
		n	%
1962—1967	501	47	9.4% (8.7%)*
1968—1973	549	50	9.1% (8.7%)
1974—1979	477	25	5.2% (4.5%)
1980—1985	570	13	2.3% (2.2%)
Total	2097	135	6.4% (6.0%)

* mortality for isolated aortic valve replacement.

Table 2. Aortic allografts: isolated aortic valve replacement ± additional surgery.

Year of operation	n	First operation Hospital deaths		n	Reoperation Hospital deaths	
		n	%		n	%
1962—1967	409	31	7.6%	64	10	15.6%
1968—1973	361	27	7.5%	112	14	12.5%
1974—1979	338	15	4.4%	59	3	5.1%
1980—1985	419	7	1.7%	73	4	5.5%
Total	1527	80	5.2%	308	31	10.1%

The differences in hospital mortality between a first operation and a reoperation (first, second, or third combined) in patients having isolated aortic allograft valve replacement with or without additional non-valve surgery is detailed in Table 2. In the 1974—1979 era, the mortality in these two subsets was virtually the same, while in the curre... era that for a first operation has fallen to 1.7% while for a reoperation the mortality remains at about 5%.

Late survival

The long-term actuarial survival is presented in a cohort of 252 patients receiving a PSKA treated allograft valve between 1968 and 1974, all of whom have been followed for a minimum of 9.5 years and a maximum of 16.5 years (mean 10.8 years). It is 77% at 5 years, 57% at 10 years and 38% at 14 years (Fig. 1). This is similar, if not slightly superior, to that achieved with prosthetic and bioprosthetic valves, although survival is known to be more dependent upon ventricular function than the type of device used for valve replacement. When late deaths due to valve failure are examined actuarially (excluding hospital mortality) the 10-year incidence is only 6% (Fig. 2), although beyond 10 years it increases somewhat. All these deaths are the result of significant allograft valve incompetence, as this device has no other

348

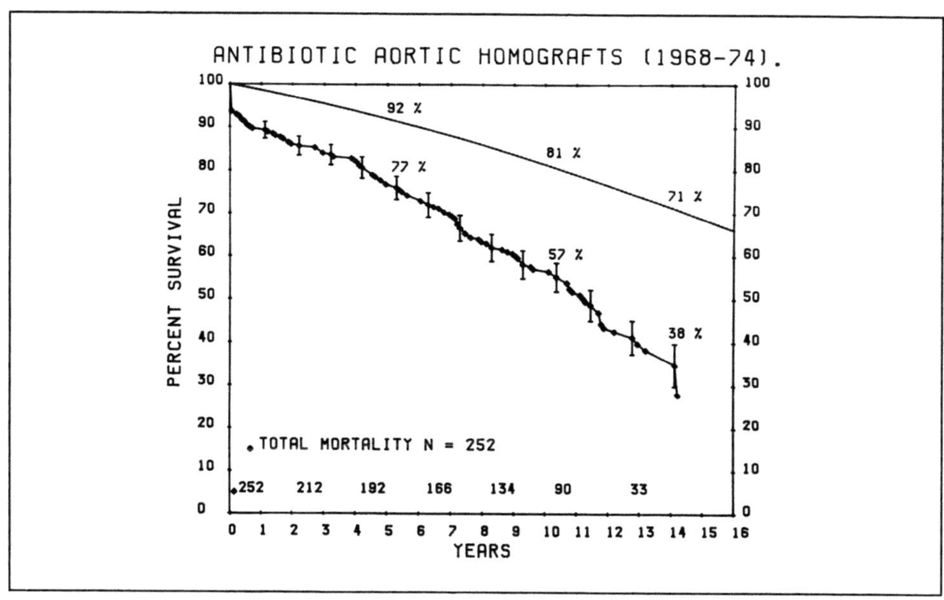

Fig. 1. Actuarial survival following isolated aortic allograft valve replacement in a subset of patients receiving PSKA treated valves and followed for a minimum of 9.5 and a maximum of 16.5 years. The upper dashed line defines survival of an age/sex matched general population. The bars define 70% confidence limits. The numbers at risk are noted.
Reproduced with permission from Barratt-Boyes et al. (5).

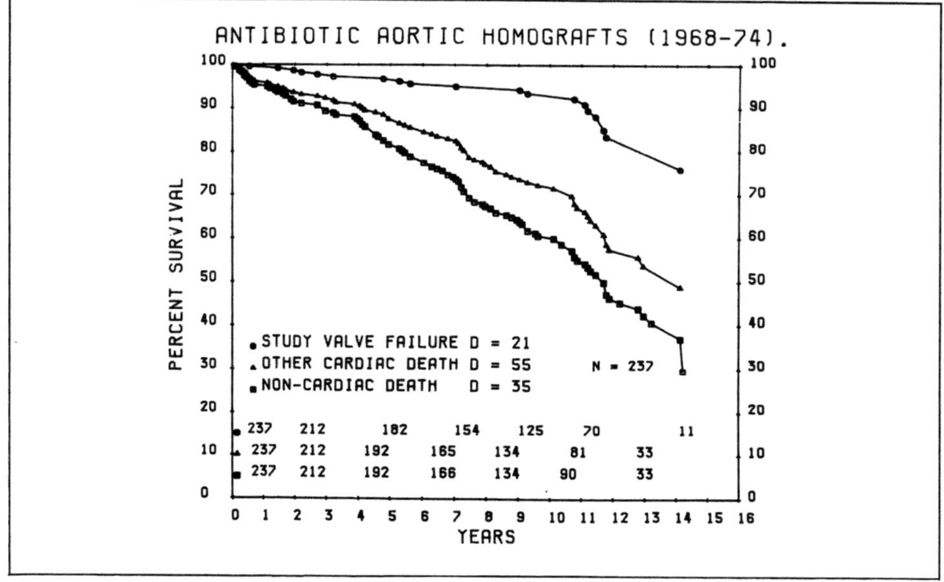

Fig. 2. Actuarial survival broken down in cumulative fashion to deaths due to allograft valve failure, other cardiac deaths, and non-cardiac deaths. The same subset as in Fig. 1 except for exclusion of the 15 hospital deaths. Thus, at 10 years, deaths due to allograft valve failure were 6%, those due to other cardiac causes were 22%, and those due to non-cardiac causes were 12%. The numbers at risk are noted.

349

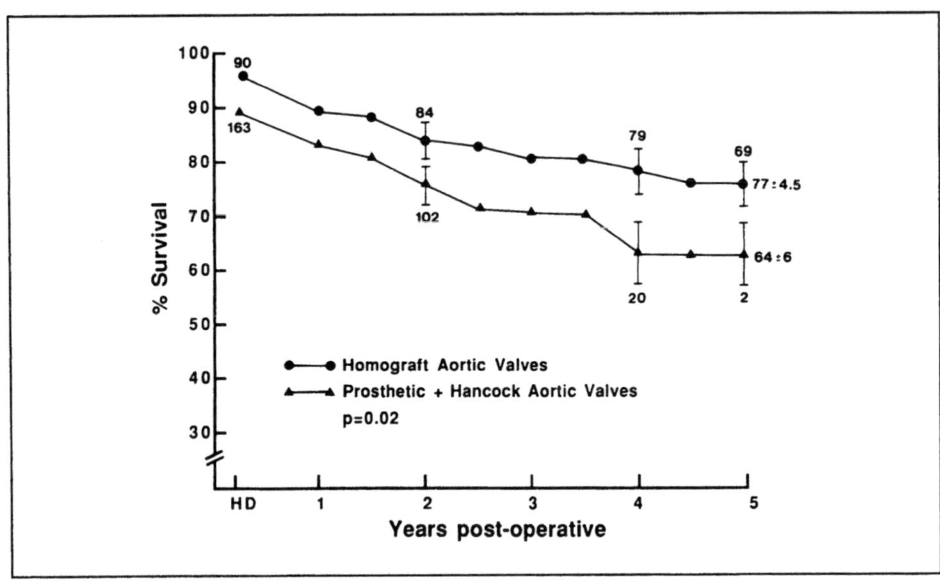

Fig. 3. Actuarial survival, including hospital deaths, in patients receiving an isolated allograft aortic valve compared to patients receiving an isolated prosthetic or bioprosthetic aortic valve. The patients were operated upon during the same time frame but were not randomised. The bars represent 70% confidence limits. The numbers at risk are noted.

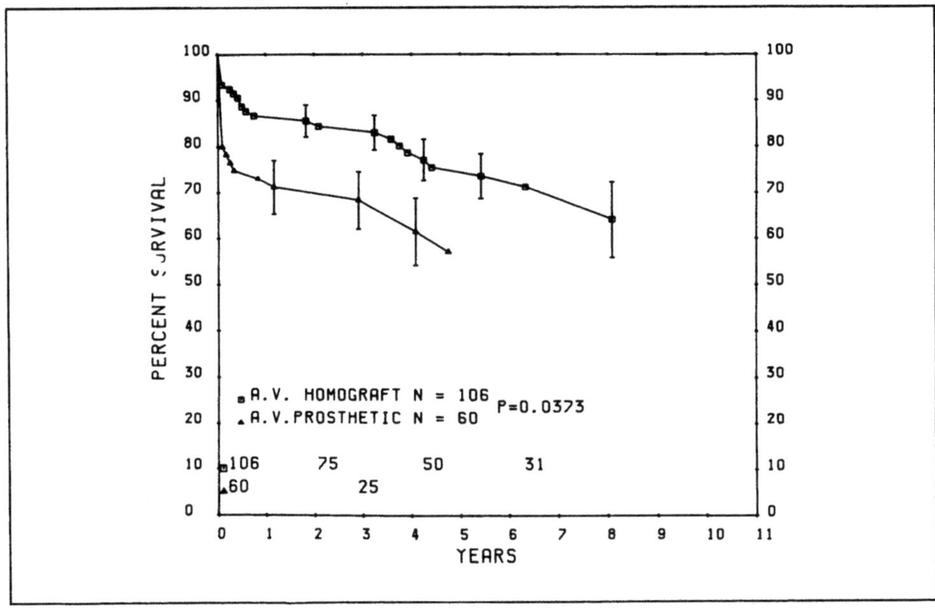

Fig. 4. Actuarial survival in patients undergoing double valve replacements (± tricuspid valve surgery) divided into those in whom the aortic valve replacement was with an allograft valve and those in whom the aortic valve replacement was with a prosthetic or bioprosthetic valve. Hospital deaths are included. The bars represent 70% confidence limits. The numbers at risk are noted. The two series were contemporaneous but were not randomised.

350

significant morbidity. They occur either at the time of reoperation, or more commonly, without reoperation in patients who are considered unsuitable because of age or frailty, or refuse reoperation, or are not referred for it by their general practitioner. Sudden deaths are not included in this category as there has never been any evidence, at numerous autopsies, of either coronary or other emboli from an allograft valve.

It is of interest that survival has been superior following allograft valve replacement compared with prosthetic or bioprosthetic valve replacement (Fig. 3), although these figures must be interpreted with caution in view of the fact that this is a retrospective, non-randomised series. The same is true for multiple valve surgery (Fig. 4), although these data are also retrospective and non-randomised. They at least allow us to state that the use of an allograft aortic valve does not compromise survival in either circumstance.

Allograft valve incompetence

It became clear early in our experience that the incidence of significant allograft valve incompetence was dependent upon the method of valve preparation, particularly the sterilisation technique. Thus, the actuarial incidence of proven cusp rupture (the most common mechanism of valve failure leading to incompetence as a result of valve wear) was unacceptably high with valves prepared by chemical sterilisation when compared with the 16 valves which we had initially used in an untreated state (Fig. 5). It was for this reason that we introduced antibiotic sterilisation in August 1968 in the hope that cusp rupture would be less frequent. This analysis of the first 114 patients with a valve so treated strongly suggested that this was the case. An update of this information is presented in Fig. 6 using significant (moderate or severe) incompetence from any cause as the marker rather than cusp rupture. The antibiotic (PKSA) treated valves are the same cohort of patients presented earlier in Fig. 1 and 2, while the chemically treated series represents a follow-up of virtually all patients who received this type of allograft valve. There is a highly significant difference between the two curves (p < 0.0001). Freedom from significant incompetence with the antibiotic preparation is much greater than with the chemical preparation during the first 9—10 years of follow-up, and thereafter the two curves become almost parallel. The difference in the incidence of significant incompetence with these two methods of preparation is due mainly to the incidence of cusp rupture. The various causes of allograft valve incompetence are listed in Fig. 7. The most common is leaflet rupture (usually in the cusp belly, sometimes adjacent to the commissure).

Endocarditis is a much less common cause as is "central leak", which can be the result of leaflet prolapse due to technical error, or to progressive dilatation of the commissural portion of the valve due to progressive dilatation of the aorta in the region of the sinuses of Valsalva, secondary usually to medionecrosis in the aortic wall, the leaflets (by definition) remaining intact. Finally, incompetence can be secondary to a peripheral (perivalvar) suture line leak. The "unknown" category includes patients in whom the mechanism could not be established as there was neither autopsy nor reoperation. Fig. 8 presents the same data for the PSKA valve and shows

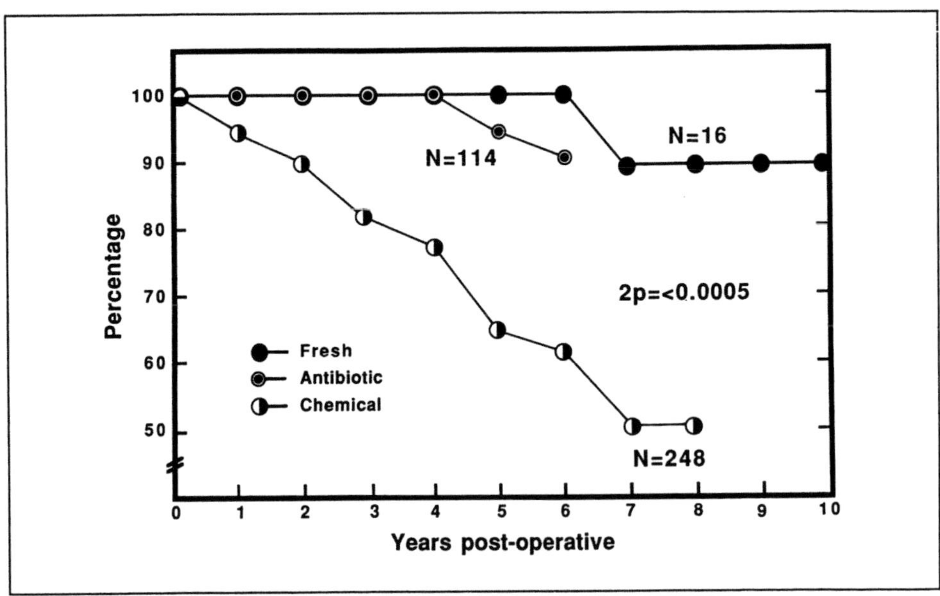

Fig. 5. Actuarial incidence of proven cusp rupture in aortic allograft valves followed postoperatively. "Fresh" valves were collected sterilely and were not treated with antibiotics — they were stored at 4 °C in Hanks' solution for short periods only prior to implantation. "Antibiotic" valves were treated with PSKA solution for 8 days at 4 °C and thereafter stored wet in Hanks' solution at 4 °C until implantation (up to 3 months). "Chemical" treated valves were sterilised using betapropiolactone and were then either stored wet in Hanks' solution at 4 °C or freeze dried (lyophilised).

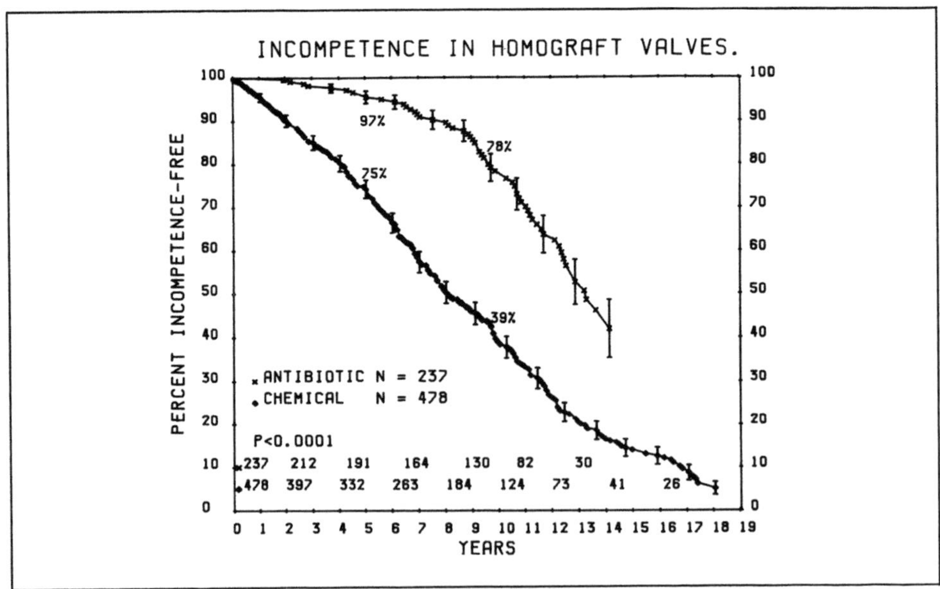

Fig. 6. Actuarial incidence of freedom from significant allograft valve incompetence (moderate or severe) in valves treated chemically (betapropiolactone or ethylene oxide) and those treated with PSKA. Bars represent 70% confidence limits. The numbers at risk are noted.
Reproduced with permission from Barratt-Boyes et al. (5).

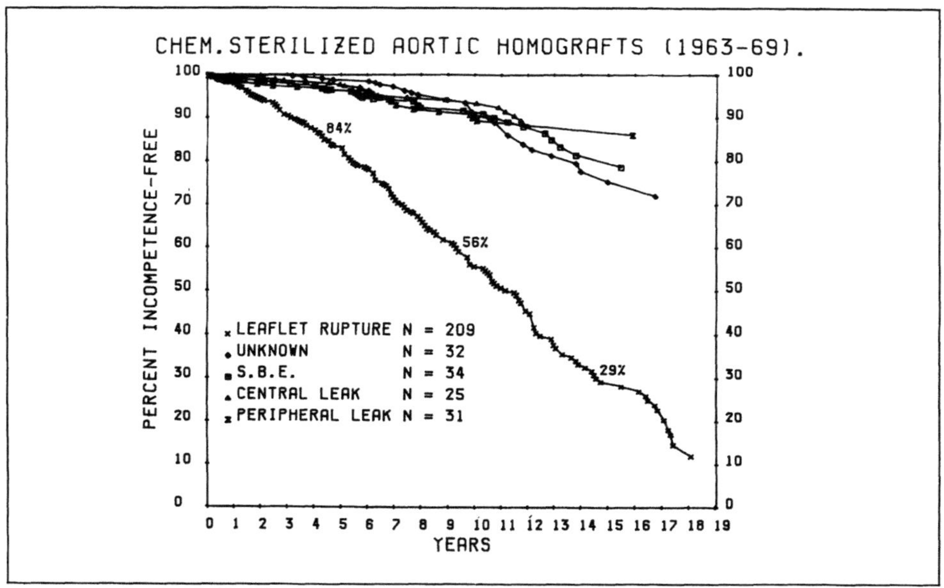

Fig. 7. Actuarial incidence of freedom from significant incompetence in chemically sterilised allograft valves followed postoperatively. The causes of incompetence are separately listed and assessed. See text.

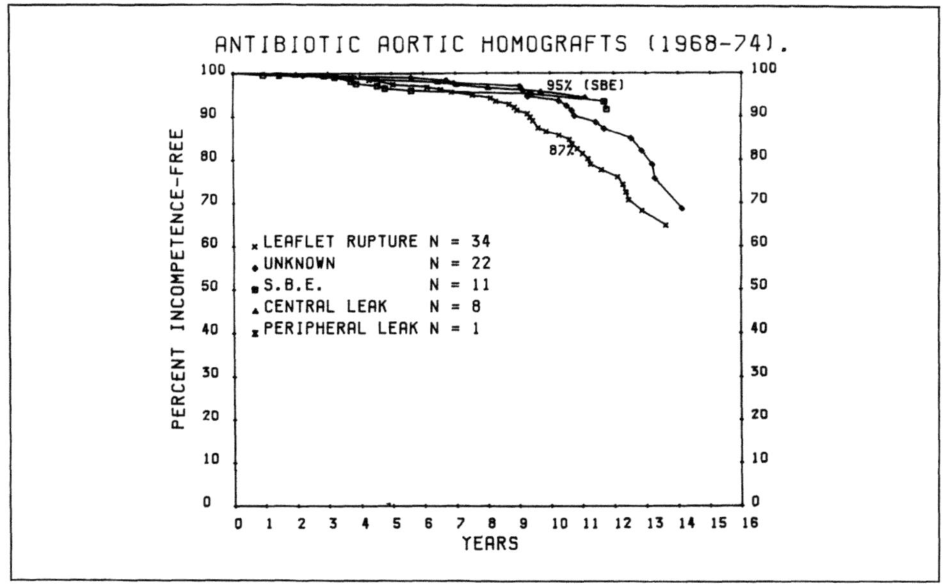

Fig. 8. Actuarial incidence of freedom from significant incompetence for allograft valves treated with PSKA and followed postoperatively. The causes of incompetence are individually assessed as for Fig. 7. The data set is the same as in Fig. 1, 2 and 6.
Reproduced with permission from Barratt-Boyes et al. (5).

353

a dramatic reduction in the incidence of cusp rupture. In addition, peripheral leak has been abolished (one proven example amongst 237 followed patients) due at least in part to the improved techniques of insertion following the introduction of vertical mattress sutures to the double suture line technique (1, 2). Endocarditis has also been an uncommon cause of significant incompetence (Fig. 8).

There is a relationship between the low incidence of allograft valve endocarditis and the absence of perivalvar leak, for the latter is much more common when a stent is present and in those circumstances is frequently complicated by infection. The absence of a stent in the freehand aortic allograft technique is thus beneficial in three ways: it minimises perivalvar leak, lessens the incidence of perioperative and late stage endocarditis, and lessens the transvalvar gradient.

Incremental risk factors for significant incompetence

It is important to look at the factors which increase the risk of significant incompetence due to valve degeneration or wear (primarily cusp rupture, but for completeness both the "unknown" cases and those when competence is thought to be due to a "central leak" are included). Incompetence due to endocarditis is excluded. The cohort of patients using this multivariate analysis is the same as that already presented in Figs. 1, 2, 6, 8, and is an essentially unselected series operated upon by five surgeons. Patient age varied from 10—76 years (mean 51 years). 61 patients had previous aortic valve surgery. The antibiotic solution used (PSKA) is shown in Table 3. The valves were collected cleanly at coroner's post mortem examinations as sterile collection had been considered too limiting when large numbers of valves were being used. Wet storage in Hanks' solution at 4 °C for periods of up to 3 months indicates from information now available that these valves were all non-viable. While we now realise that this non-viable valve almost certainly behaves less well than the so-called "viable" valve, which we and others are now using, much can be learnt from this analysis.

The total incidence of significant allograft valve incompetence from all causes in this cohort is presented in Fig. 6. The time of censoring in this series was reoperation or death from significant (moderate or severe) incompetence or, in patients still alive and not reoperated upon, the status in this regard at last follow-up. If the time of appearance of significant incompetence is used for censoring, the curve moves to the left. We have not used this because it has not been possible to review every patient and assess the degree of incompetence at yearly intervals, and because the

Table 3. PSKA antibiotic solution.

Penicillin	50 µg/ml
Streptomycin	1000 µg/ml
Kanamycin	1000 µg/ml
Amphotericin	25 µg/ml

In TC 199 or Hanks' solution; clean collection stored at 4 °C for 8 days.

354

Table 4. Significant allograft valve incompetence due to valve wear. Cox proportional hazards model (n = 228).

Incremental risk factor	Coefficient ± SD	P value
Donor age > 50 yr	1.12 ± 0.30	0.0002
*Aortic root diameter > 30 mm	1.39 ± 0.41	0.0007
Recipient age < 15 yr	2.03 ± 0.61	0.0008

* Corresponds to allograft valve internal diameter > 28 mm.

initial onset of moderate incompetence is seldom associated with symptoms or disability. Clearly, reoperation alone is not a satisfactory censoring point.

The Cox proportional hazards model analysis of incremental risk factors in relation to significant homograft valve incompetence due to valve degeneration or wear are listed in Table 4. Both donor age and aortic root diameter are also significant as continuous variables but are most significant when categorised as in Table 4. An aortic root diameter > 30 mm corresponds to an allograft valve internal diameter > 28 mm. This factor loses significance when a large aortic root is reduced in diameter to > 30 mm by excision of a segment of the non-coronary aortic sinus extending downwards into the adjacent mitral leaflet (aortic root tailoring) (3). Aortic root tailoring is performed only when root tissues are strong and not when there is medionecrosis. It is particularly useful in rheumatic chronic severe aortic incompetence when the aortic ring diameter may be 34 mm or more in association with a still normal ascending aortic diameter (24 mm or so). If aortic root tailoring is not performed, this particularly deserving group of patients is excluded. The final variable, patient age, is not significant in this data set as a continuous variable but only when the patient is < 20 years and most significantly, when < 15 years (children). However, as there were only five children in the set, the information remains suspect. A similar analysis reported by O'Brien et al. (4) also showed that donor age and patient age were significant factors. Aortic root diameter did not appear, however, perhaps because there were few, if any, large aortic roots.

Low risk and high risk groups

When patients are categorised into low risk and high risk groups according to whether all the risk factors are absent or one or more are present (5) (Fig. 9), it can be seen that in the low risk group, which comprises the majority of the patients (n = 144), there was only a 2 % incidence of significant incompetence at 5 years and 6% at 9 years. After 9—10 years however, the rate increases more dramatically. To obtain the total incidence of significant incompetence, that due to endocarditis must be added (Fig. 10). This increases the incidence by about 3%.

There is one other report in the literature (6) which analyses an 11-year follow-up of antibiotic sterilised allograft aortic valves inserted in patients with aortic roots < 28 mm and donors < 50 years of age (corresponding therefore to our low risk group). Of the 194 patients there were only three reoperations for cusp rupture. The

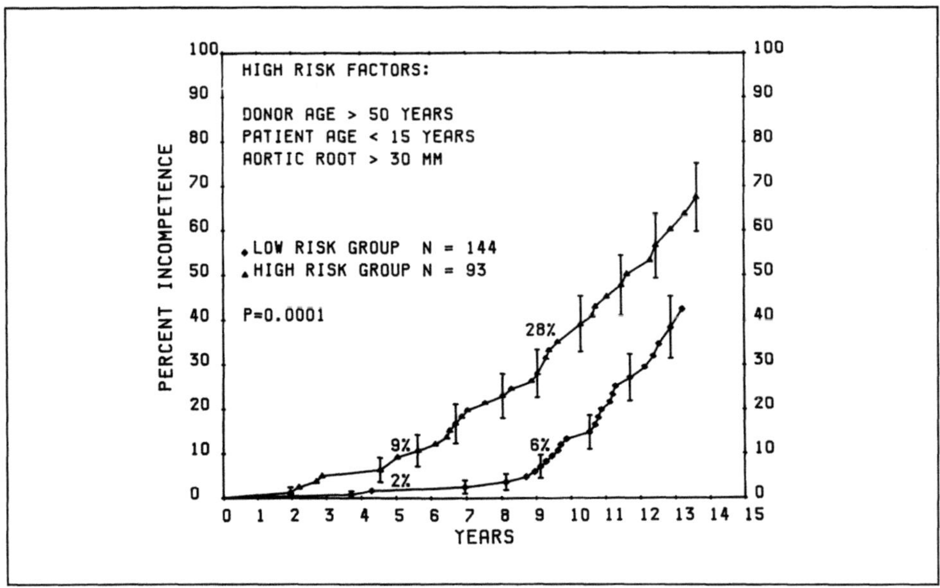

Fig. 9. Actuarial incidence of significant incompetence in PSKA treated allograft valves according to whether the incremental risk factors are included (high risk group) or excluded (low risk group). The bars represent 70% confidence limits.

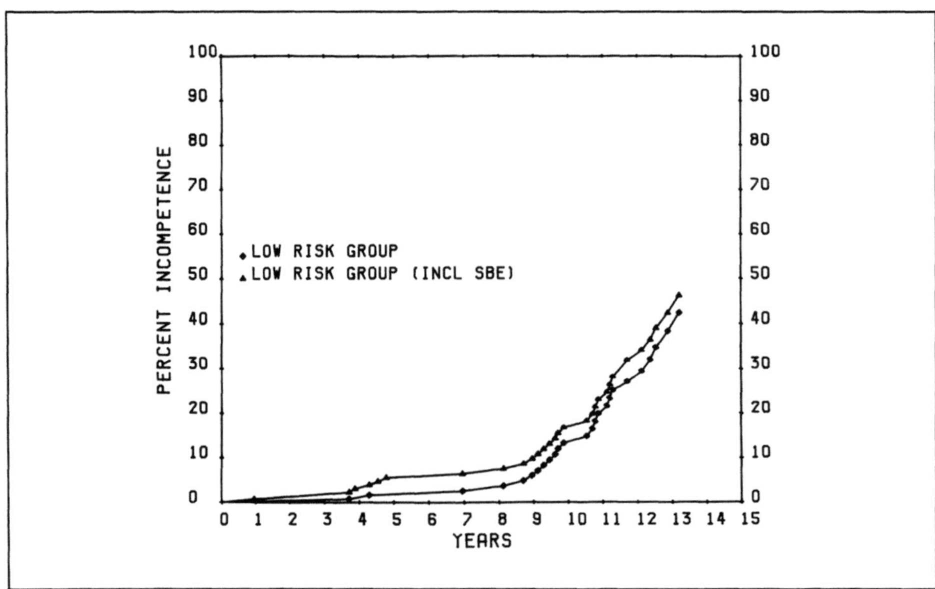

Fig. 10. Actuarial incidence of significant incompetence in allograft valves treated with PSKA in the low risk group with and without the addition of endocarditis.

356

actuarial incidence of reoperation at 10 years was approximately 9%. In comparison, the reoperation incidence in the "viable" valve series recently reported by O'Brien et al. (4) was also 9% at 10 years. There is thus no significant difference between these two series and our own. However, O'Brien's analysis failed to reveal any example of cusp rupture in the reoperated patients, a finding which may be of considerable significance. The histological findings in the viable valves (vide infra) would suggest that this valve will behave considerably better beyond 10 years than the PSKA non-viable valve.

The effect of valve sterilisation and storage on graft changes post-implantation

This discussion is based mainly on our own data supplemented by other reports in the literature where appropriate. There are five GLH published studies which are particularly pertinent to this matter. The first is that by Girinath et al. (7) which reports the results of *tissue culture studies* on dogs' antibiotic-treated (PSKA) aortic valves stored in nutrient medium at 4 °C for varying periods (Table 5). The point of most interest is the finding that a positive growth was present after 1 week's storage in 62% of valves. Electron microscopy performed prior to mincing the specimens, showed lethal damage to many of the cells at 24 h and almost all at 1 week. However, not all the cells showed similar changes, emphasising that tissue culture is not quantitative. Moreover, cellular viability does not recognise damage to the leaflet ground substance which is probably more important in altering the host reaction than fibroblast viability. It is known from other studies that after 1 week in PSKA all the cells die after implantation and the ground substance is so altered that minimal host ingrowth occurs.

The next study details the *electron microscopy findings* in the fibroblasts of canine heart valves with and without antibiotic treatment (Table 6) (8). In comparison with

Table 5. Dog valve tissue culture studies. Antibiotic-treated (PSKA) stored in TC 199 at 4 °C.

n	storage time	+ve growth
60	24 h	93%
60	1 week	62%
60	2 weeks	15%
60	3 weeks	Nil

Salvage time < 2 h.

Table 6. Dog valve electron microscopy studies.

1. Immediate fixation
2. Storage in Hanks' without antibiotics*
3. Storage in Hanks' with PSKA*
4. Storage in TC 199 with PSKA*
5. Storage in TC 199 with Angell soln*

* Examined after 1, 2 and 3 weeks storage at 4 °C.

357

Table 7. Dog implant studies: Stented aortic allografts in mitral position.

1. Sterile collection — Hanks' only — implanted after 1—2 days;
   n = 13
2. Antibiotic (PSKA) in Hanks' — implanted after 1—32 weeks;
   n = 26
   Salvage time < 2 h
   Explanted serially from 2d — 522d
   Light and electron microscopy

the control normal leaflet fixed immediately after removal from the donor dog, leaflets stored in Hanks' solution only for 1 week show only minor reversible changes and were therefore viable, while by 2 weeks there was lethal damage in many cells. When antibiotics were aded, lethal changes were present at 1 week and there was no difference whether the PSKA treated valve was stored in Hanks' solution or TC199. However, when Angell's less concentrated antibiotic solution was used (9), the onset of lethal changes was delayed compared with PSKA. These findings re-emphasise that both the concentration of the antibiotics and the time they are in contact with the valve, influence fibroblast viability.
In the next study (10) (Table 7), *dog aortic allograft valves were implanted into the mitral position mounted on stents.* They were either viable or nonviable at implan-

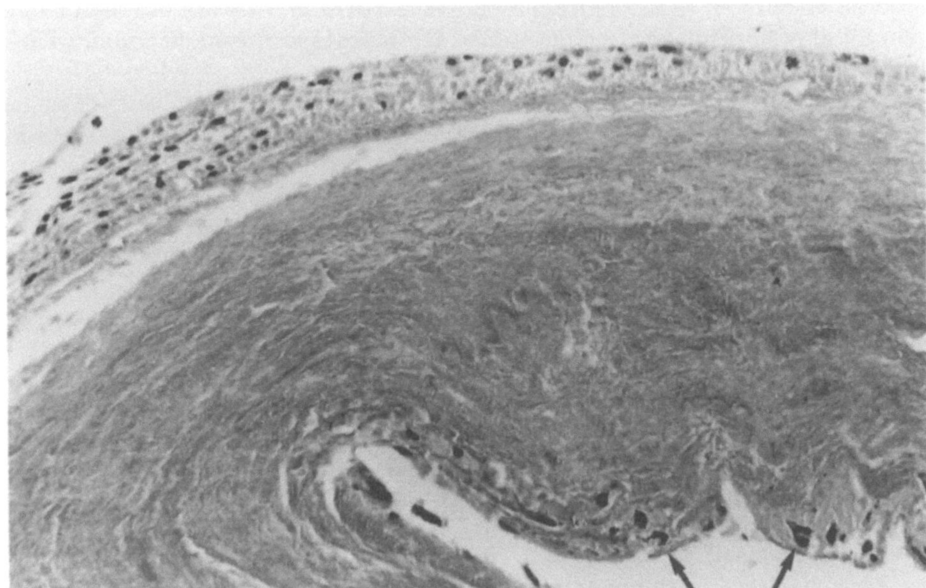

Fig. 11. The cusp of PSKA treated aortic valve allograft explanted 129 days from the dog after insertion on a stent into the mitral position. The cusp is acellular apart from the intimal fibrous sheath (above) which tapers onto it from its base, and a few leucocytes which are trapped in surface deposits of fibrin (arrows). van Gieson, × 360.
Reproduced with permission from Gavin et al. (10).

tation and were explanted serially from 2 days to 1.4 years and then submitted to light and electron microscopy. The PSKA non-viable valve leaflets rapidly became acellular and remained essentially acellular as the host intimal fibrous sheath was poorly developed and there was minimal or absent host tissue ingrowth into the leaflet (Fig. 11). The viable valves initially behaved similarly as they also rapidly became acellular. Thus (Fig. 12) after 1 week the fibroblasts were pyknotic on light microscopy and electron microscopy confirmed they were dead or dying. Within a month or so, all were devoid of typical donor cells, but as with the PSKA leaflet the intimal fibrous sheath extended irregularly across the leaflet, usually for greater distances than with the antibiotic leaflet. The importance of the host intimal fibrous sheath cannot be over-emphasised for we believe it plays a very important in the subsequent behaviour of the cusp. This host reaction was well described by Mohri et al. (11) (Fig. 13) and is often easily seen in the gross specimen. Unfortunately, it does not form as a continuous sheet, but rather as a fingerlike process extending both from the base, and also from the commissural areas along the free edge in some instances, but leaving areas of cusp uncovered (Fig. 14). The essential difference between the so-called viable valve and the PSKA treated valve is that in the viable valve there is ingrowth into the leaflet of cells from the sheath, perhaps supplemented in the hinge area by direct ingrowth from the adjacent host tissue. The initial ingrowth appears to be by macrophages which sometimes form giant cells and can be seen often with clear spaces around them, suggesting that they are digesting the acellular, rather homogenous collagenous ground substance of the cusp. Beneath the macrophages, immature fibroblasts are seen forming new cellular cusp tissue (Fig. 15). A bizarre example of this process is seen in Fig. 16 which is a section from a viable dog allograft valve explanted at 1.4 years. There is abundant loose fibrous connective tissue increasing the leaflet thickness to three or four times the normal.

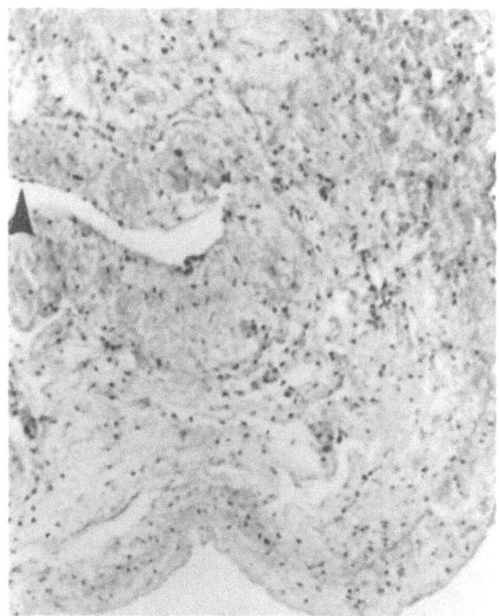

Fig. 12. The cusp of an untreated (viable) aortic allograft valve explanted after one week. Some endothelial cells persist (arrow) but most have been lost and the fibroblasts are pyknotic. H and E, × 50.
Reproduced with permission from Gavin et al. (10).

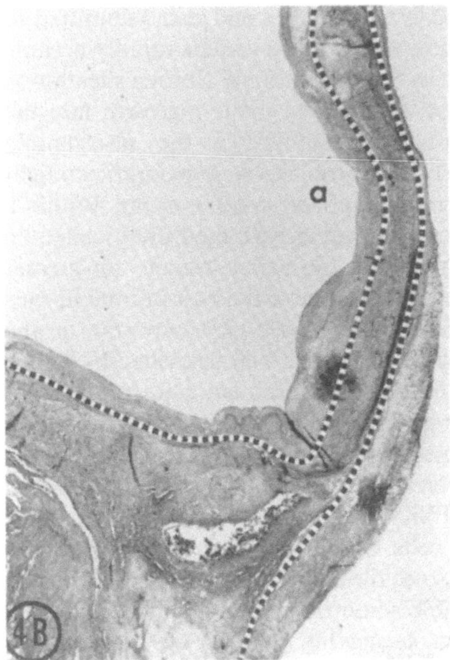

Fig. 13. An untreated (viable) dog aortic allograft valve explanted after 23 months. It shows prominent thickening of the valve leaflet due to extension of a connective tissue sheath (intimal fibrous sheath) along both surfaces of the leaflet. The sheath is more extensive on the aortic side (a). The extent of the original graft is outlined. Verhoeff-van Gieson stain × 4.
Reproduced with permission from Mohri et al. (11).

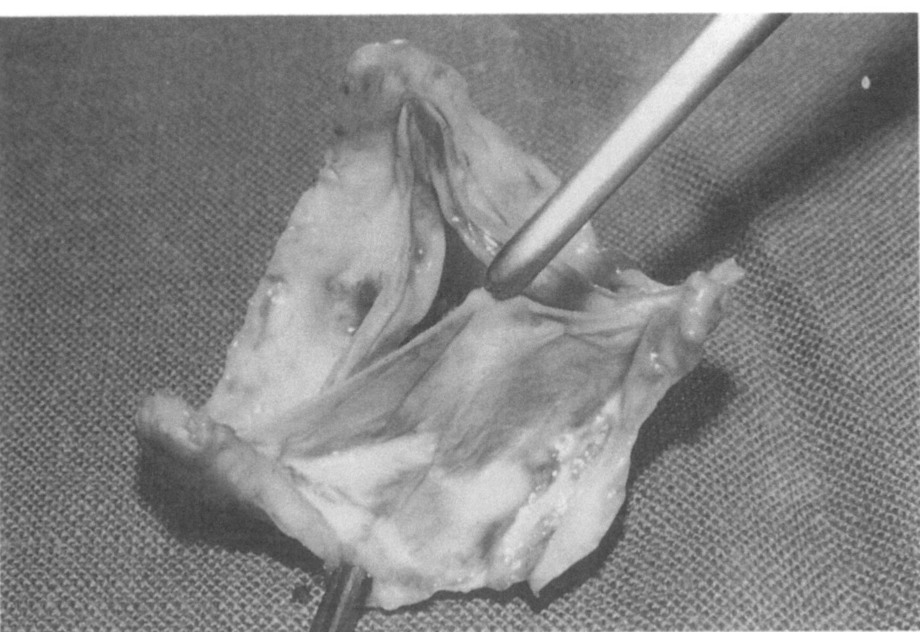

Fig. 14. Gross specimen of a human PSKA treated allograft valve removed at 10 months because of central incompetence due to progressive dilatation of the host aortic sinuses and root. The intimal fibrous sheath can be seen extending on the aortic aspect of the leaflet as a fingerlike process maximal in the hinge area.

360

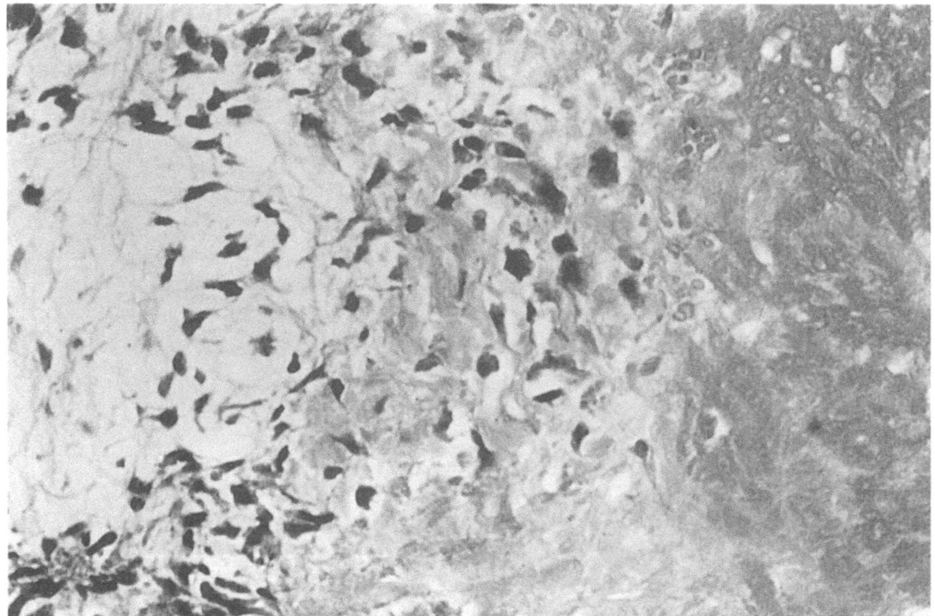

Fig. 15. Untreated (viable) fresh dog allograft valve removed at approximately 4 months. This section demonstrates the classical macrophage reaction characteristic of grafts in which the ground substance of the leaflet has not been importantly damaged by the method of sterilisation and preservation. The dense amorphous acellular collagenous tissue of the graft lies to the right. To the left is an area of young fibrous tissue containing fibroblasts (stellate cells) and between these two zones an area containing plump macrophages, many of which are surrounded by clear spaces. It is presumed that the macrophages are ingesting the collagenous tissue of the cusp and that this is gradually replaced by the advancing edge of new fibrous tissue. H and E × 650.

It is well known that these histological changes are much more rapid and florid in the dog model than in the human allograft valve.

This difference in the ingrowth pattern between the viable graft and the PSKA graft has led us to postulate that the antibiotics (as well as various chemicals and irradiation) not only kill the fibroblasts but also damage the leaflet ground substance. Otherwise, why sould the host cells not repopulate the PSKA leaflets?

The fourth study concerns the *histological findings in the GLH untreated viable human allograft valve series.* Four of this original series of 16 such valves that were unquestionably viable at insertion (on the basis of the evidence already presented in Table 6) have become available for histological study (Table 8). They show essentially the same features as the dog valves although slower to develop and less florid. Thus, the specimen stored for 3 days and explanted at 9 months shows a fairly well marked intimal fibrous sheath (Fig. 17), with a commencing ingrowth pattern (Fig. 18). The specimen stored for 5 days and explanted at 5 years (Fig. 19) shows an extensive intimal fibrous sheath which covers the whole surface of the leaflet except for the extreme tip and is associated on its deep surface with excessive production of new fibrous tissue containing an excess of acid mucopolysaccharide ground sub-

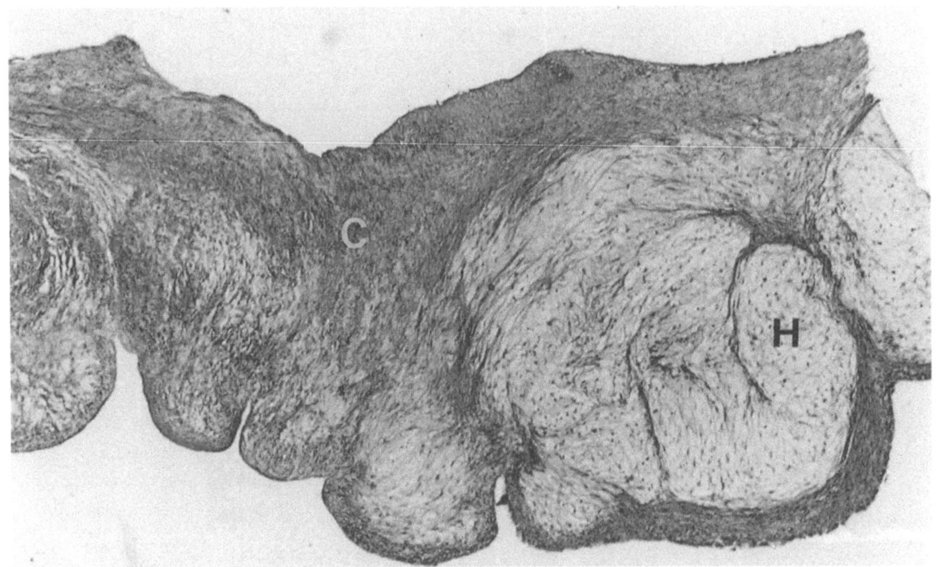

Fig. 16. Untreated fresh (viable) aortic allograft valve explanted after 522 days from the dog. The cusp (C) shows infiltrations and nodular thickening by immature, cellular host tissue (H). van Gieson, × 125.
Reproduced with permission from Gavin et al. (10).

Table 8. Human untreated allograft valves.

Storage time (h)	Months in recipient
3	9
4	42
5	65
3	110

Salvage time < 24 h; sterile collection Hanks' solution without antibiotics.

stance. The entire leaflet is highly cellular and potentially a permanent graft, although the structure is not that of a normal leaflet. The interface between the intimal fibrous sheath and the underlying graft tissue shows the usual macrophages (Fig. 20).
Unfortunately there are few other studies of late histological findings in human viable grafts. Material recently published by O'Brien (4, 13) is similar as it also shows loss of donor cells with collagenous acellular tissue and significant leaflet thickening. O'Brien's demonstration at 9 years in one explanted valve of surviving donor fibroblasts, using sex chromatin studies to establish this (4, 13) indicates that donor fibroblasts can occasionally survive. Presumably this depends upon the host rejection response, which may rarely be absent. The canine studies undertaken by Mohri

362

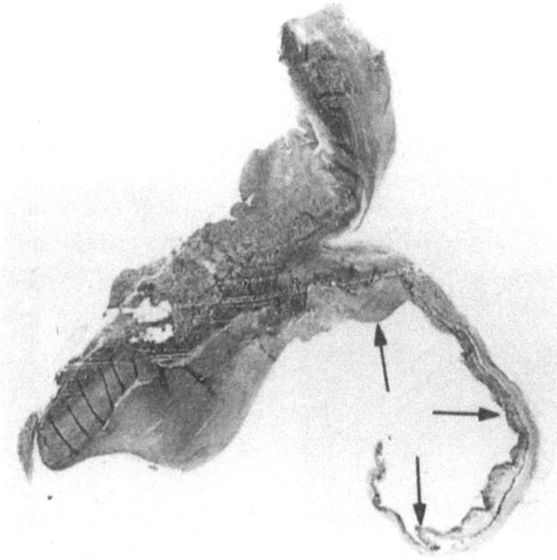

Fig. 17. Untreated fresh (viable) human allograft aortic valve explanted after 36 weeks. An intimal fibrous sheath (arrows) thickens the proximal two-thirds of the cusp. H and E × 9.
Reproduced with permission from Gavin et al. (12).

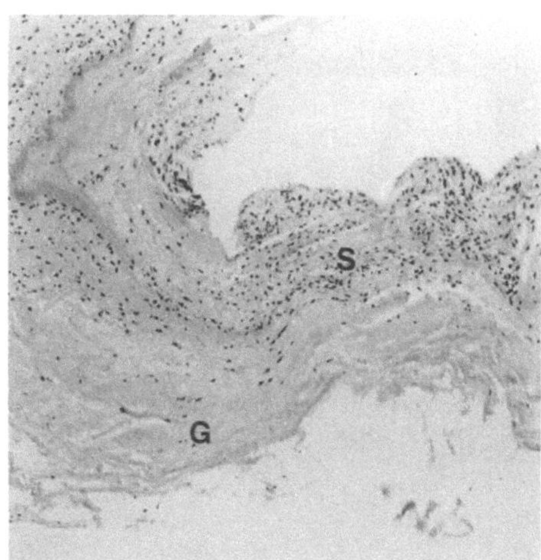

Fig. 18. The same cusp as in Fig. 17 examined under higher magnification. Fibroblasts from the more cellular intimal fibrous sheath above (S) extend into the less cellular graft beneath (G). H and E × 165.
Reproduced with permission from Gavin et al. (12).

et al. (11, 14) appear to show progressive loss of donor fibroblasts such that by 2 months 30% of the cells were sex chromatin positive but by 6 months only 15% could be so identified.

The final GLH study addresses the vitally important question as to whether the antibiotic solution can be modified so that it will not damage the leaflet ground substance and thereby allow host tissue ingrowth to occur. This question is important because a bacteriologically competent non-toxic antibiotic solution would allow us to disinfect valves harvested cleanly at post mortem examination by the pathologist, rather than confine ourselves only to valves obtained by sterile techniques, and would thereby increase the number of valves available for a valve bank, particularly now that cryopreservation techniques appear to allow indefinite preservation of leaflet integrity.

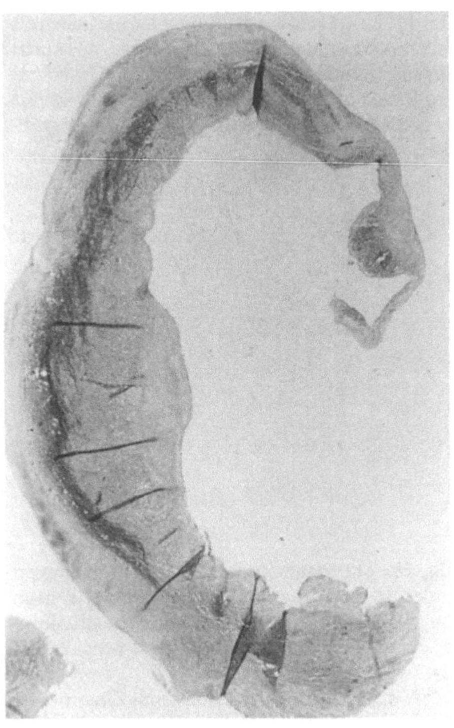

Fig. 19. Untreated, fresh (viable) human allograft valve explanted after 262 weeks. A bulky intimal fibrous sheath covers virtually the entire length of the ventricular side of the cusp (to the left) and is less extensive on the aortic side (to the right). The extreme tip of the cusp is not covered by intimal fibrous sheath and is much thinner. The acid mucopolysaccharide ground substance is plentiful. The entire leaflet is cellular. See text. Alcian blue × 5.

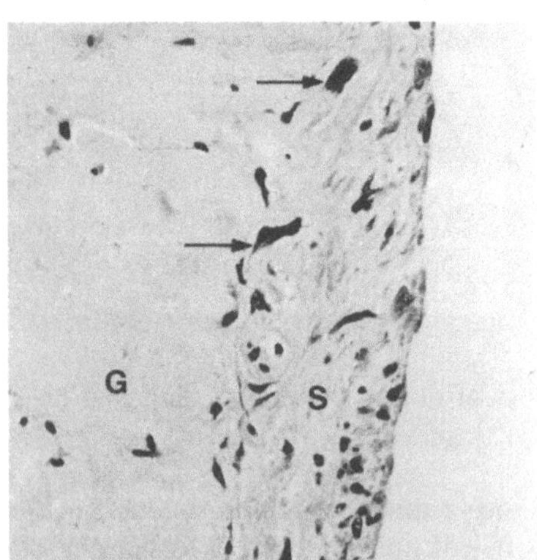

Fig. 20. The same specimen as in Fig. 19. The interface between the intimal fibrous sheath (S) and the underlying much less cellular cusp (G) of the allograft is well displayed. Macrophages (arrows) are prominent along this interface. H and E × 650.
Reproduced with permission from Gavin et al. (12).

The solution used by O'Brien, which contains penicillin 50 units/ml, streptomycin 5 μg/ml and amphotericin 10 μg/ml in TC199 will not disinfect valves harvested cleanly at post mortem examination and stored at 4 °C. It was for this reason that our PSKA solution contained antibiotics in higher concentration, including kana-

mycin, and remained in contact with the tissue for 8 days, rather than the 24 h at
37 °C used by O'Brien. However, as we have demonstrated, this methodology results
in an acellular valve prone to cusp rupture, and is therefore unacceptable. Dr. Seelye,
a biochemist in our department, postulated that the beta-lactam ring of penicillin
causes cross-linkage of the collagen fibres similar to that produced by glutaraldehyde, and that the strongly basic aminoglycosides, streptomycin and kanamycin,
combine with the acid mucopolysaccharide ground substance. There could be other
mechanisms which alter the ground substance and prevent host tissue ingrowth into
the graft. Accordingly, we set about formulating a bacteriologically competent antibiotic solution which avoided penicillin and aminoglycosides, was much less concentrated, and required only a short exposure time (48 h). After extensive testing of
many solutions, "CLPVA" was selected (Table 9). To assess whether this solution
would result in a host reaction similar to that produced by an untreated completely
fresh allograft, a series of implant studies using single aortic allograft cusps were
commenced in the dog in 1976. The protocol used in these studies is summarised
in Table 10 (16). All these leaflets were explanted at 4 months and examined blindly
by the pathologist to assess leaflet cellularity with the various types of preimplant
preparation. The results can be summarised by stating that the untreated leaflet
implanted immediately (the control group), the untreated leaflets stored in Hanks'
at 4 °C for 6 days, and the CLPVA leaflet which was immersed in the antibiotic for
2 days and then in Hanks' without antibiotic for a further 4 days, all showed an
identical degree of leaflet cellularity when examined at 4 months (Fig. 21, 22, 23).
The cryopreserved untreated leaflets were also similar, the cellularity being perhaps
a little less than the other three groups but without any statistically significant dif-

Table 9. CLPVA antibiotic solution.

Cefoxitin	240 µg/ml
Lincomycin	120 µg/ml
Polymyxin B	100 µg/ml
Vancomycin	50 µg/ml
Amphotericin B	25 µg/ml

In Hanks' solution
Clean collection
Stored at 4 °C for 48 h

Table 10. Dog implant studies: Freehand single aortic allograft cusp in aortic position.

1. Untreated (viable) — immediate implantation   n = 6
2. Untreated. Hanks' 4 °C for 6 days   n = 4
3. Untreated. Cryopreservation within 24 h   n = 5
4. Antibiotic (PSKA) Hanks' 4 °C for 8 days   n = 7
5. Antibiotic (CLPVA) Hanks' 2 days + Hanks' alone 4 days   n = 7

Explanted at 4 months
Examined by light microscopy to assess ingrowth pattern
Salvage time < 2 h

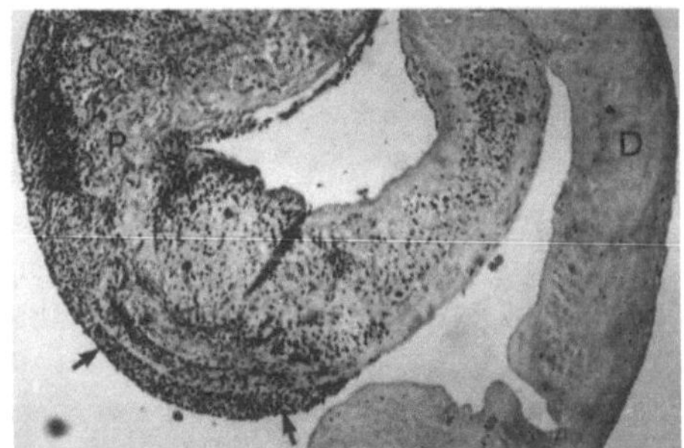

Fig. 21. Untreated fresh (viable) dog allograft leaflet explanted at 4 months. The section shows a cellular proximal hinge region (P) and a largely acellular, apparently structureless distal region (D). The cellular elements of the former are derived from ingrowth of host tissue both into and onto (arrows) the base of the grafted leaflet. The arrows depict the surface of the intimal fibrous sheath. H and E × 50.
Reproduced with permission from Armiger et al. (16).

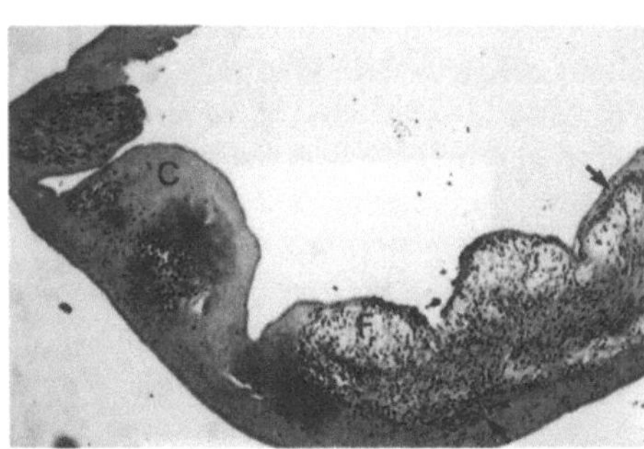

Fig. 22. Untreated fresh dog leaflet stored for 6 days in sterile Hanks' solution at 4 °C prior to implantation. The section examined at 4 months shows lack of endothelium and an amorphous appearance of the original connective tissue (C) which is being progressively replaced by loosely organised, proliferating host fibrous tissue (F) with peripheral infiltrates consisting largely of macrophages (arrows). The large focus of fibrous tissue extended throughout the proximal half of the leaflet and the ingrowth pattern was therefore classed as good and comparable to that with the fresh leaflet (Fig. 21). H and E × 50.
Reproduced with permission from Armiger et al. (16).

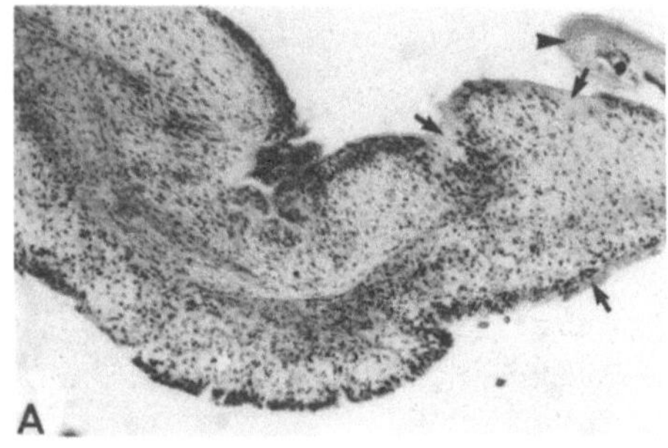

Fig. 23. CLPVA treated dog allograft leaflet examined at 4 months showing particularly good ingrowth of host element.
(A) Shows the distal half of the leaflet. There is only a narrow rim of uncolonised tissue (arrows) persisting adjacent to the completely uncolonised free edge (arrow head) at the extreme tip of the leaflet. H and E × 50.
(B) Detail of parts of another leaflet showing macrophages (arrows) lying between the uncolonised tissue (U) and the loosely organised endothelialised (arrow head) fibrous connective tissue (F) occupying the remainder of the cusp. H and E × 150.
Reproduced with permission from Armiger et al. (16).

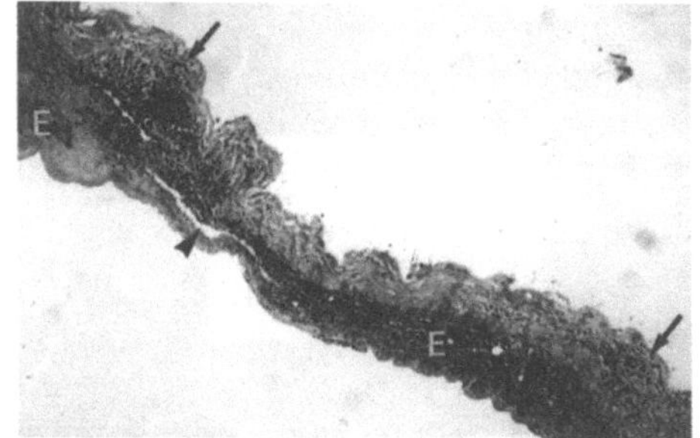

Fig. 24. PSKA treated allograft dog leaflet examined at 4 months. This proximal portion of the leaflet shows aggregates of red blood cells (E) present in two still uncolonised areas. A cellular infiltrate focally mixed with varying amounts of young, proliferating fibrous connective tissue (arrows) extends irregularly through the leaflet. Two large rents (arrow heads) are present in this area and the uncolonised connective tissue of the upper surface shows marked separation of its collagenous components. The degree of fibrous tissue ingrowth is poor. H and E × 50.
Reproduced with permission from Armiger et al. (16).

ference. In contrast, the PSKA treated leaflet (Fig. 24) showed much less cellularity, a less well-developed host intimal fibrous sheath, areas of separation of the collagen bundles and foci of intracusp haemorrhage. On the basis of our earlier experiments already outlined, we interpret these changes as a host ingrowth pattern into the donor leaflet. As all these leaflets were explanted at 4 months we do not know what they were like at 1 month but we can safely assume that they were then largely acellular. Whether the cellularity at 4 months is indeed persistence of donor cells or a host ingrowth phenomenon is however of little moment practically. The important point is that the CLPVA treated leaflet is apparently identical to the so-called "viable" leaflet. On the basis of these animal experiments, all human allograft tissue is now treated using the CLPVA solution which remains in contact with the cusp for 48 h at 4 °C. Thereafter the leaflet is transferred to TC199 without antibiotics and is stored at 4 °C until cryopreserved. Ideally, cryopreservation is performed within 72 h of collection from the cadaver but up to 5 days is considered acceptable. (The CLPVA valves implanted in the dog studies had been stored at 4 °C for 6 days but the salvage time for these valves was very short, whereas the salvage time in the human cadaver valves extends occasionally up to 36 h but is usually less than 24 h).

Conclusions

The following conclusions would appear to be justified:
1. Fibroblast viability as assessed by tissue culture is a useful yardstick of leaflet integrity but does not guarantee it. Thus it does not assess the status of the ground substance.
2. Donor fibroblasts usually die within months of implantation whether the fibroblasts are viable at implantation or not.
3. The leaflet is repopulated with fibroblasts largely from the host. In rare instances donor cells may possibly contribute.
4. Antibiotics must be in low concentration and in contact for no more than a few days to prevent damage to the leaflet ground substance.

367

5. CLPVA solution allows clean collection of autopsy specimens (98% are disinfected) and does not damage the leaflet if immersion is limited to 48 h at 4 °C.
6. Storage by cryopreservation at 3—5 days from the time of collection does not further damage leaflet integrity significantly and allows more or less indefinite storage.

Acknowledgements

It is not possible to mention the names of all the surgeons, cardiologists and research personnel who have contributed to this work over the 25-year period. However, I would particularly like to thank Drs. John Gavin and Lois Armiger and Ms. M. Strickett for their contributions to the pathology and microbiology studies. Thanks are also due to Mr. D. Brown for the photography and Ms. K. Martin for typing the manuscript.

References

1. Gonzalez-Lavin L, Barratt-Boyes BG (1969) Surgical considerations in the treatment of ventricular septal defects associated with aortic valvular incompetence. J Thorac Cardiovasc Surg 57: 422
2. Brandt PWT, Roche AHG, Barratt-Boyes BG, Lowe JB (1969) Radiology of homograft aortic valves. Thorax 24: 129
3. Barratt-Boyes BG (1965) A method for preparing and inserting a homograft aortic valve. Br J Surg 52: 847
4. O'Brien MF, Stafford EG, Gardner MAH, Pohlner PG, McGiffin DC A comparison of aortic valve replacement with viable cryopreserved and fresh allograft valves with a note on chromosomal studies. J Thorac Cardiovasc Surg (in press)
5. Barratt-Boyes BG, Roche AHG, Subramanyan R, Pemberton JR, Whitlock RML (1987) Long-term follow up of patients with the antibiotic sterilised aortic homograft valve inserted freehand in the aortic position. Circulation 75: 768
6. Virdi IS, Monro JL, Ross JK (1968) Aortic valve replacement with antibiotic sterilised homograft valves: 11 year experience at Southampton, In: Bodner E, Yacoub M (eds) Biologic and Bioprosthetic Valves. Yorke Medical Books, USA, Chapt 5
7. Girinath MR, Gavin JB, Strickett MG, Barratt-Boyes BG (1974) The effects of antibiotics and storage on the viability and ultrastructure of fibroblasts in canine heart valves prepared for grafting. Aust NZ J Surg 44: 170
8. Gavin JB, Monro JL, Wall FM, Chalcroft SCW (1973) Fine structural changes in the fibroblasts of canine heart valves prepared for grafting. Thorax 28: 748
9. Angell WW, Shumway NE, Kosek JC (1972) A 5 year study of viable aortic valve homografts. J Thorac Cardiovasc Surg 64: 329
10. Gavin JB, Monro JL (1974) The pathology of pulmonary and aortic valve allografts used as mitral valve replacements in dogs. Pathology 6: 119
11. Mohri H, Reichenbach DD, Barnes RW, Merendino KA (1968) Homologous aortic valve transplantation. Alterations in viable and non-viable valves. J Thorac Cardiovasc Surg 56: 767
12. Gavin JB, Barratt-Boyes BG, Hitchcock GC, Herdson PB (1973) Histopathology of "fresh" human aortic valve allografts. Thorax 28: 482
13. O'Brien MF, Stafford G, Gardner M, Pohlner P, McGiffin D, Johnston N, Brosnan A, Duffy P (1987) The viable cryopreserved allograft aortic valve. J Cardiac Surg 1: 153
14. Mohri H, Reichenbach DD, Barnes RW, Merendino KA (1967) A biologic study of the homologous aortic valve in dogs. J Thorac Cardiovasc Surg 54: 622

15. Strickett MG, Barratt-Boyes BG, MacCulloch D (1983) Disinfection of human heart valve allografts with antibiotics in low concentration. Pathology 15: 457
16. Armiger LC, Gavin JB, Barratt-Boyes BG (1983) Histological assessment of orthotopic aortic valve leaflet allografts: its role in selecting graft pretreatment. Pathology 15: 67

Author's address:
Brian Barratt-Boyes, M.D.
Cardiothoracic Surgical Unit
Green Lane Hospital
Auckland, New Zealand

Panel Discussion

Chaired by: W. W. Angell, J. Somerville

Panelists:
B. Barratt-Boyes, New Zealand
R. Hetzer, Germany
J. Kirklin, USA
M. O'Brien, Australia
A. C. Yankah, Germany

ANGELL:

We would like to use the panel for two purposes: One is to answer the questions from the audience, and the other is to have the panelists sum up their opinions on the results of the information which has been made available to them during the conference.

BANK:

Question to Sir Brian Barratt-Boyes: As regards your examination of Dr. O'Brien's antibiotic solution for the autopsy valve specimens, I imagine that there are quite a number of breakthroughs. Would these breakthroughs be due to the presence of penicillin or R-factor containing microbes or was it simply a generalized failure due to insufficient strength of the antibiotics? Did you test for a specific resistence to those antibiotics?

BARRATT-BOYES:

The microbiologists tested pulmonary valves collected cleanly at autopsy and used a number of solutions to see whether they could sterilise them. The solution of Dr. O'Brien's will not sterilise valves collected in this way.

BANK:

Did they test to see whether the bacteria present in the autopsy specimens were resistent specifically to the penicillin? There are a number of R-factors which can force simultaneous resistence.

BARRATT-BOYES:

You'd have to ask the microbiologists that question. I do not know.

SOMERVILLE:

I think there are a number of problems which need to be considered. I would like to ask the panel what they think the role of the pulmonary autograft should be. Provided you know how to put it in without regurgitation and you avoid the large aortic root it does seem to be the valve that is living and does not fail other than from endocarditis.

BARRATT-BOYES:

I feel guilty that I cannot or have not done this operation and that Donald Ross does that so well, because there is no question, it is a very good operation. We have used pulmonary valve in many situations but never for aortic valve replacement. I suppose it is a question of "grabbing the nettle" and trying it. If we are going to move in that direction there will be significant mortality and morbidity until the technique is learned. I think that is what puts most of us off and Mr. Ross too, had a significant mortality and morbidity in the early stages. We would all agree that it is more difficult to put in. It is anatomically a different valve than the homograft.

SOMERVILLE:

I can confirm that the mortality was high in the first 20 patients. It was quite frightening. Part of that mortality related to inadequate myocardial protection and long bypass times. It is a technically more demanding and difficult operation. In the last 50 cases, complications were higher than with other aortic valve replacement but I think it is acceptable, bearing in mind the good long-term results. The learning curve is very difficult.

BODNAR:

Over the past 11 years there were 65 patients operated on. All 65 are alive today. There was zero operative mortality, zero post-operative mortality, and five patients had to be reoperated, one for right-sided homograft failure, one for an infective endocarditis, and three we believe for technical problems.

BARRATT-BOYES:

There is one other point which I want to mention. The curves of significant incompetence from your institution for that valve are no better than the curves of significant incompetence that many people have presented today. There are significant technical problems which are not necessarily evident initially but which produce incompetence. The etiology must be different, but it is certainly not free of significant late incompetence. Is that correct?

BODNAR:

Yes. But those curves which you have seen were spanning over a 20-year period, and I was referring to the last 10 years.

SOMERVILLE:

It is true that there is more aortic regurgitation than in the aortic homograft. Mild to moderate aortic regurgitation does not require reoperation. A progressive condition is a problem and that has to be accepted.

O'BRIEN:

I am not too sure that we should accept it, Dr. Somerville. It is a wonderful valve and I think it is perhaps the ideal valve for a young woman of childbearing age. But if the learning curve is going to be so difficult then are we justified in doubling the mortality in a young person when we know the allograft can be re-operated in a second decade. I am not sure we can double our mortality to go through a learning curve. We have to be assured of doing 10 or 20 a year. I have been challenged often about whether I should commence using autografts and I have not made a decision. If I did, I would spend a lot of time in the autopsy room and with animal specimens doing the exact operation. Probably in that way the learning curve may be improved.

TRENKNER:

A few years ago we investigated the pulmonary valve in a laboratory study in vitro. There are several factors that may contribute to success, in the early post-operative period. First of all, the pulmonary leaflet has exactly the same breaking strength as the aortic leaflet, even though it is half as thick as the aortic leaflet. Secondly the pulmonary valve distensibility is at the lowest level of the leaflet attachment. It is less than the distensibility of the aortic valve at the same pressure. It reaches a plateau at approximately 20—30 mmHg while the aortic ring at this level reaches a plateau at pressures above 30 mmHg. So, even if it is not contained in the aortic root, this feature prevents leaking from central incompetence. At the level of commissures, the pulmonary valve is much more distensible than the aorta and this contributes to the lifting of the free margin of the leaflets, increases the coaptation area and makes the valve more competent at higher aortic pressures. Thirdly, the geometry of the pulmonary valve, when loaded with the aortic pressure three times higher than pulmonary assumes the geometry of the aortic valve and the forces acting upon the leaflet are roughly the same. Thus there is the same breaking strength of the leaflet and the same forces acting to balance the situation. Finally, by extrapolation of our study, the dynamic load of the valve transplanted from the pulmonary orifice to the aortic orifice has a similar dP/dt, unlike in the mitral position where the rise in the ventricular pressure is very sharp.

GONZALEZ-LAVIN:

Just a word of encouragement for Sir Brian and Dr. O'Brien and all of you who have experience with homograft aortic valve replacement. I have performed about 20 pulmonary valve switches into the aortic position. I helped Mr. Ross with quite a few cases and mortality at that time was 8%. Most of the patients have done very well, as reported by Dr. Bodnar.

KIRKLIN:

Do you currently do this operation?

GONZALEZ-LAVIN:

I am not planning to continue this procedure even though this is probably the best valve for a young patient.

SOMERVILLE:

It is currently done fairly routinely in the Heart Hospital for young patients. In some cases, we find a pulmonary valve that is bicuspid. In my opinion it is the valve of choice, provided the aortic root is not too dilated, in young patients, provided Mr. Ross is available to do it.

O'BRIEN:

It is very difficult to justify this procedure in a young person when aortic valve replacement mortality should be less than 1% in this group.

ANGELL:

Have you considered this procedure in Alabama?

KIRKLIN:

No, we have not. There has been consideration of it, but none of us has taken the step to do it. In the young patient you would expect an operative mortality which approaches zero. In our homograft experience since 1981, we have a zero hospital mortality for isolated primary aortic valve replacement. We have been a bit reluctant to embark on this procedure when we believed the operative risk would be tripled. Perhaps, however, we are wrong.

SOMERVILLE:

At Alabama, you took a long time to change from the atrial buffle for transposition of the great arteries before you switched the great arteries for exactly the same reasons. Now everyone who is able is switching the great arteries. It is the same philosophy on switching to the pulmonary autograft. There is the moment when you may have to take courage, even if we have not arrived at the justification on the basis of improved results. Improvement must be judged not only in terms of mortality and morbidity at the beginning, but also the complications and need for timing and problems of reoperation in long term survivors.

KIRKLIN:

I might argue that I am not sure that by placing an aortic valve homograft, the patient's life expectancy is reduced. Even if he requires three operations over a lifetime it is not the same as the difference between atrial baffle and aortic switch.

SOMERVILLE:

You may be right. I was referring to the concept of change.

BODNAR:

This slide from Mr. Ross is a homograft which is clearly non-viable. This by contrast is how a viable cusp looks 3 years after surgery in a pulmonary switch patient who died in an accident.

ELLIOTT:

Would someone comment on the possibility of the pulmonary autograft growing as Mr. Ross briefly mentioned yesterday in his presentation?

SOMERVILLE:

It is a dream that the pulmonary autograft might grow. We have no evidence that it does. It does, having living cells, and must have the potential to do so. Patients have not had the operation under 5 years followed for a decade or more. We also have no evidence to say it does not grow. I know Mr. Ross wants to do it in infants to see and have already done the operation in infant aortic stenosis. I wonder if it would be timely to mention the place of the inverted homograft in the mitral position. The subject has been alluded to, I would like to know what the panel feeling is about the use of the homograft in the mitral position. I know there were many techniques.

374

ANGELL:

We have a large series of these patients. The use of the stented homograft is an easy operation. Personally, I would like to wait until a few more of the answers on viable homografts before embarking on any substantial move back towards that technique. The survival of the homograft valve is not better than the pig valve in the mitral position. This series applies to patients of all ages. If you ask the same question about a 15-year-old patient the stimulus to get re-involved with stented homografts is greater. I personally would like to wait just a little bit longer and see whether these frozen viable grafts will have a mean survival of 15 or 20 years. We can then look at the comparison with the pig valve again.

BARRATT-BOYES:

I still regard the homograft stented valve to be the best valve in the mitral position in children and use it for that purpose. We know it will fail, but the failure mode is very benign. It does not calcify and we have patients in whom it has lasted for 10, 15 years. It is particularly valuable, too, in our sort of population where the patients cannot take anticoagulants: that is our Polynesian and Maori population. So, all the islanders who come over to Auckland and have mitral valve replacement receive a homograft valve. They do not need anticoagulants. The valve will last 10 to 15 years. For children and young adults who come from the island, we would use stented homograft. I think it does have a place and the reason we do not use it in other patients is because in our experience the failure mode is increased by detachment of the pillars of the antibiotic treated valve from the stent.

SOMERVILLE:

Our experience agrees with Brian in the young patient. I must say the ones not on the semi-rigid stent but in the top hat, of dacron has lasted well and don't need anticoagulants. Magdi Yacoub has a large series and still uses the technique in special cases.

GONZALEZ-LAVIN:

What is your experience at the National Heart with the viable homografts in mitral position?

BODNAR:

I said yesterday that I believe our valves were not viable. Now, as far as the inverted homografts in the mitral position are concerned, there are two distinct series: In one, the valve was mounted on rigid titanium stents and they failed at 7 years, or earlier. In the other series, the stent is called a "top hat", with the homograft within a fully flexible Dacron graft segments diagonal tube on flexible polypropylene stents. There was a big difference between the two curves, in favour of the flexible stent. The top hat series is being reevaluated now.

SOMERVILLE:

We don't have very many patients, young patients now. It is not like it was in the old days. The spectrum of mitral valve disease has changed so much and the demand to have this has changed dramatically in the last ten years. I don't know if that is your experience. I mean, we do not see bad rheumatic mitral disease in the young except from the Middle East and occasionally from endocarditis or congenital mitral abnormality. Always valve conservation has been practised in the National Heart Hospital by Yacoub and Ross, often successfully. Thus it has then been relatively infrequent to require mitral replacement, in children and adolescents.

HETZER:

We do have some mitral disease in young patients, usually from the foreign workers. In almost all children and young adults you can perform a reconstructive mitral valve procedure, with a low risk of re-operation. When the individual reaches an adult age you can perform a replacement on a more secure basis.

SOMERVILLE:

So you think it is the case for going back to the inverted homograft? I believe it is something to be considered, but the technique of mounting is of paramount importance.

DAVIS:

Since 1973, we have had a small experience with 7 mitral homografts treated with antibiotics, which were mounted on rigid titanium frames. Two of these were explanted at 10 and 11 years. One is still functioning at 15 years. I have attended Sir Brians' talks before where he has demonstrated that the aortic wall dehisces. In 1979 we started mounting valve on a polypropylene frame and they are doing very well. 2 weeks ago we had a woman who died and at post mortem we inspected her mitral valve, which had been functioning well, by echo two weeks prior to her death. It looks as if the same mode of failure occurred. We have also done a small number of glutaraldehyde homografts to see whether this will strengthen the aortic wall. On this valve the aortic wall on two of the stent legs came away freely. The quality control of the valves was not very good. We used to put a suture transversely above the commissure, and it has cut through the aorta. We were disappointed to see this because the polypropylene frame was very flexible. We are investigating ways to cause collagen cross-linking in the aortic wall and preserve the natural flexibility of the cusps.

ANGELL:

We did not see this problem in our series of mounted homografts. One thing that is strikingly different is that, we were religious about using the tough fibrous tissue that is behind the commissure in the back of this maximum stress point. This will anchor the back part of the homograft to the stent. Also, the sutures that we placed in the aortic cuff came all the way in to the tissue that builds up for the commissural attachment. I think there is a striking difference in the way we mounted the homografts.

BARRATT-BOYES:

Have you actually used a biostrip?

DAVIS:

On the original rigid frame we had no biostrip. But since 1979 on the polypropylene frame we used the biostrip of dacron.

BARRATT-BOYES:

We have not seen this erosion. On the contrary, our experience is very different. When we used a simple over-and-over suture on the solid frame, the commissure did dehisce from the top of the pillar. When we switched to the biostrip which is like a glutaraldehyde treated valve mounting technique, and put them on a flexible frame, they dehisced even more quickly. On electron microscopy the tissue underneath the biostrip seems to liquify. It is my impression that the biostrip is contraindicated and that valve mounting is better without it.

376

SOMERVILLE:

It seems to be very important how one makes this valve. Our series is much better with the "top hat". Sir Brian, are you still continuing to use mounted homografts and do you think there is a place for them?

BARRATT-BOYES:

There is a place for mounted homografts and there is a lot to be learned and it is essential that we continue to investigate them.

DAVIS:

We agree and are hoping to increase the number we implant because at present our results are better than the porcine valve.

ANGELL:

For young people or for everyone?

DAVIS:

Everyone. We have had early calcification in porcine valves in middle-aged people.

SOMERVILLE:

How does the panel feel about which valve they put in the tricuspid area?

BARRATT-BOYES:

Our experience has been published. We have followed up a series of 80 triscupid valve stented replacements. In the days before we had an annulus operation, we used a series of these. The data are clear that it is the best valve replacement in the tricuspid position. It does not come off the frame in the tricuspid position because the pressure is low, and there is absolutely no gradient across it.

SOMERVILLE:

If you have to replace the tricuspid valve, after 8 or 9 years, the few we have calcified, became stenotic and they had to be replaced.

BARRATT-BOYES:

We have not had that experience.

GONZALEZ-LAVIN:

Brian has shown that you do not need a very large sized homograft to replace the tricuspid valve. What size do you use for a tricuspid valve replacement?

BARRATT-BOYES:

What we usually used was a 28-mm homograft which mounts on a 31 to 33 mm external diameter stent. There is no gradient across that sized valve. There is no difference in the incidence of failure of aortic or pulmonary valves and the pulmonary valve is desirable because it is larger.

SOMERVILLE:

Much of this conference has been devoted to the significance of viability and immunology. I wonder if not viability is correctly equated with durability. Perhaps viable cells might stimulate more immunogenic reaction, and it is better if the tissue has no viable cells. How would you feel about that, Dr. Yankah?

YANKAH:

According to the series from Dr. O'Brien, a cryopreserved valve will survive beyond the 10 year mark, after which degenerative changes are observed. After studying his explanted valves 10 years post-operatively, living fibroblasts were present which were supposed to be donor origin according to sex chromosome analysis, in contrast to the animal experimental findings of Sir Brian, in which host specific fibroblasts were found. I am worried about the specificity of these findings. Currently we have reliable methods to study the origin of cellular components of grafts, i.e. by immunochemistry using the monoclonal antibodies. We have also the possibility of identifying the endothelial cells of the allografts by identifying factor VIII antigens and the fibroblasts can be identified morphologically by transmission electron microscopy. We should also be aware that macrophages of hosts are permanently present in the allografts so long as tissue degeneration and inflammation take place. How can you reconcile your findings without these technical possibilities?
We need a systematic study to answer the question of whether the cellular components persist or die away and whether they are replaced by host cells.
Thinking in immunological terms, how can one maintain these cells in vivo? We now know that the endothelial cells are antigenic but not necessarily immunogenic. If the cells of the allografts are viable and are cryopreserved, they will maintain their viability and antigenicity, and thus induce immunologic reactions postoperatively. According to our experimental work, in order to maintain the viable cells in vivo, it was necessary to have them compatible with the host cells. Incompatible allografts lost their cellular components gradually, late post-operatively, and eventually became acellular.
These findings were also observed clinically in our Kiel series from explants 16 weeks after transplantation, as reported by Prof. Müller-Hermelink. Focal infiltrations of macrophages were the prominent findings. Our extensive studies, both in animal experiments and clinical studies, revealed neither reendothelialisation after loss by endothelial cells nor fibroblasts.
The fate of incompatible freshly cryopreserved allografts seems to be marked with acellularity or nonviability. The factors which might prolong durability of incompatible allografts are: (1) temperature and time of procurement to avoid autolysis and (2) cryopreservation. To enhance the durability and long-term survival of the cardiac valve allografts, ABO compatibility at least, or histocompatibility, is the logical way of reducing immune response of the allografts.

SOMERVILLE:

I am not yet convinced with respect to Dr. O'Brien's curves. Am I right, Mark, in thinking you call it a technical fault when there are three thick cusps requiring reoperation at several years? You do not call it a degenerative fault?

O'BRIEN:

To me, a technical fault is an obvious one. Immediately after the operation there is a moderate degree of incompetence. We felt a diastolic murmur on the operating room table, and the patient went on

378

for a number of years, then required reoperation. It was immediate. Anything we label technical, would have to have a significant diastolic murmur and a wide pulse pressure in the hospital.

SOMERVILLE:

But those patients from whom you subsequently remove the valves because they are thickened, don't you also call them technical faults?

O'BRIEN:

The valve that I showed in my paper was explanted 9 years after surgery. From the beginning there was malposition of the leaflets producing incompetence.

SOMERVILLE:

Because there are only 30 patients at the end. How do we know that those valves are not thick because they have cells in them.

O'BRIEN:

We would hope that the viable valves do thicken. They may all become acellular eventually but if the valve is thicker it will not perforate. Dr. Angell will confirm that the viable valve does not perforate. That is different from non viable aortic valve, which should not be used in this day and age. We are pleased that we gave it up in 1975. Brian's new antibiotic valve may well be superior to any other dead valve, but we must wait for the clinical results of his data.

BODNAR:

In our past 5 years' homograft experience, the results are 100%. I believe that these are viable valves and we have changed very little in the method of preservation. Patient selection is good and we used an interrupted suture technique. Only exceptional people can collect homografts under sterile conditions, and the rest of us are left with the ordinary mortuary material. We wish to introduce Sir Brian's sterilising method in London in order to achieve better results. The chemical structure of the antibiotics from the Heart Hospital and Sir Barratt-Boyes are very similar. The Heart Hospital antibiotics are much more concentrated. Our normal routine over the years is to work with 3 or 4% rejection for contamination. With the Barratt-Boyes solution, we had a 62% positive culture. We evaluated the difference in toxicity of the two antibiotics. The Barratt-Boyes solution is less toxic than the Heart Hospital antibiotics but both were within the same range. So as far as ultimate viability is concerned, the difference is not significant because both of them will be toxic.

ANGELL:

In the United States, CryoLife is acting very much like a blood bank. I believe that we need a separate organization. It could be a non-profit valve bank organization. The tissue bank technicians can go into the post mortem room, prepare the chest and take the heart out, under virtually sterile conditions. This can be done easily as they procure the cornea, which they get 10 to 100-fold the number of heart valves that are taken. Once valves are available under these conditions, then strictly physiologic doses of antibiotics can be used to sterilise them.
I disagree strongly that we have to use strong antibiotic solutions. The whole solution to this problem lies in the procurement system. One more thing about the CryoLife Company is, they have made valves available to non-procuring centers. You don't need to have a complex system in order to use homografts. You can call the company and say "Do you have homografts?" and if they have them

available, they will make them available to you. This is a very substantial change from several years ago or perhaps from the situation that exists in Europe where you need to have a very complicated system to obtain valves.

YANKAH:

There are two types of homografts: the viable and non-viable. The viable homografts ("allovital") are those which we procure sterilely within 12 h post mortem from the transplantation program. These valves are viable and can be cryopreserved within 1 h of procurement. Valves procured from the mortuary are not sterile and must be treated with antibiotic solution for 1 day. We must differentiate between the two types of allografts. The allovital valves can be cryopreserved, and stored without antibiotic solution, avoiding damage by the antibiotics. These have viable cells which will induce immunologic reactions. As has been shown, the allografts become non-viable and acellular after a period of time. What does this tell us? Which factors cause this acellularity. The immunological factors have to be considered when one is using the fresh allovital allografts. The antibiotic-treated valves at 4 °C are mostly non-viable, which affects their antigenicity. In summary, these are the two valve types which will dictate long-term post-operative results.

ANGELL:

One of the things we need to know is whether the homograft should be matched for ABO compatibility or not. We need a consensus opinion.

O'BRIEN:

In a fresh, non-viable series, we did a multivariant analysis, and ABO compatibility was not a factor. Yes, we try and match for ABO compatibility.

BARRATT-BOYES:

We have never done ABO matching.

KIRKLIN:

I would encourage people not to attempt the ABO compatibility with the cryopreserved grafts. The ABO compatibility has not been demonstrated to be a risk factor for these valves. I would be inclined not to do ABO matching in advance and hope that retrospectively the comparison might give some useful information.

YANKAH:

I would like to ask Mark to define the causative factors leading to degeneration, when does degeneration occur, and when do you diagnose it?

O'BRIEN:

I agree with Sir Brian. When a valve which was previously not incompetent, suddenly becomes significantly incompetent, that is due to valve failure. At autopsy, one has an obvious macroscopic and histological diagnosis if the valve becomes acellular and perforates. At reoperation, the diagnosis also becomes evident. There will be people who die with mild valve incompetence, and an autopsy has not been carried out. This is the problem I find in my own series. In those that have gone over 10 years, there were seven who have died and had no autopsy.

BARRATT-BOYES:

The mode of failure of the antibiotic PSK valve that we have talked about is very clearly defined. Most of it is due to cusp rupture. The mode of failure of the "viable" valve is not defined and is probably different. We have to be very careful of these failures that Mark is calling "technical". That may be the mode of failure of this particular device, it may be different and I suspect that it is going to be different. One interesting point of Dr. O'Brien's material is that in the more recent series of "viable" valves, there are many more technical failures than in the early series. That is very strange. We would have expected it to be the other way around because one becomes more competent at the operation. I suspect, and your material would support, that this is the mode of failure of this valve. The question is when is it going to occur? I hope it is going to be delayed, I am also not convinced that the valves are all acellular, as you have shown, but many of them are going to be.

O'BRIEN:

The four technical failures were early except for one. I do not think that is a factor at all. I agree that the viable frozen values are going to fail in a different way, they are not going to rupture, but rather thicken, shrink, and finally calcify. I would not be surprised that this will happen in 15 to 20 years.

BARRATT-BOYES:

Two of our initial 16 clearly viable grafts did rupture. I do not think even viable valves are going to be devoid of rupture because the whole leaflet is not covered adequately. It will be less common, I agree but will occur.

BODNAR:

There is an immunological factor which is common in viable and non-viable valves, that is calf serum. We are talking about ABO matching and tissue typing and with the exception of Sir Brian, everyone has been soaking the homologous tissue in a heterologous antigen, called calf serum.

O'BRIAN:

We have never used it.

BODNAR:

We have formel in animal experiments that the heat-treated fetal calf serum is very seriously antigenic. We provoked second set reactions. The material is not limited to the surface but penetrates all layers of the aortic wall and cusp. The natural antigenicity is mainly limited to the surface and the endothelial cells but the calf serum is everywhere. One of our keen Japanese fellows started checking incoming heart surgical patients for anti-calf antibodies. Eight of 27 had anti-calf antibodies. We abandoned calf serum at the National Heart Hospital. We are presently keeping fresh 4 °C valves in TC 199 without human serum. When I asked Cryolife why are they using fetal calf serum they said it was because Dr. O'Brien recommeded its.

O'BRIEN:

We have never used it. 17 years ago, the advice we got was that it can be toxic to cells and that was the reason why we did not use it. I subsequently was aware of your work with its antigenicity, so we never used it.

KIRKLIN:

What is your freezing solution, Dr. O'Brien?

O'BRIEN:

It consists of TC 199 plus DMSO.

KIRKLIN:

Sir Brian uses the same?

BARRATT-BOYES:

Yes.

YANKAH:

We were using fetal calf serum but now we have changed to human serum because of the role of calf serum in perpetuating antigenic response.
In our research laboratory, we had similar findings as Endre. The only time when calf serum is used to enhance the nutrient medium at a pH between 7.2 and 7.6 is when the tissue cultures are necessary for non-immunological studies.

BANK:

As the techniques become optimized for cryopreservation, we no longer simply optimize the viability of the fibroblast but also improve the viability of the endothelial cells, provided trauma doesn't scrape the cells off. We may find that it becomes an increasing problem because the ABO receptors do lie on the endothelial cells. I have done work with an immunologist and in his patient population, 87% have anticalf antibodies. These are not people with heart problems. These antigens occur after exposure to egg and milk. To one knows whether this adversely affects long-term viability. I have asked the same question of Cryolife about 30 times: It the fetal calf serum used in the dilution procedure, in order to minimize the dilution shock of the dimethyl sulphoxide and not in the freezing procedure?

KIRKLIN:

At the University of Alabama we definitely have used it as part of the freezing solution.

McNALLY:

Fetal calf serum is used during the freezing process, as well as during the thawing dilution. We have an active program to look for substitutes that will relieve the osmostic properties during thawing.

We have been attending these meetings over the last few years and have heard the same comment by Dr. Bodnar before. We are independently evaluating it.

HETZER:

There are other widely used substitutes and I am still not sure what the place of the homograft is. I have not seen age-related valve degeneration curves. Dr. Bodnar talks about proper patient selection. What is that? I understand that in Sir Brian Barratt-Boyes unit, there are not only homografts being implanted, I cannot imagine that in Alabama only homografts are implanted. Furthermore, I see Dr. Miller from Stanford who has a huge experience with heterografts and is using homografts now. Which patients do you think will do better with a homograft? Those questions have not been answered, and I think it would be very important for us to know that. Is it only the young patients? Is it the ones with renal failure and calcium disorders?

ANGELL:

If the patients are under 65 and do not have complex disease, and we can safely put in a free aortic homograft, then that is our first choice. In other cases we do not use it.

SOMERVILLE:

Is calcification age-related? Brian has very good data on this.

BARRATT-BOYES:

Calcification is not present in the childhood valves. Calcification in our experience was commoner with the chemically treated valve. With the antibiotic treated valve it can occur but is never a cause of obstruction, it is a cause of rupture. As the data would still suggest, and Dr. O'Brien's multivariant analysis also suggests, age of the patient is a factor. The younger the patient, the more likely there is to be failure. This data indicated that this is a continuous variable as does the analysis of UAB. Our data does not show that. We looked very carefully and there is not a continuous variable in our data. Age does come into it, somewhere. In fact, you are never going to be able to use the homograft in a significant number of cases, unless you alter your preparation techniques. The only way you are going to be able to use it as we have used it, is to salvage the valves cleanly at autopsy. I would like to go back to Dr. Bodnar's comments about his inability to repeat our 98% sterility (disinfection) of valves using CUPYA solution. This is due to the way they are collected at autopsy. It is vitally important, and as Dr. Angell has said, you have to train the people and if you do not, you will have a significant wastage. If you don't do a clean collection, you are wasting your time.

CRAIG MILLER:

These are precious resources. You have to be selective and it is foolhardy to think of homografts for everybody. For some of our mitral valve patients, 15 years might be several lifetimes. We do not have to have every valve in every patient last 15 or 20 years. We used a lot of xenografts and very few mechanical valves. We do not have a good option in the young adults and particularly females and children. We feel strongly that the allograft is preferable. The other category of patients is adults with prosthetic aortic valve endocarditis. An allograft may give these patients an edge in terms of a lower incidence of recurrent endocarditis.

ANGELL:

It is very clear that we all are looking primarily at durability of the homograft and that we are seeking the truth. We are looking very hard, all of us, to determine exactly what the true invidence of valve failure is. In my opinion. the technique by which valves are inserted may well be a significant factor in determining their short- and long-term durability.

Summary

W. W. Angell

This International Symposium marks the 25th anniversary of the use of human valves by Sir Brian Barratt-Boyes and Mr. Donald Ross. The use of allografts was based upon the pioneering work of Lam (1952) and Heimbecker and Murray (1956) who implanted sleeves of fresh aortic allograft valves in the descending thoracic aorta for aortic insufficiency. In 1960, Duran and Gunning described the dissection and preparation of the aortic allograft valve and the surgical technique for subcoronary insertion. In 1967, on the basis of animal work by Braunwald and Welden, Angell reported the first successful use of premounted aortic allografts for mitral and tricuspid valve replacement.

Initially, aortic valves were taken directly from cadavers under sterile conditions with minimal physical damage and implanted within hours without exposure to toxic agents. Some of these allografts may well have been viable at the time of implantation. However, the logistic problems of this technique subsequently led to removal of the valve under clean conditions and sterilisation by one of several modes. The early use of ethylene oxide, betapropiolactone and irradiation of freeze-dried valves all rendered the allograft nonviable with decreased tensile strength and durability. When early clinical failures were observed, all groups changed to antibiotic sterilization in combination with hypothermic storage. Most of the early antibiotic concentrations were cytotoxic. The issue of the significance of homograft viability was raised by O'Brien and Angell who, between 1972 and 1974, jointly described the experimental basis for and then the clinical application of the antibiotic sterilized frozen viable grafts. The issues concerning the feasibility and importance of viability have persisted until today and were the subject of argument and discussion during this symposium. Viability, therefore, becomes the primary topic in the summarization of data presented.

Viability is important as it relates to the metabolic activity and reproductive capacity of the three primary cell elements: fibroblasts, endothelium and elastin-producing cells. Viability is defined as the persistence and documented combined metabolic and structural function of these cells after implantation in experimental animals or man. The normal function of these cells over weeks, months and years is related to the post-operative reaction, as determined largely by the immunogenicity of the donor tissue and rejection by the host. Therefore, whereas viable grafts provide the only possibility for permanent valve replacement, the immunologic reaction becomes the key to achieving this ultimate goal. With optimal treatment, the allograft appears to have a mean valve survival of 15—20 years, but failure of the graft is inevitable. This is not true for the immunogenetically identical autograft valve. Preimplant viability assays include: (1) light and electron microscopic morphology after 24 h in whole graft tissue culture, (2) cell suspension tissue culture with uptake of isotope labelled proteins or thymidine and (4) supravital stains with immunofluorescence of monoclonal antibodies.

Methods of valve preparation for subcoronary insertion

1. Allovital allografts and isografts

These grafts are inserted by immediate transfer of the donor valve to the patient within a minutes or hours. These allovital grafts are certainly viable at implantation and definitely contain Class I and II antigens in the endothelial and stroma cells. These grafts provide maximum antigenic stimulus for both graft and host reaction post implantation. Morphology of both autograft and allovital allografts was examined. Autografts have the persistence of all cell components long-term. The persistence of viable allograft cellularity is quantitative and does not persist long-term.

2. Viable preserved allografts

These grafts are prepared with short-term storage or cryopreservation and have proven viability of at least the fibroblast cell component. Cusp fibroblasts can be shown to produce collagen, as evidenced by a gradual thickening of the collagen stroma over weeks to months postoperatively. Probably the function of endothelial and elastin cells is insignificant after implantation. The antigenicity of endothelial Class I antigens is significantly altered as compared to allovital implants.

There is great controversy over whether the cells in valves explanted are host or donor in origin. Ross and Barratt-Boyes believe all cells die after implantation and that cusp repopulation is from the donor sheath or pannus cells. Similar findings were observed in ABO incompatible allografts but without re-endothelisation by Müller-Hermelink and Yankah. Evidence from the experience of O'Brien and Angell suggests that donor cells persist in some grafts and are the source of new valve cusp collagen which thickens, strengthens and can repair the valve after implantation. This controversy remains unresolved, but is a pivotal issue in the methodology of valve procurement, sterilization, preparation and storage. Both Ross and Barratt-Boyes agree with O'Brien and Angell that viability testing at implantation is desirable. This is based, however, on the belief that viability determines optimal preservation of the structural components of the cusp and that the function of the viable fibroblasts is not important.

3. Fresh non-viable allografts

These are valves treated with high-dose antibiotics or maintained in long-term 4 °C storage until all cell components are clearly non-viable at the time of implantation. Except for O'Brien's series, there is no clinical evidence that these grafts are less durable than viable grafts. Barratt-Boyes and Ross show no difference in significant valve insufficiency between the viable and fresh non-viable grafts. Angell's early frozen series shows no difference between frozen viable and fresh grafts.

4. *Preserved non-viable allografts*

These valves were implanted primarily in the mid-1960s by Ross, Malm and Kirklin after being treated with betapropriolactone or ethylene oxide and freeze-dried or irradiated. There was concern over the protection of structural elements, but poor control with the result that many of the grafts suffered from early failure with stretching, thinning, fenestration and prolapse of leaflets. Ross's data questions whether some of these failures were not more related to the recipient/patient selection than to the processing techniques. This suggests that the incidence of graft failure is not different from that experienced with the antibiotic (fresh) valves. All other groups however, conclude that these grafts, both experimentally and clinically, have unacceptably short mean survival times of about 7 or 8 years and are significantly less durable than the fresh frozen or viable grafts. Three series by Ross, Kirklin and the Mayo Clinic quote mean survival times of 5.5, 6.7 and 7.5 years respectively.

Valve durability

With both the scalloped subcoronary valve and the intact aortic root, valve failure is the "end point" to be measured when comparing allograft series or comparing allografts with xenografts or mechanical prostheses. The character of allograft valve failure may be different when comparing viable and nonviable grafts as cusp rupture is unlikely in grafts that were viable at implantation. Allograft valve failure must be defined as significant valve insufficiency, whether documented clinically by echocardiogram, explantation or postmortem examination. The index or measure of valve failure can be expressed as an actuarial freedom from valve failure curve, a Hazard function curve or the mean interval to valve failure.

Immunology

The immunologists, both surgical and medical, agree upon the importance of antigenicity, immunogenicity and immunogenetic response to the maintenance of viability after implantation. Hypocellular response, loss of cellularity, loss of endothelium, alteration in fibroblasts, monocytic infiltration and macrophage digestion of structural collagen can all be implicated as immunogenetically mediated phenomena. Preventing these reactions in order to prolong graft survival is an obvious goal and may be the only way by which the allograft can achieve permanency and therefore have the potential self-regenerative processes commensurate with a persistently viable organ transplant. There are three possibilities, outlined by Müller-Ruchholtz:
1. To reduce immunogenicity of the graft by matching or altering the antigenic incompatibility
2. To reduce the host immunogenic response by diffuse immunosuppression with Prednisone, Imuran and Cyclosporine
3. To achieve specific graft immunotolerance with suppression of the low grade response.

Yacoub and Yankah have described the antigenicity of cellular components as documented by immunofluorescent monoclonal antibodies. The antigenicity of endothelial cells after 24 h preservation at 4 °C in antibiotic solution is shown to decrease. The rat model accelerated response after a second challenge with skin grafts documented immunogenic antigenicity in vivo. Endothelial cells first, and then fibroblasts, were seen to deteriorate. The viability and immunogenic response to cellularity is documented by examination of clinically explanted valves with electron microscopy and immunohistology. Yacoub reported no differences in valve failure with or without ABO compatibility at 7 years or after postoperative treatment with low dose immunosuppression. Blind clinical trials were suggested to establish the need for tissue matching and the relationship between the viable grafts and the immunogenetic importance of matching or immunosuppression.

Right ventricular outflow tract reconstruction

It was generally accepted that the homograft is the conduit of choice in infants and children due to the ease of insertion and the low calcification rate, as compared to xenografts. Durability of the conduit may be greater than that of the free aortic subcoronary grafts; however, the data is not conclusive and in some series there was no difference. It was suggested that the ideal pulmonary annulus patch is one containing an allograft valve cusp. It was accepted that pulmonary allografts are the valve of choice in reoperation for tetralogy of Fallot with symptomatic pulmonary insufficiency. Meisner demonstrated the allograft inlay technique to reduce postoperative valve incompetence.

Aortic root replacement

The allograft as an aortic root implant was also the general choice for aortic atresia. There is a question of this application in patients with subvalvular aortic stenosis. Clark's technique involves the use of a "Konno" like procedure with allograft aortic root, coronary implantation and the use of allograft aorta for the right ventricular patch. Clark feels that the extended root replacement is appropriate for tunnel aortic atresia while Barratt-Boyes and Ross feel that this is too radical and that the proper technique is subvalvular ventricular resection.

The aortic sleeve graft with coronary implantation was compared to annulus narrowing or annulus widening procedures with standard allograft valve insertion. Long-term results with frozen valves are necessary before wider applications of these techniques can be recommended. The use of the aortic allograft root for infective endocarditis was felt to be the method of choice. Yacoub reported 130 patients with aortic root replacement and a valve failure incidence *less* than that with subcoronary aortic valve replacement. This raises the question of the influence of technical factors on valve failure with the standard subcoronary allograft method.

Techniques

The basic method of implantation is a scalloped aortic valve secured in the subcoronary position with two suture lines, the inferior one being below the valve cusp attachment of the recipient. Experts can implant a valve in the subcoronary position in approximately 1 h, but those learning this method should allow as much as 2 h. Proper orientation and handling of the tissue at surgery probably affects the valve failure incidence.

The technique of pulmonary autotransplantation continues to be done only by Ross. Other experts in the field appear to be reluctant to use this technique. There is some question of the short- and long-term valve failure rates with the use of autografts. The unsupported pulmonary valve in the right ventricular outflow tract has an increased risk of leakage. For pulmonary insufficiency and pulmonary branch stenosis after tetralogy repair, the pulmonary allograft allows extension to the pulmonary arteries. Stenosis occurred in 5% and pulmonary insufficiency in 7% in Meisner's series at the Munich Heart Center. This agrees with the Great Ormond Street and Boston Children's Hospital experiences. There is little requirement for repeat valve surgery or removal of the allograft. The allograft is also the choice for right ventricular outflow tract reconstruction in truncus arteriosus. It is not felt that valves are necessary for the present Fontan reconstruction and that direct connection without valves is the technique of choice. The allograft is used for Rastelli reconstruction, although freedom from reoperation, as published to date, is no different than with the use of xenografts.

Conclusions

It was agreed that for aortic valve replacement in children and young adults, the use of allografts is the technique of choice. The allograft is also preferred for right ventricular outflow tract reconstruction, aortic root hypoplasia and aortic root infection. The autograft is used only by one surgeon and should be further evaluated. The significance of graft viability is the primary area of disagreement with the use of the allograft valve. Viability affects (1) immunogenicity, (2) antigenicity, (3) morphology of valve stroma, endothelium and collagen deposition, (4) type and incidence of valve failure and (5) is an indicator of optimal valve preparation. If viability adversely affects immunogenicity and is only a marker for adequate structural preservation and not critical to long-term function, then perhaps this is better measured in other ways. Also, if early viability only increases collagen deposition and the valve subsequently becomes acellular there may be a better way to strengthen nonviable tissue.

There is, at present, no proof that any allograft remains viable long-term, and there is good evidence that even valves that were viable at implantation become primarily acellular with no repair of cellular components functioning in a beneficial way several years after implantation. O'Brien has one frozen valve with persistent donor cells 9 years after implantation, but the architecture is disarranged with little evidence that the donor cells are functioning. He also reports a series of 34 patients from 1975 to 1977 with 23 survivors, all over 10 years, with two valve failures for a 10-year valve failure rate of less than 10%. This suggests that the frozen viable grafts have a different and slower failure mode, possibly due to viable donor cells.

This experience is contradicted by Angell's series of 23 frozen viable valves implanted from 1972 to 1974 with a valve failure the same as with the fresh grafts. Barratt-Boyes' selected patients with a small aortic root from his fresh valve series and reports a mean valve survival of 15 years, suggesting that long-term function is also possible with fresh non-viable grafts from young donors implanted into patients with a small recipient aortic root. Proof of the importance of the frozen viable graft lies in (1) longer follow-up with O'Brien's series, (2) documentation of valve failure rates, (3) morphology of long-term valves and (4) confirmation of results from other centers.

Author's address:
William W. Angell, M.D.
Division of Cardiac Surgery
Scripps Clinic and Research Foundation
La Jolla, California
U.S.A.

Closing Remarks

J. Somerville

It is perhaps appropriate to say thank you to Dr. Yankah and Dr. Hetzer for having the courage and foresight and excellent planning to organise this meeting. I think this meeting has shown the point we have arrived at in the use of this valve and there is still much work to be done. It is interesting that 25 years on after Mr. Donald Ross and Sir Brian Barratt-Boyes implanted the first aortic homografts that they are really still here to stay. Also thanks to Sir Brian Barratt-Boyes. Personally I would like to say his lecture was sparkling and interesting and shows how much science he has introduced into the surgery of the homograft.

There is a newcomer in the field, and that is commerce. That has its advantages and possibly its disadvantages. It is interesting that commerce can sell something that it has not bought but nevertheless, if there is a market for it, I think that this is extremely useful. I hope that it won't interfere with the culling of homografts by private banks, and that there won't be legal patenting to stop those who run private banks. There is now a trade organisation heavily involved in the big commercial venture of marketing homograft valves.

It would be appropriate to say thank you very much to all of you. We from the National Heart Hospital would like to say that we feel we have never left our homograft. We are very grateful now that you "swallows" who have been and gone, have now returned to the use of the homograft and we hope you don't bring a vulture with it!

Author Index

Subject Index

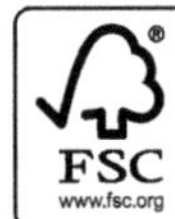
FSC
www.fsc.org
MIX
Papier aus verantwortungsvollen Quellen
Paper from responsible sources
FSC® C105338